Essential Obstetrics and Gynaecology

To our families

Commissioning Editor: Ellen Green
Project Development Manager: Janice Urquhart
Project Manager: Frances Affleck
Designer: Judith Wright

Essential Obstetrics and Gynaecology

E. Malcolm Symonds

MD MB BS FRCOG FFPHM FACOG(Hon) FRANZCOG(Hon)
Professor Emeritus in Obstetrics and Gynaecology, University of Nottingham, Nottingham, UK

Ian M. Symonds

MD MB BS BMedSci MRCOG ILTM
Senior Lecturer and Honorary Consultant in Obstetrics and Gynaecology, Derby City General Hospital, Derby, UK

FOURTH EDITION

Illustrated by
Robert Britton, Diane Mercer, Amanda Williams

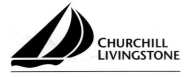

CHURCHILL
LIVINGSTONE

EDINBURGH LONDON NEW YORK OXFORD PHILADELPHIA ST LOUIS SYDNEY TORONTO 2004

CHURCHILL LIVINGSTONE
An imprint of Elsevier Limited

First edition 1987
Second edition 1992
Third edition 1998
Fourth edition 2004

ISBN 978 0 443 07147 8
  Reprinted 2005, 2006, 2007, 2008
International edition 978 0 443 07148 5
  Reprinted 2005, 2006

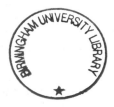

British Library Cataloguing in Publication Data
A catalogue record for this book is available from the British Library

Library of Congress Cataloging in Publication Data
A catalog record for this book is available from the Library of Congress

Notice
Medical knowledge is constantly changing. Standard safety precautions must be
followed, but as new research and clinical experience broaden our knowledge, changes
in treatment and drug therapy may become necessary or appropriate. Readers are
advised to check the most current product information provided by the manufacturer
of each drug to be administered to verify the recommended dose, the method and
duration of administration, and contraindications. It is the responsibility of the
practitioner, relying on experience and knowledge of the patient, to determine dosages
and the best treatment for each individual patient. Neither the Publisher nor the
authors assumes any liability for any injury and/or damage to persons or property
arising from this publication.
The Publisher

Cover image credit: BSIP, Veronique Estiot/Science Photo Library

Printed in China

Preface

When the first edition of this book was published in 1987, the concept was based on having a text with simple line drawings to reinforce and simplify the content of each chapter. This principle was maintained for the next two editions.

In this edition, we have changed the presentation to include both grey scale and colour images. Many of the illustrations have been taken from *Diagnosis in Color*, a joint publication with Dr. Marion MacPherson, and we wish to acknowledge our gratitude to her for her previous efforts in obtaining these images. We also wish to thank Dr. Graham Robinson for his assistance in preparing some of the histopathology material and Dr. Rajakumar for providing the images of pelvic infections.

All of the chapters have been either re-written or re-edited to bring the contents into line with evidence-based medicine and with currently accepted methods of clinical practice.

Obstetrics and gynaecology, as a discipline practised in the UK, is becoming increasingly fragmented, with growing separation between the practice of obstetrics and of gynaecology. With the domination of the subject by sub-specialist groups, it has become increasingly difficult for students to achieve an overview of the broad field of pregnancy and its complications as well as the various aspects of human reproduction and diseases of the female genital tract.

To this end, we have tried to keep a balance in this edition with emphasis on common disorders and problems without attempting in any way to make the book encyclopaedic. Once again, we are indebted to Dr. Margaret Oates for her important contributions on the subject of psychiatric disorders in obstetrics and gynaecology.

We have expanded the number of case studies included in the text as we believe that such case material can add to the coherence of the text. As with previous editions, we have deliberately not included our reference sources in the text. However, the sources of much of our material can be found in the additional reading lists included at the end of this edition.

Finally, we wish to thank the publishers and our panel of expert reviewers for their help in the production of this fourth edition.

E. Malcolm Symonds
Ian M. Symonds

International Panel of Reviewers

Professor Shaughn Brennecke, Head of Clinical School, Melbourne University, Department of Obstetrics and Gynaecology, Royal Women's Hospital, Melbourne, Australia

Professor Allan Chang, Director of Obstetrics and Gynaecology, Kevin Ryan Centre, Mater Mothers Hospital, Brisbane, Australia

Professor Diane Fraser, Reader and Head of Division, Academic Division of Midwifery, University of Nottingham, Queen's Medical Centre, Nottingham, UK

Professor Chris Haines, Reader, Department of Obstetrics and Gynaecology, The Chinese University of Hong Kong, Prince of Wales Hospital, Hong Kong, China

Professor P. M. Shaughn O'Brien, Professor and Head, Academic Department of Obstetrics and Gynaecology, Maternity Unit, City General Hospital, Stoke on Trent, UK

Mr Mahmood Shafi, Consultant in Gynaecology, Birmingham's Women's Hospital, Birmingham, UK

Contents

SECTION 1
Essential reproductive science

1 Anatomy of the female pelvis

Knowledge of the major features of the female pelvis is essential to the understanding of the processes of reproduction and childbearing and to the effect that various pathological processes may have on the pelvic organs and on the health of the woman.

The structure and function of the genital organs vary considerably with the age of the individual and her hormonal status, as will be apparent in various chapters that specifically relate to puberty and the menopause. This chapter aims to outline the major structures contained in the female pelvis and predominantly in the sexually mature female.

THE EXTERNAL GENITALIA

The term *vulva* is generally used to describe the female external genitalia and includes the mons pubis, the labia majora, the labia minora, the clitoris, the external urinary meatus, the vestibule of the vagina, the vaginal orifice and the hymen (Fig. 1.1).

The **mons pubis**, sometimes known as the *mons veneris*, is composed of a fibrofatty pad of tissue that lies above the pubic symphysis and in the mature female is covered with dense pubic hair. The upper border of this hair is usually straight or convex upwards and differs from the normal male distribution. Pubic hair begins to appear between the ages of 11 and 12 years.

The **labia majora** consist of two longitudinal cutaneous folds that extend downwards and posteriorly from the mons pubis anteriorly to the perineum posteriorly. The labia are composed of an outer surface covered by hair and sweat glands and an inner smooth layer containing sebaceous follicles. The labia majora enclose the pudendal cleft into which the urethra and vagina open.

Posterior to the vaginal orifice, the labia merge to form the posterior commissure and the area between this structure and the anterior verge of the anus constitutes the obstetric perineum.

The labia majora are homologous with the male scrotum.

3

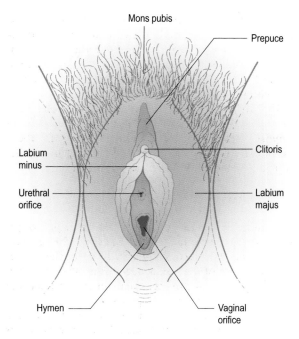

Fig. 1.1 External genital organs of the female.

The **labia minora** are enclosed by the labia majora and are cutaneous folds that enclose the clitoris anteriorly and fuse posteriorly behind the vaginal orifice to form the posterior fourchette or posterior margin of the vaginal introitus. Anteriorly, the labia minora divide to enclose the clitoris, the anterior fold forming the prepuce and the posterior fold the frenulum. They are richly vascularized and innervated and are erectile. They do not contain hair but are rich in sebaceous glands.

The **clitoris** is the female homologue of the penis and is situated between the anterior ends of the labia minora. The body of the clitoris consists of two corpora cavernosa of erectile tissue enclosed in a fibrous sheath. Posteriorly, these two corpora divide to lie along the inferior rami of the pubic bones. The free end of the clitoris contains the glans, which is composed of erectile tissue covered by skin and is richly supplied with sensory nerve endings and hence is very sensitive. The clitoris plays an important role in sexual stimulation and function.

The **vestibule** consists of a shallow depression lying between the labia minora. The external urethral orifice opens into the vestibule anteriorly and the vaginal orifice posteriorly. The ducts from the two Bartholin's glands drain into the vestibule at the posterior margin of the vaginal introitus and the secretions from these glands have an important lubricating role during sexual intercourse.

Skene's ducts lie alongside the lower 1 cm of the urethra and also drain into the vestibule. Although they have some lubricating function, it is minor compared to the function of Bartholin's glands.

The **bulb of the vestibule** consists of two erectile bodies that lie on either side of the vaginal orifice and is in contact with the surface of the urogenital diaphragm. The bulb of the vestibule is covered by a thin layer of muscle known as the bulbocavernosus muscle.

The **external urethral orifice** lies 1.5–2 cm below the base of the clitoris and is often covered by the labia minora, which also function by directing the urinary stream. In addition to Skene's ducts, there are often a number of paraurethral glands without associated ducts and these sometimes form the basis of paraurethral cysts.

The **vaginal orifice** opens into the lower part of the vestibule and, prior to sexual activity, is partly covered by the hymenal membrane. The **hymen** is a thin fold of skin attached around the circumference of the vaginal orifice. There are various types of opening within the hymen and the membrane varies in consistency. Once the hymen has been penetrated, the remnants are represented by the *carunculae myrtiformes*, which are nodules of fibrocutaneous material at the edge of the vaginal introitus.

Bartholin's glands are a pair of racemose glands located at either side of the vaginal introitus and measuring 0.5–1.0 cm in diameter. The ducts are approximately 2 cm in length and open between the labia minora and the vaginal orifice. Their function is to secrete mucus during sexual excitement. Cyst formation is relatively common but is the result of occlusion of the duct, with fluid accumulation in the duct and not in the gland.

Although it does not strictly lie within the description of the vulva, the **perineum** as described in relation to obstetric function is defined as the area that lies between the vaginal fourchette anteriorly and the anus posteriorly; it lies over the perineal body, which occupies the area between the anal canal and the lower one third of the posterior vaginal wall.

THE INTERNAL GENITAL ORGANS

The internal genitalia include the vagina, the uterus, the fallopian tubes and the ovaries. Situated in the pelvic cavity, these structures lie in close proximity to the urethra and urinary bladder anteriorly and the rectum, anal canal and pelvic colon posteriorly (Fig. 1.2).

The vagina

The vagina is a muscular tube some 6–7.5 cm long in the mature female. It is lined by non-cornified squamous epithelium and is more capacious at the vault than at the introitus. In cross-section, the vagina is H-shaped and it is capable of considerable distension, particularly during parturition when it adapts to accommodate the passage of the fetal head. Anteriorly, it is intimately related to the trigone of the urinary bladder and the urethra. Posteriorly, the lower part of the vagina is separated from the anal canal by the perineal body. In the middle third, it lies in apposition to the ampulla of the rectum and in the upper segment it is covered by the peritoneum of the rectovaginal pouch.

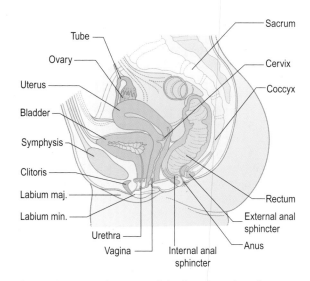

Fig. 1.2 Sagittal section of the female pelvis showing the relationship of the pelvic organs with surrounding structures.

The uterine cervix protrudes into the vaginal vault. Four zones are described in the vaginal vault: the anterior fornix, the posterior fornix and the two lateral fornices. The lateral fornices lie under the base of the broad ligament in close proximity to the point where the uterine artery crosses the ureter.

The pH of the vagina in the sexually mature non-pregnant female is between 4.0 and 5.0. This has an important antibacterial function that reduces the risk of pelvic infection. The functions of the vagina are copulation, parturition and the drainage of menstrual loss.

The uterus

The uterus is a hollow, muscular, pear-shaped organ situated in the pelvic cavity between the bladder anteriorly and the rectum and pouch of Douglas posteriorly. The size of the uterus depends on the hormonal status of the female. In the sexually mature female, the uterus is 7.5 cm long and approximately 5 cm across at its widest point. The uterus normally lies in a position of *anteversion* such that the uterine fundus is anterior to the uterine cervix. In about 10% of women, the uterus lies in a position of *retroversion* in the pouch of Douglas. The uterus may also be curved anteriorly in its longitudinal axis, a feature that is described as *anteflexion.*

It consists of a body or corpus, an isthmus and a cervix.

The **corpus uteri** consists of a mass of smooth muscle cells arranged in three layers. The external layers contain smooth muscle cells that pass transversely across the uterine fundus into the lateral angles of the uterus, where the muscle fibres merge with the outer layers of the smooth muscle of the fallopian tubes and the ovarian and round ligaments. The muscle fibres in the middle layer are arranged in a circular manner and the inner layer contains some longitudinal fibres but also with some circular and oblique muscle cells.

The cavity of the uterus is triangular in shape and is flattened anteroposteriorly so that the total volume of the cavity in the non-pregnant state is approximately 2 ml. It is lined by endometrium that consists on the surface of mucus-secreting columnar epithelium. The nature of the endometrium depends on the phase of the menstrual cycle. Following menstruation, the endometrium in the proliferative phase is only 1–2 mm thick and grows to a thickness of up to 1 cm by the second half or secretory phase of the cycle.

The endometrial cavity is in contact with the vaginal cavity inferiorly via the cervical canal and superiorly with the peritoneal cavity through the fallopian tubes.

The **cervix** is a barrel-shaped structure that extends from the external cervical os, opening into the vagina at the apex of the vaginal portion of the cervix, to the internal cervical os in the supravaginal portion of the cervix, opening into the uterine cavity through the isthmus of the uterus.

The cervical canal is fusiform in shape and is lined by ciliated columnar epithelium that is mucus-secreting. The transition between this epithelium and the stratified squamous epithelium of the vaginal ectocervix forms the squamocolumnar junction and the site of this junction is related to the hormonal status of the woman. Some of the cervical glands in the endocervical lining are extensively branched and mucus-secreting. If the opening to these glands becomes obstructed, small cysts may form, known as *nabothian follicles*.

The muscle layers of the cervix consist of circular bundles of smooth muscle cells and fibrous tissue. The outer longitudinal layer merges with the muscle layer of the vagina.

The **isthmus** of the uterus joins the cervix to the corpus uteri and in the non-pregnant uterus is a narrow, rather poorly defined area some 2–3 mm in length. In pregnancy, it constitutes the zone that will go on to form the lower uterine segment. Functionally, it becomes an extension of the birth canal and does not contribute significantly to the expulsion of the fetus.

Supports and ligaments of the uterus

The uterus and the pelvic organs are supported by a number of ligaments and fascial thickenings of various strengths and importance. The pelvic organs also depend on the integrity of the pelvic floor: a particular feature in the human female is that, an upright posture having been adopted, the pelvic floor has to contain the downward pressure of the viscera and the pelvic organs.

The **anterior ligament** is a fascial condensation along with the peritoneal fold that forms the uterovesical fold and extends from the anterior cervix of the uterus across the superior surface of the bladder to the anterior pelvic peritoneal covering. It has a weak supporting role.

Posteriorly, the **uterosacral ligaments** play a major role in supporting the uterus and the vaginal vault. These ligaments and their peritoneal covering form the lateral boundaries of the rectouterine pouch, otherwise known as the pouch of Douglas. The ligaments contain a considerable amount of fibrous tissue and non-striped muscle and extend from the cervix onto the anterior surface of the sacrum.

Laterally, the **broad ligaments** are reflected folds of peritoneum that extend from the lateral margins of the uterus to the lateral pelvic walls. They cover the fallopian tubes and the round ligaments, the blood vessels and nerves that supply the uterus, tubes and ovaries, and the mesovarium and ovarian ligament that suspend the ovaries from the posterior surface of the broad ligament. Like the uterovesical ligament, the broad ligament plays only a weak supportive role.

The **round ligaments** are two fibromuscular ligaments that extend from the anterior surface of the uterus. In the non-pregnant state, they are a few millimetres thick and are covered by the peritoneum of the broad ligaments. They arise from the anterolateral surface of the uterus just below the entrance of the tubes and extend diagonally and laterally for 10–12 cm to the lateral pelvic walls, where they cross the pelvic brim and enter the abdominal inguinal canal, and then to the labia majora. These ligaments have a weak supporting role for the uterus but do play a role in maintaining its position. In pregnancy, they become much thickened and strengthened and during contractions may pull the uterus anteriorly and align the long axis of the fetus in such a way as to improve the direction of entry of the presenting part into the pelvic cavity.

The **cardinal ligaments** form the strongest supports for the uterus and vaginal vault and are dense fascial thickenings that extend from the cervix to the fascia over the obturator fossa on each side. Medially, they merge with the mass of fibrous tissue and some smooth muscle cells that encloses the cervix and the vaginal vault and is known as the *parametrium*. Both the uterosacral ligaments and the cardinal ligaments merge with the parametrium. Close to the cervix, it contains the uterine arteries, nerve plexuses and the ureter passing through the ureteric canal to reach the urinary bladder. Lower down, the muscular activity of the pelvic floor muscles and the integrity of the perineal body play a vital role in preventing the development of uterine prolapse.

The Fallopian tubes

The Fallopian tubes or uterine tubes are the oviducts. They extend from the superior angle of the uterus, where the tubal canal at the tubal ostium opens into the lateral and uppermost part of the uterine cavity. The tubes are approximately 10–12 cm long and lie on the posterior surface of the broad ligament, extending laterally in a convoluted fashion so that, eventually, the tubes open into the peritoneal cavity in close proximity to the ovaries.

The tubes are enclosed in a mesosalpinx, a superior fold of the broad ligament, and this peritoneal fold, apart from containing the tube, also contains the blood vessels and nerve supply to the tubes and the ovaries. It also houses various embryological remnants such as the epoophoron, the paroophoron, Gartner's duct and the hydatid of Morgagni. These embryological remnants are significant in that they may form para-ovarian cysts, which are difficult to differentiate from true ovarian cysts. They are generally benign.

The tube is divided into four sections:

- The *interstitial portion* lies in the uterine wall.
- The *isthmus* is a constricted portion of the tube extending from the emergence of the interstitial portion until it widens into the next section. The lumen of the tube is narrow and the longitudinal and circular muscle layers are well differentiated.
- The *ampulla* is a widened section of the tube and the muscle coat is much thinner. The widened cavity is lined by thickened mucosa.
- The *infundibulum* of the tube is the outermost part of the ampulla; it terminates at the abdominal ostium, where it is surrounded by the fimbriae, the longest of which is attached to the ovary.

The tubes are lined by a single layer of columnar epithelium, some of the cells of which are ciliated and serve to assist the movement of the oocyte down the tube, while some are non-ciliated and serve a secretory function. The tubes are richly innervated and have an inherent rhythmicity that varies according to the stage of the menstrual cycle and whether or not the woman is pregnant.

The ovaries

The ovaries are paired organs that serve both reproductive and endocrine functions.

They are almond-shaped organs approximately 2.5–5 cm in length and 1.5–3.0 cm in width. They lie on the posterior surface of the broad ligaments in a shallow depression known as the ovarian fossa in close proximity to the external iliac vessels on the lateral pelvic walls and over the ureters. Each ovary has a medial and lateral surface, an anterior border that joins

with the mesovarium, a posterior border that lies free in the peritoneal cavity, an upper or tubal pole and a lower or uterine pole.

The ovary is attached to the posterior layer of the broad ligament by a fold in the peritoneum known as the *mesovarium*. This fold contains the blood vessels and nerves supplying the ovary. The tubal pole of the ovary is attached to the pelvic brim by the *suspensory ligament* of the ovary. The lower pole is attached to the lateral border of the uterus by a musculofibrous condensation known as the *ovarian ligament*.

The surface of the ovary is covered by a cuboidal or low columnar type of germinal epithelium. This surface opens directly into the peritoneal cavity.

> **!** The development of malignant disease in the ovary leads to the shedding of malignant cells directly into the peritoneal cavity as soon as the tumour breaches the surface of the ovary. The disease is silent and often asymptomatic and thus presents late. As a result of these characteristics, the prognosis is generally poor unless the disease is diagnosed when it has not extended beyond the substance of the ovary.

Beneath the germinal epithelium is a layer of dense connective tissue that effectively forms the capsule of the ovary; this is known as the **tunica albuginea**. Beneath this layer lies the **cortex** of the ovary, formed by stromal tissue and collections of epithelial cells that form the **graafian follicles** at different stages of maturation and degeneration. These follicles can also be found in the highly vascular, central portion of the ovary, the **medulla**. The blood vessels and nerve supply enter the ovary through the medulla.

THE BLOOD SUPPLY TO THE PELVIC ORGANS

Internal iliac arteries

The major part of the blood supply to the pelvic organs is derived from the internal iliac arteries (sometimes known as the hypogastric arteries), which originate from the bifurcation of the common iliac vessels into the external iliac arteries and the internal iliac vessels (Fig. 1.3).

The internal iliac artery arises at the level of the lumbosacral articulation and passes over the pelvic

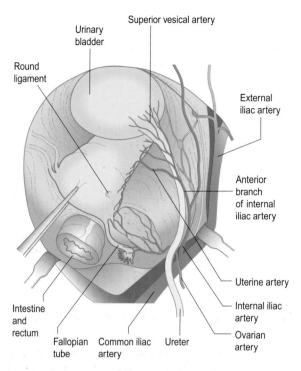

Fig. 1.3 Major blood vessels of the female pelvis.

superior and middle branches, having passed medially to the lateral and superior surfaces of the bladder, anastomose with branches from the contralateral vessels and with the branches of the uterine and vaginal arteries.

It also forms the middle haemorrhoidal artery.

The uterine artery becomes the major vascular structure arising from this division during pregnancy, when there is a major increase in uterine blood flow. It initially runs downward in the subperitoneal fat under the inferior attachment of the broad ligament towards the cervix.

The artery crosses the ureter shortly before that structure enters the bladder approximately 1.5–2 cm from the lateral fornix of the vagina. At the point of contact with the vaginal fornix, it gives off a vaginal branch that runs downwards along the lateral vaginal wall. The main uterine artery then follows a tortuous course along the lateral wall of the uterus, giving off numerous branches into the substance of the uterus and finally diverging laterally into the broad ligament to anastomose with the ovarian artery, thus forming a continuous loop that provides the blood supply for the ovaries and the tubes as well as the uterine circulation.

There are also parietal branches of the anterior division of the internal iliac artery and these include the obturator artery, the internal pudendal artery and the inferior gluteal artery.

brim, continuing downward on the posterolateral wall of the cavity of the true pelvis beneath the peritoneum until it crosses the psoas major and the piriformis muscles. It then reaches the lumbosacral trunk of the sacral plexus of nerves and, at the upper margin of the greater sciatic notch, it divides into anterior and posterior divisions. It then continues as the umbilical artery, which shortly after birth, becomes obliterated to form the lateral umbilical ligament. Thus, in fetal life, this is the major vascular network, which delivers blood via the internal iliac anterior division and its continuation as the umbilical artery to the placenta.

The branches of the two divisions of the internal iliac artery are as follows.

Anterior division

The anterior division provides the structure for the umbilical circulation as previously described. It also provides the superior, middle and inferior vesical arteries that provide the blood supply for the bladder. The

> **!** The ureters are particularly vunerable to surgical damage at two sites in the pelvis. One is the point at which the ureter enters the pelvis under the lateral origin of the infundibulopelvic fold, particularly at the time of removal of a large ovarian tumour, where clamping of the fold may incorporate the ureter as the tumour is pulled medially and the ureter is lifted off the lateral pelvic wall. Second, the ureter may be damaged where it passes under the uterine artery during a hysterectomy, when the parametrium is clamped or during dissection of the ureteric tunnel under the uterine artery.

Posterior division

The posterior division divides into the iliolumbar branch and the lateral sacral and superior gluteal branches and does not play a major function in the blood supply to the pelvic organs.

The ovarian vessels

The other important source of blood supply to the pelvic organs are the ovarian arteries. These arise from the front of the aorta between the origins of the renal and inferior mesenteric vessels. They descend behind the peritoneum on the surface of the corresponding psoas muscle until they reach the brim of the pelvis, where they cross into the corresponding infundibulo-pelvic fold and from there to the base of the meso-varium and on to anastomose with the uterine vessels. Both the uterine and ovarian arteries are accompanied by a rich plexus of veins.

 The richness of the anastomosis of the uterine and ovarian vessels means that it is possible to ligate both internal iliac arteries and reduce bleeding from the uterus and yet still maintain the viability of the pelvic organs by expanding the blood flow through the ovarian vessels.

THE PELVIC LYMPHATIC SYSTEM

The lymphatic vessels follow the course of the blood vessels but have a specific nodal system that is of particular importance in relation to malignant disease of the pelvis (Fig. 1.4).

The lymphatic drainage from the lower part of the vagina, the vulva and the perineum and anus passes to the superficial inguinal and adjacent superficial femoral nodes.

The superficial inguinal nodes lie in two groups with an upper group lying parallel to the inguinal ligament and a lower group situated along the upper part of the great saphenous vein.

Some of these nodes drain into the deep femoral nodes, which lie medial to the upper end of the femoral vein.

One of these nodes, known as the gland of Cloquet, occupies the femoral canal.

There are also pelvic parietal nodes grouped around the major pelvic vessels. These include the common iliac, external iliac and internal iliac nodes, which subsequently drain to the aortic chain of nodes.

The lymphatics of the cervix, the uterus and the upper portion of the vagina drain into the iliac nodes whereas the lymphatics of the fundus of the uterus, the fallopian tubes and the ovaries follow the ovarian

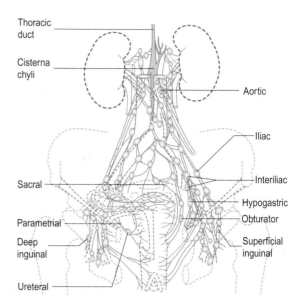

Fig. 1.4 Lymphatic drainage of the female pelvis.

vessels to the aortic nodes. Some of the lymphatics from the uterine fundus follow the round ligament into the deep and superficial inguinal nodes.

NERVES OF THE PELVIS

The nerve supply to the pelvis and the pelvic organs has both a somatic and an autonomic component. While the somatic innervation is both sensory and motor in function and relates predominantly to the external genitalia and the pelvic floor, the autonomic innervation provides the sympathetic and parasympathetic nerve supply to the pelvic organs (Fig. 1.5).

Somatic innervation

The somatic innervation to the vulva and pelvic floor is provided by the pudendal nerves which arise from the S2, S3 and S4 segments of the spinal cord. These nerves include both efferent and afferent components.

The pudendal nerves arise in the lumbosacral plexus and leave the pelvis under the sacrospinous ligament to enter Alcock's canal and pass through the layers of the wall of the ischiorectal fossa to enter the perineum. Motor branches provide innervation of the external anal sphincter muscle, the superficial perineal muscles and the external urethral sphincter.

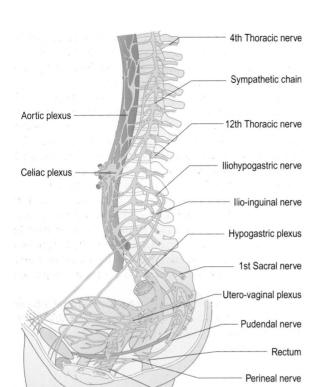

Fig. 1.5 Nerve supply of the pelvis.

Sensory innervation is provided to the clitoris through the branch of the dorsal nerve of the clitoris. The sensory innervation of the skin of the labia and of the perineum is also derived from branches of the pudendal nerves. Additional cutaneous innervation of the mons and the labia is derived from the ilioinguinal nerves (L1) and the genitofemoral nerves (L1, L2) and to the perineum through the posterior femoral cutaneous nerve from the sacral plexus (S1, S2 and S3).

Autonomic innervation

Sympathetic innervation arises from preganglionic fibres at the T10/T11 level and supplies the ovaries and tubes through sympathetic fibres that follow the ovarian vessels.

The body of the uterus and the cervix receive sympathetic innervation through the hypogastric plexus, which accompanies the branches of the iliac vessels, and also contain fibres that signal stretching.

The parasympathetic innervation to the uterus, bladder and anorectum arises from the S1, S2 and S3 segments; these fibres are important in the control of smooth muscle function of the bladder and the anal sphincter system.

Uterine pain is mediated through sympathetic afferent nerves passing up to T11/T12 and L1/L2; the pain is felt in the lower abdomen and the high lumbar spine.

Cervical pain is mediated through the parasympathetic afferent nerves passing backwards to S1, S2 and S3; perineal pain is felt at the site and is mediated through the pudendal nerves.

THE PELVIC FLOOR

The pelvic floor provides a diaphragm across the outlet of the true pelvis that contains the pelvic organs and some of the organs of the abdominal cavity. The integrity of the pelvic floor is naturally breached by the passage of the vagina, the urethra and the rectum. It plays an essential role in parturition and in urinary and faecal continence (Fig. 1.6). The principal supports of the pelvic floor are the constituent parts of the levator ani muscles. These are described in three sections.

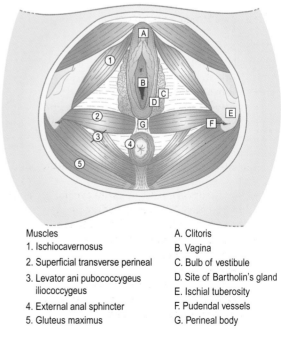

Muscles	
1. Ischiocavernosus	A. Clitoris
2. Superficial transverse perineal	B. Vagina
3. Levator ani pubococcygeus iliococcygeus	C. Bulb of vestibule
4. External anal sphincter	D. Site of Bartholin's gland
5. Gluteus maximus	E. Ischial tuberosity
	F. Pudendal vessels
	G. Perineal body

Fig. 1.6 Muscles of the pelvic floor.

- The iliococcygeus muscle arises from the parietal pelvic fascia, extends from the posterior surface of the pubic rami to the ischial spines and is inserted into the anococcygeal ligament and the coccyx.
- The puborectalis muscle arises from the posterior surface of the pubic rami and passes to the centre of the perineal body anterior to the rectum, with some decussation with muscle fibres from the contralateral muscle.
- The pubococcygeus muscle has a similar origin and passes posteriorly to the sides of the rectum and the anococcygeal ligament.

These muscles play an important role in defecation, coughing, vomiting and parturition.

THE PERINEUM

The perineum is the region defined as the inferior aperture of the pelvis and consists of all the pelvic structures that lie below the pelvic floor. The area is bounded anteriorly by the inferior margin of the pubic symphysis, the subpubic arch and the ischial tuberosities. Posteriorly, the boundaries are formed by the sacotuberous ligaments and the coccyx.

The whole region is divided into **anterior** and **posterior triangles** by a line drawn between the two ischial tuberosities. The anterior portion is known as the urogenital triangle and includes part of the urethra. The posterior or anal triangle includes the anus, the anal sphincter and the perineal body. The two triangles have their base on the deep transverse perineal muscles.

The **ischiorectal fossa** lies between the anal canal and the lateral wall of the fossa formed by the inferior ramus of the ischium covered by obturator internus muscle and fascia. Posteriorly, the fossa is formed by the gluteus maximus muscle and the sacrotuberous ligament and anteriorly by the posterior border of the urogenital diaphragm.

The pudendal nerve and internal pudendal vessels pass through the lateral aspect of the fossa enclosed in the fascial layer of Alcock's canal.

ESSENTIAL INFORMATION

The external genitalia

- The term *vulva* includes:
  - Mons pubis
  - Labia majora
  - Labia minora
  - Clitoris
  - External urinary meatus
  - Vestibule of the vagina
  - Vaginal orifice and the hymen
- Appearance dependent on age and hormonal status
- Labia majora homologous with the male scrotum
- Clitoris female homologue of the penis
  - Important role in sexual stimulation
- The vestibule contains openings of:
  - Urethral meatus
  - Vaginal orifice
  - Skene's and Bartholin's ducts
- Hymen thin fold of skin attached around the margins of the vaginal orifice

The internal genital organs

- The internal genitalia include:
  - Vagina
  - Uterus
  - Fallopian tubes
  - Ovaries

Vagina

- Muscular tube lined by squamous epithelium
- H-shaped in cross-section
- Capable of considerable distension
- Related
  - Anteriorly with urethra and bladder
  - Posteriorly with anus, perineal body, rectum, pouch of Douglas and pelvic colon

Uterus

- Cervix
  - Musculofibrous cylindrical structure

- – Vaginal portion and supravaginal portion
- – Canal lined by columnar epithelium
- – Ectocervix lined by stratified squamous epithelium
- – External os opens into vagina
- – Internal os opens into uterine cavity
- Isthmus
  - – Junctional zone between cervix and corpus uteri
  - – Forms lower segment in pregnancy
- Corpus uteri
  - – Three layers of smooth muscle fibres:
    External transverse fibres
    Middle layer circular fibres
    Inner layers longitudinal fibres
  - – Cavity lined by endometrium
  - – Tall columnar epithelium and stromal layers
  - – Change with stage of cycle

Supports of the uterus

- Direct supports
  - – Weak: Round ligaments
    Broad ligaments
    Pubocervical ligaments
  - – Strong: Uterosacral ligaments
    Transverse cervical ligaments
- Indirect supports – the pelvic floor
  - – Levator ani muscles
  - – Perineal body
  - – Urogenital diaphragm

Fallopian tubes (oviducts)

- Thin muscular tubes
- Lined by ciliated columnar epithelium
- Consist of four sections:
  - – Interstitial (intramural)
  - – Isthmus
  - – Ampulla
  - – Infundibulum (fimbriated ends)

The ovaries

- Paired almond-shaped organs
- Surface lies in peritoneal cavity
- Capsule of dense fibrous tissue (tunica albuginea)
- Cortex stroma and epithelial cells

Blood supply

Internal iliac arteries

- Anterior division: Visceral
  Parietal
  - – Visceral: Three vesical branches
    Uterine arteries
  - – Parietal: Obturator artery
    Internal gluteal artery
- Posterior division
  - – Iliolumbar branch
  - – Lateral sacral arteries
  - – Inferior gluteal branches

Ovarian arteries

- From aorta below renal arteries
- Rich anastomosis with uterine vessels

Pelvic lymphatic system

- Lymphatic vessels follow blood vessels
- Inguinal nodes (superficial and deep) drain lower vagina, vulva, perineum and anus
- Iliac and then aortic nodes drain cervix, lower part uterus, upper vagina
- Uterine fundus, tubes and ovaries drain to aortic nodes
- Some drainage follows round ligaments to inguinal nodes

Innervation

- Somatic innervation – pudendal nerves from S2, S3, S4
- Autonomic innervation
  - – Sympathetic outflow T10, T11, T12, L1, L2
  - – Parasympathetic outflow S1, S2, S3
- Pain fibres through T11, T12, L1, L2, S1, S2, S3

Perineum

- Anterior triangle – urogenital triangle includes passage of urethra
- Posterior triangle – includes anus, anal sphincters, perineal body

2 Conception and nidation

OOGENESIS

Primordial germ cells originally appear in the yolk sac and can be identified by the fourth week of fetal development (Fig. 2.1). These cells migrate through the dorsal mesentery of the developing gut and finally reach the genital ridge between 44 and 48 days post-conception. Migration occurs into a genital tubercle consisting of mesenchymal cells that appears over the ventral part of the mesonephros. The germ cells form sex cords and become the cortex of the ovary.

The sex cords subsequently break up into separate clumps of cells and by 16 weeks these clumped cells become primary follicles, which incorporate central germ cells.

These cells undergo rapid mitotic activity and, by 20 weeks of intrauterine life, there are about 7 million cells, known as *oogonia*. After this time, no further cell division occurs and no further ova are produced. At birth, the oogonia have begun the first meiotic division and have become primary oocytes. The number of oocytes falls to 1 million by birth and 0.5 million by puberty.

Meiosis

The chromosome number of gametes is half that of normal cells. With the fusion of egg and sperm, the chromosome count is returned to the normal count of 46 chromosomes. In meiosis, two cell divisions occur in succession, each of which consists of prophase, meta-phase, anaphase and telophase. However, the first of the two cell divisions is a reduction division and the second is a modified mitosis in which the prophase is usually lacking (Fig. 2.2). At the end of the first meiotic prophase, the double chromosomes undergo synapsis, producing a group of four homologous chromatids called a *tetrad*.

The two centrioles move to opposite poles. A spindle forms in the middle and the membrane of the nucleus disappears. As the cell enters the metaphase of the first meiotic division, the tetrads line up around the equator of the spindle.

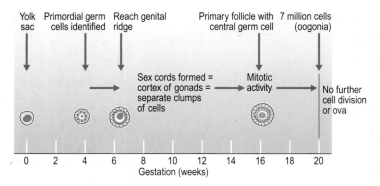

Fig. 2.1 Embryonic and fetal development of oogonia.

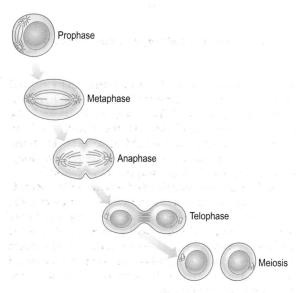

Fig. 2.2 Primary oocytes remain in suspended prophase. Meiotic division resumes under stimulation by LH.

Primary oocytes remain in suspended prophase until sexual maturity is reached. Meiotic division resumes as the dominant follicle is triggered by luteinizing hormone (LH) to commence ovulation. In anaphase, the daughter chromatids separate and move towards opposite poles.

Thus, the nuclear events in oogenesis are the same as in spermatogenesis but cytoplasmic division is unequal, resulting in one secondary oocyte. This small cell consists almost entirely of a nucleus and is known as the first polar body. As the ovum enters the fallopian tube, the second meiotic division occurs and a secondary oocyte forms, with the development of a small second polar body.

Follicular development in the ovary

The gross structure and the blood supply and nerve supply of the ovary have been described in Chapter 1. However, the microscopic anatomy of the ovary is important in understanding the mechanism of follicular development and ovulation.

The surface of the ovary is covered by a single layer of cuboidal epithelium. The cortex of the ovary contains a large number of oogonia surrounded by follicular cells that become *granulosa* cells. The remainder of the ovary consists of a mesenchymal core. Most of the ova in the cortex never reach an advanced stage of maturation and become atretic early in follicular development. At any given time, follicles can be seen in various stages of maturation and degeneration (Fig. 2.3).

The first stage of development is characterized by enlargement of the ovum with the aggregation of stromal cells to form the thecal cells. The innermost layers of granulosa cells adhere to the ovum and form the *corona radiata*. A fluid-filled space develops in the granulosa cells and a clear layer of gelatinous material collects around the ovum, forming the *zona pellucida*. The ovum becomes eccentrically placed and the graafian follicle assumes its classic mature form. The mesenchymal cells around the follicle become differentiated into two layers, forming the *theca interna* and the *theca externa*.

As the follicle enlarges, it bulges towards the surface of the ovary and the area under the germinal epithelium

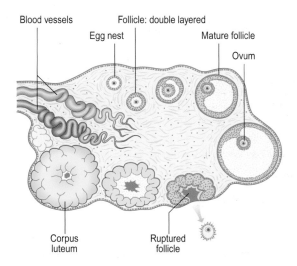

Fig. 2.3 Development and maturation of the graafian follicle.

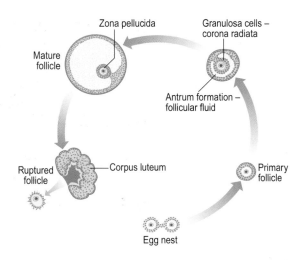

Fig. 2.4 Ovulation and corpus luteum formation.

thins out. Finally, the ovum with its surrounding investment of granulosa cells escapes through this area at the time of ovulation.

The cavity of the follicle often fills with blood but, at the same time, the granulosa cells and the theca interna cells undergo the changes of luteinization to become filled with yellow carotenoid material. The corpus luteum in its mature form shows intense vascularization and pronounced vacuolization of the theca and granulosa cells with evidence of hormonal activity. This development reaches its peak approximately 7 days after ovulation and thereafter the corpus luteum regresses unless implantation occurs. This degeneration is characterized by increasing vacuolization of the granulosa cells and the appearance of increased quantities of fibrous tissue in the centre of the corpus luteum. This finally develops into a white scar known as the *corpus albicans* (Fig. 2.4).

HORMONAL EVENTS ASSOCIATED WITH OVULATION

The maturation of oocytes, ovulation and the endometrial and tubal changes of the menstrual cycle are all regulated by a series of interactive hormonal changes (Fig. 2.5).

The process is initiated by the release of LH-releasing hormone, a major neurosecretion produced in the median eminence of the hypothalamus. It has been isolated in many sites in the central nervous system and may act as a neurotransmitter. The hormone is a decapeptide and is released from axon terminals into the pituitary portal capillaries. As the release of both follicle-stimulating hormone (FSH) and LH are stimulated by this hormone, it is more appropriately designated gonadotrophin-releasing hormone (GnRH).

GnRH is released in episodic fluctuations but there is no definite association between these surges and LH release. However, there is an increase in the number of surges associated with the higher levels of plasma LH and there is evidence of a decline in the GnRH content of the hypothalamus in mid-cycle in women. Continued ongoing GnRH action is required to initiate the oestrogen-induced LH surge.

The three major hormones involved in reproduction are produced by the anterior lobe of the pituitary gland or adenohypophysis, and include FSH, LH and prolactin. Blood levels of both FSH and LH appear to remain at a relatively constant level in the first half of the cycle. There is a marked surge of LH 35–42 hours before ovulation and a smaller coincidental FSH peak (Fig. 2.5). The LH surge is, in fact, made up of two proximate surges and a peak in plasma oestradiol precedes the LH surge. This surge may be a factor that stimulates the hypothalamus to release GnRH. Plasma LH and FSH levels are slightly lower in the second half of the cycle than in the preovulatory phase. Pituitary gonadotrophins influence the activity of the hypothalamus by a short-loop feedback system.

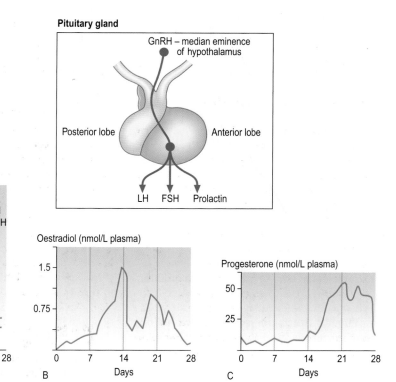

Fig. 2.5 The hormonal regulation of ovulation. GnRH stimulates the release of gonadotrophins from the anterior lobe of the pituitary. Blood levels of (a) LH, FSH, (b) oestradiol, (c) progesterone during a 28-day menstrual cycle.

✓ There is a feedback mechanism that regulates the release of FSH and LH by oestrogens produced by the ovaries. In the presence of ovarian failure as seen in the menopause, the gonadotrophin levels become markedly elevated.

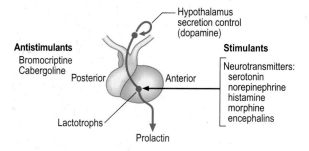

Fig. 2.6 Factors regulating the release of prolactin.

Prolactin is secreted by lactotrophs in the anterior lobe of the pituitary gland. Prolactin levels rise at mid-cycle and remain elevated during the luteal phase and tend to follow the changes in plasma oestradiol-17β. Prolactin tends to control its own secretion through a short-loop feedback on the hypothalamus, which produces the prolactin-inhibiting factor, dopamine, and probably by the production of a hypothalamic releasing factor (Fig. 2.6). Oestrogen appears to stimulate prolactin release and various neurotransmitters, such as serotonin, noradrenaline (norepinephrine), morphine and enkepha-

lins, also stimulate prolactin release by a central action on the brain. Antagonists to dopamine such as phenothiazine, reserpine and methyltyrosine also stimulate the release of prolactin, whereas dopamine agonists such as bromocriptine and cabergoline have the opposite effect.

Hyperprolactinaemia inhibits ovulation and is an important cause of secondary amenorrhoea and infertility.

The action of gonadotrophins

FSH stimulates follicular growth and development and binds exclusively to granulosa cells in the growing follicle. Of the 30 or so follicles that begin to mature in each menstrual cycle, one becomes pre-eminent. The granulosa cells produce oestrogen, which feeds back on the pituitary to suppress FSH release. At the same time, FSH stimulates receptors for LH.

LH stimulates and sustains development of the corpus luteum; receptors for LH are found in the theca and granulosa cells and in the corpus luteum. There is a close interaction between FSH and LH in follicular growth and maturation. The corpus luteum produces progesterone until it begins to deteriorate in the late luteal phase (Fig. 2.4). Prolactin appears to exert a direct effect on the follicle and to play a role in the initiation and maintenance of luteinization. It stimulates the development of LH receptors and thus supports the production of high levels of progesterone.

THE ENDOMETRIAL CYCLE

The normal endometrium responds in a cyclical manner to the fluctuations in ovarian steroids. The endometrium consists of three zones and it is the two outer zones that are shed during menstruation (Fig. 2.7).

The basal zone (*zona basalis*) is the thin layer of the compact stroma that interdigitates with the myometrium and shows little response to hormonal change. It is not shed at the time of menstruation. The next adjacent zone (*zona spongiosa*) contains the endometrial glands which are lined by columnar epithelial cells surrounded by loose stroma. The surface of the endometrium is covered by a compact layer of epithelial cells (*zona compacta*) that surrounds the ostia of the endometrial glands. The endometrial cycle is divided into four phases:

1. **Menstrual phase.** This occupies the first 4 days of the cycle and results in shedding of the outer two layers of the endometrium. The onset of menstruation is preceded by segmental

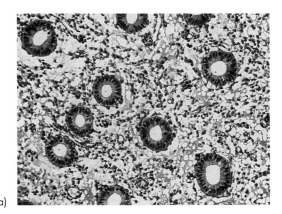
(a)

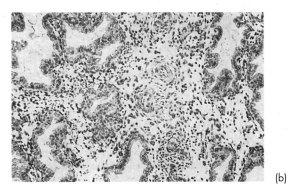
(b)

Fig. 2.7 Cyclical changes in the normal menstrual cycle. (a) Proliferative phase. (b) Mid-luteal phase. (c) Menstrual phase.

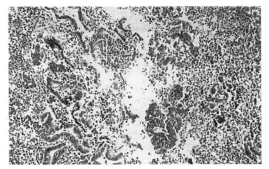
(c)

vasoconstriction of the spiral arterioles. This leads to necrosis and shedding of the functional layers of the endometrium. The vascular changes are associated with a fall in both oestrogen and progesterone levels but the mechanism by which these vascular changes are mediated is still not understood.

2. **Phase of repair.** This phase extends from day 4 to day 7 and is associated with the formation of a new capillary bed arising from the arterial coils and with the regeneration of the epithelial surface.

3. **Follicular or proliferative phase.** This is the period of maximal growth of the endometrium and is associated with elongation and expansion of the glands and with stromal development. This phase extends from day 7 until the time of ovulation on day 14.

4. **Luteal or secretory phase.** This follows ovulation on day 14 and continues until day 28 when menstruation starts again. During this phase, the endometrial glands become convoluted and 'saw-toothed' in appearance. The epithelial cells exhibit basal vacuolation and, by day 20 of the cycle, there is visible secretion in these cells. The secretion subsequently becomes inspissated and, as menstruation approaches, there is oedema of the stroma and a pseudodecidual reaction. Within 2 days of menstruation, there is infiltration of the stroma by leukocytes.

It is now clear that luteinization of the follicle can occur in the absence of the release of the oocyte, which may remain entrapped in the follicle. This condition is described as *entrapped ovulation* or the LUF (luteinized unruptured follicle) syndrome and is associated with

normal progesterone production and an apparently normal ovulatory cycle. Histological examination of the endometrium generally enables precise dating of the menstrual cycle and is particularly important in providing presumptive evidence of ovulation.

PRODUCTION OF SPERM

Spermatogenesis

The testis provides the dual function of spermatogenesis and androgen secretion. FSH is predominantly responsible for stimulation of spermatogenesis and LH for the stimulation of Leydig cells and the production of testosterone.

The full maturation of spermatozoa takes 64 days (Fig. 2.8). All phases of maturation can be seen in the testis. The spermatogonia divide and give rise to primary spermatocytes that have a diploid number of chromosomes. These cells undergo maturation division to secondary spermatocytes (2N haploid) and, finally, reduction division to form the haploid spermatids that develop into the mature spermatozoa.

Structure of the spermatozoon

The spermatozoon consists of a head, neck and tail (Fig. 2.9). The head is flattened and ovoid in shape and is covered by the acrosomal cap, which contains several lysins.

The nucleus is densely packed with the genetic material of the sperm. The neck contains two centrioles, proximal and distal, which form the beginning of the

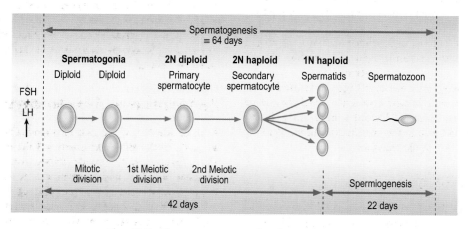

Fig. 2.8 The maturation cycle of spermatozoa.

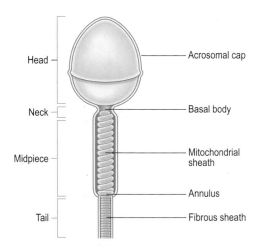

Fig. 2.9 Structure of the mature spermatozoon.

tail. The distal centriole is vestigial in mature spermatozoa but is functional in the spermatid. The body contains a coiled helix of mitochondria that provides the 'powerhouse' for sperm motility.

The tail consists of a central core of two longitudinal fibres surrounded by nine pairs of fibres that terminate at various points until a single ovoid filament remains. These contractile fibres propel the spermatozoa.

Seminal plasma

Spermatozoa carry little nutritional reserve and therefore depend on seminal plasma for nutritional support. Seminal plasma originates from the prostate, the seminal vesicles, the vas deferens and the bulbourethral glands. There is a high concentration of fructose, which is the major source of energy for the spermatozoa. The plasma also contains high concentrations of amino acids, particularly glutamic acid and several unique amines such as spermine and spermidine.

Seminal plasma also contains high concentrations of prostaglandins, which have a potent stimulatory effect on uterine musculature. Normal semen clots shortly after ejaculation but liquifies within 30 minutes through the action of fibrinolytic enzymes.

FERTILIZATION

The process of fertilization involves the fusion of the male and female gametes to produce the diploid genetic complement from the genes of both partners.

Sperm transport

Following the deposition of semen near the cervical os, migration occurs rapidly into the cervical mucus. The speed of this migration depends on the presence of receptive mucus in mid-cycle. During the luteal phase, the mucus is not receptive to sperm invasion and therefore very few spermatozoa reach the uterine cavity. Under favourable circumstances, sperm migrate at a rate of 6 mm/minute. This is much faster than could be explained by the motility of the sperm and must therefore also be dependent on active support within the uterine cavity. Only motile spermatozoa reach the fimbriated end of the tube.

Capacitation

During their passage through the fallopian tubes, the sperm undergo the final stage in maturation (capacitation), which enables penetration of the zona pellucida. It seems likely that these changes are enzyme-induced and enzymes such as β-amylase or β-glucuronidase may act on the membranes of the spermatozoa to expose receptor sites involved in sperm penetration. In addition, various other factors that may be important in capacitation have been identified, such as the removal of cholesterol from the plasma membrane and the presence of α- and β-adrenergic receptors on the spermatozoa. Until recently, it was thought that capacitation occurred only in vivo in the fallopian tubes. However, it can also be induced in vitro by apparently non-specific effects of relatively simple culture solutions.

Inhibitory substances in the plasma of the cauda epididymis and in seminal plasma can prevent capacitation and these substances also exist in the lower reaches of the female genital tract. It seems likely that these substances protect the sperm until shortly before fusion with the oocyte.

Fertilization and implantation

A small number of spermatozoa reach the oocyte in the ampulla of the tube and surround the zona pellucida. The adherence of the sperm to the oocyte initiates the *acrosome reaction*, which involves the loss of plasma membrane over the acrosomal cap (Fig. 2.10a).

The process allows the release of lytic enzymes, which facilitates penetration of the oocyte membrane. The sperm head fuses with the oocyte plasma membrane

(a)

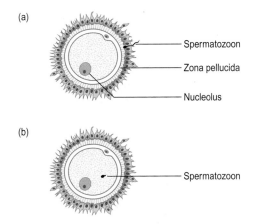

— Spermatozoon

— Zona pellucida

— Nucleolus

(b)

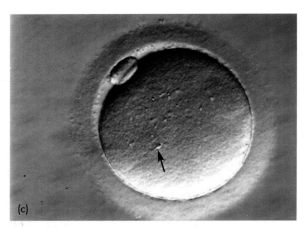

— Spermatozoon

(c)

Fig. 2.10 (a) Adherence of the sperm to the oocyte initiates the acrosome reaction. (b, c) Syngamy involves the passage of the nucleus of the sperm head into the cytoplasm of the oocyte with the formation of the zygote.

and by phagocytosis the sperm head and midpiece are engulfed into the oocyte.

The sperm head decondenses to form the male pronucleus and eventually becomes apposed to the female pronucleus in the female egg to form the *zygote*. The membranes of the pronuclei break down to facilitate the fusion of male and female chromosomes. This process is known as *syngamy* (Fig. 2.10b, c) and is followed almost immediately by the first cleavage division.

During the 36 hours after fertilization, the conceptus is transported through the tube by muscular peristaltic action. The egg undergoes cleavage and at the 16-cell

stage, becomes a solid ball of cells known as a *morula*. A fluid-filled cavity develops within the morula to form the *blastocyst* (Fig. 2.11). Six days after ovulation, the embryonic pole of the blastocyst attaches itself to the endometrium, usually near to the mid-portion of the uterine cavity. By the seventh day, the blastocyst has penetrated deeply into the endometrium.

Endometrial cells are destroyed by the cytotrophoblast and the cells are incorporated by fusion and phagocytosis into the trophoblast. The endometrial stromal cells become large and pale; this is known as the *decidual reaction*.

The process of fertilization and implantation is now complete.

THE PHYSIOLOGY OF COITUS

Normal sexual arousal has been described in four levels in both the male and the female. These levels consist of excitement, plateau, orgasmic and resolution phases. In the male, the *excitement phase* results in compression of the venous channels of the penis, resulting in erection. This is mediated through the parasympathetic plexus through S2 and S3. During the *plateau phase*, the penis remains engorged and the testes increase in size, with elevation of the testes and scrotum. Secretion from the bulbourethral glands results in the appearance of a clear fluid at the urethral meatus. These changes are accompanied by general systemic features including increased skeletal muscle tension, hyperventilation and tachycardia.

> ❗ Erectile dysfunction may result from neurological damage to the spinal cord or the brain and is seen as a result of spina bifida, multiple sclerosis and diabetic neuropathy. However, there are over 200 prescription drugs that are known to cause impotence and these account for some 25% of all cases. Recreational drugs such as alcohol, nicotine, cocaine, marijuana and LSD may also cause impotence.

The *orgasmic phase* is induced by stimulation of the glans penis and by movement of penile skin on the penile shaft. There are reflex contractions of the bulbocavernosus and ischiocavernosus muscles and ejaculation of semen in a series of spurts. Specific musculoskeletal activity occurs that is characterized by

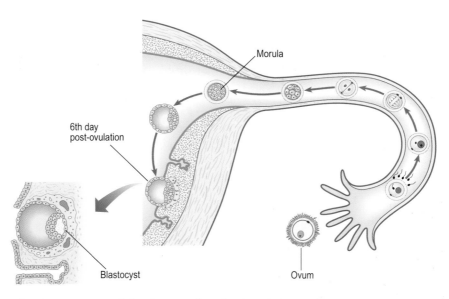

Fig. 2.11 Stages of development from fertilization to implantation.

penile thrusting. The systemic changes of hyperventilation and rapid respiration persist.

 Seminal emission depends on the sympathetic nervous system. Expulsion of semen is brought about by contraction of smooth muscle within the seminal vesicles, ejaculatory ducts and prostate.

During the *resolution phase*, penile erection rapidly subsides, as does the hyperventilation and tachycardia. There is a marked sweating reaction in some 30–40% of individuals. During this phase, the male becomes refractory to further stimulation. The plateau phase may be prolonged if ejaculation does not occur.

In the female, the *excitement phase* involves nipple and clitoral erection, vaginal lubrication, resulting partly from vaginal transudation and partly from secretions from Bartholin's glands, thickening and congestion of the labia majora and the labia minora and engorgement of the uterus. Stimulation of the clitoris and the labia results in progression to the *orgasmic platform*, with narrowing of the outer third of the vagina and ballooning of the vaginal vault. The vaginal walls become congested and purplish in colour and there is a marked increase in vaginal blood flow. During orgasm, the clitoris retracts below the pubic symphysis and a succession of contractions occur in the vaginal walls and pelvic floor approximately every second for several seconds. At the same time, there is an increase in pulse rate, hyperventilation and specific skeletal muscular contractions. Blood pressure rises and there is some diminution in the level of awareness. Both intravaginal and intrauterine pressures rise during orgasm.

The *plateau phase* may be sustained in the female and result in multiple orgasm. Following orgasm, resolution of the congestion of the pelvic organs occurs rapidly, although the tachycardia and hypertension accompanied by a sweating reaction may persist.

Factors that determine human sexuality are far more complex than the simple process of arousal by clitoral or penile stimulation. Although the frequency of intercourse and orgasm declines with age, this is in part mediated by loss of interest by the partners. The female remains capable of orgasm until late in life but her behaviour is substantially determined by the interest of the male partner. Sexual interest and performance also decline with age in the male and the older male requires more time to achieve excitement and erection. Ejaculation may become less frequent and forceful.

Common sexual problems are discussed in Chapter 19.

ESSENTIAL INFORMATION

Oogenesis

- Primordial germ cells appear in the yolk sac
- By 20 weeks, there are 7 million oogonia
- Number of oocytes falls to 1 million by birth
- Number falls to 0.5 million by puberty
- Chromosome number of gametes half that of normal cells
- Primary oocyte remains in suspended prophase
- The second meiotic division occurs as the ovum enters the tube

Follicular development in the ovary

- Most ova never reach advanced maturity
- Aggregation of stromal cells around follicles become thecal cells
- Innermost layers of granulosa cells form the corona radiata
- After ovulation, the corpus luteum is formed

Hormonal events and ovulation

- FSH stimulates follicular growth
- FSH stimulates LH receptor development
- LH stimulates and sustains development of the corpus luteum
- Follicles produce oestrogen
- Corpus luteum produces progesterone

The endometrial cycle

- Menstrual phase – shedding of functional layer of endometrium
- Phase of repair – day 4–7 of cycle
- Follicular phase – maximum period of growth of endometrial glands

- Luteal phase – 'saw-toothed' glands, pseudodecidual reaction in stroma

Spermatogenesis

- Full maturation takes 64 days
- Mature sperm arise from haploid spermatids

Structure of spermatozoon

- Head is covered by acrosomal cap
- Body contains helix of mitochondria
- Tail consists of two longitudinal fibres and nine pairs of fibres

Seminal plasma

- Originates from the prostate, seminal vesicles and bulbourethral glands
- High concentration of fructose provides energy for sperm motility
- High concentration of prostaglandins

Sperm transport

- Rapid migration into receptive cervical mucus
- Sperm migrate at 6 mm/min
- Only motile sperm reach the fimbriated ends of the tubes

Capacitation

- Final sperm maturation occurs during passage through the oviduct
- Inhibitory substances produced in caudo-epididymis and in seminal plasma

Fertilization

- Small number of sperm reach oocyte
- Adherence of sperm initiates acrosome reaction
- Sperm head fuses with oocyte plasma membrane
- Sperm head and midpiece engulfed into oocyte
- Fusion of male and female chromosomes is known as syngamy
- 36 hours after fertilization, morula is formed
- 6 days after fertilization, implantation occurs

Physiology of coitus

- Penile erection results from compression of venous channels
- Ejaculation mediated by contractions of bulbo- and ischiocavernosus
- Female excitation results in nipple and clitoral erection
- Lubrication comes from vaginal transudation, Bartholin's glands secretions
- Orgasm results in clitoral retraction and contractions of pelvic floor muscles

3 Physiological changes in pregnancy

The recognition of abnormal events in pregnancy demands a clear understanding of the normal processes of maternal adaptation. These changes affect all systems to varying degrees and may be influenced within a physiological range by factors such as age, parity, multiple pregnancy, socioeconomic status and race.

In all mammalian species, there are extensive biochemical, physiological and structural changes during pregnancy and the puerperium. These changes start as early as the luteal phase of a conceptual menstrual cycle.

From a teleological point of view, there are two main reasons for these changes:

- To provide a suitable environment for the nutrition, growth and development of the fetus
- To protect and prepare the mother for the process of parturition and subsequent support and nurture of the newborn infant.

The changes that occur in pregnancy are both visible and subtle.

MATERNAL WEIGHT GAIN

Of the physical changes that occur, the most obvious are the enlargement of the abdomen and the increase in body weight. An important part of this increase in all systems is the retention of water; the mean total increase is about 8.5 litres. The same increase in total body water occurs in both primigravid and multiparous women.

There are no reliable data available for weight gain in the first 12 weeks of pregnancy. Many women during this time do not gain any weight because of reduced food intake associated with loss of appetite and morning sickness. However, in normal pregnancy, the average weight gain is 0.3 kg/week up to 18 weeks, 0.45 kg/week from 18 to 28 weeks and thereafter a slight reduction with a rate of 0.36–0.41 kg/week until term (Fig. 3.1).

Weight gain is 12.5 kg in primigravidae and about 0.9 kg less in multigravidae. Increased weight gain is commonly associated with oedema and fluid retention. However, overall weight gain has a positive association with birthweight and, although acute excessive weight

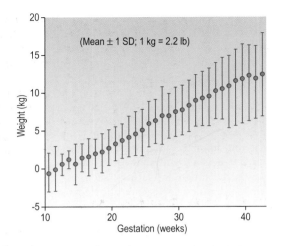

Fig. 3.1 Maternal weight gain (mean ± 1 SD) in normal pregnancy. (With permission from James et al. 1994 High risk pregnancy: management options. Baillière Tindall, London.)

gain may be associated with the development of pre-eclampsia, mild oedema is associated with a good fetal outcome.

Far more sinister is failure to gain weight, which may be associated with impaired fetal growth and an adverse outcome.

Contributions to weight gain

Weight gain in pregnancy is derived from both maternal and fetoplacental sources. Water is retained in all systems of the body and the increased hydration of connective tissue results in laxity of the joints, particularly in the pelvic ligaments and the pubic symphysis.

Pregnancy is an anabolic state and thus results in an increase in body fat and protein and the growth of the breasts and the uterus (Fig. 3.2). The breasts account for 0.4 kg and the uterus for 0.9 kg. Body fat increases by 4 kg and most of this accumulates during the second trimester. Blood volume expands by 1.2 kg and a further contribution of 1.2 kg occurs as a result of the expansion of extracellular fluid.

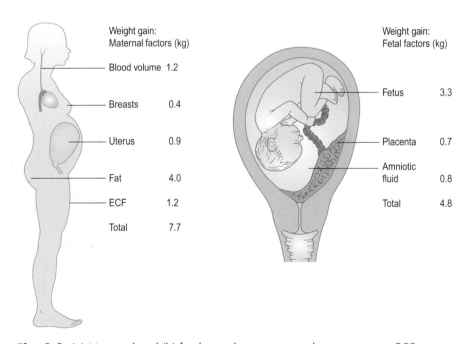

Fig. 3.2 (a) Maternal and (b) fetal contributions to weight gain at term. ECF, extracellular fluid.

> ! Acute excess weight gain indicates fluid retention. Poor weight gain is associated with fetal growth restriction.

The fetus, placenta and amniotic fluid contribute to some 40% of the weight gain, with 3.3 kg from the fetus, 0.7 kg from the placenta and 0.8 kg from amniotic fluid.

Poor weight gain is associated with an increased incidence of low-birthweight infants, reduced amniotic fluid volume and reduced placental size.

The range of maternal weight gain in normal pregnancy may vary from near zero to twice the mean weight gain as a result of variation in the multiple contributory factors.

Although there have been conflicting reports about the status of protein storage in human pregnancy, it seems likely that no more protein is laid down than can be accounted for by fetal and placental growth and by the increase in size in specific target organs such as the uterus and the breasts.

The increase in fat storage in normal pregnancy occurs principally in the second trimester, mainly over the back, the upper thighs, the buttocks and the abdominal wall. Surprisingly, the correlation between energy intake and maternal weight gain is poor and it is generally not advisable to inhibit weight gain or attempt to promote weight loss in pregnancy, as it may result in a parallel restriction of essential nutrients and this in turn may have undesirable effects on fetal growth and development.

Postpartum weight

Immediately following delivery, there is a weight loss of some 6 kg, which is accounted for by water and fluid loss and by the loss of the products of conception. Body weight then remains constant, or may rise, over the next 3 days and then falls by approximately 0.3 kg/day until day 10, stabilizing by the 10th week after delivery with a positive gain from the prepregnant weight of 2.25 kg (Table 3.1). This positive balance is 0.7 kg in women who are continuing to lactate.

Diuresis occurs during the puerperium, removing the water retained in all tissues during pregnancy. In women who are not oedematous the diuresis commences 3–4 days after delivery and continues for 2 weeks. If oedema is present, fluid loss commences immediately after delivery.

CHANGES IN THE BREASTS

Some of the first signs and symptoms of pregnancy are exhibited in the breasts and these include breast tenderness, an increase in size, enlargement of the nipples and increased vascularity and pigmentation of the areola.

The areola contains sebaceous glands that hypertrophy during pregnancy and are called Montgomery's tubercles. The areola is richly supplied with sensory nerves and this ensures that suckling sends impulses to the hypothalamus and thus stimulates the release of oxytocin from the posterior lobe of the pituitary gland and the expulsion of milk.

Breast anatomy

The breasts consist of variable amounts of adipose tissue, glandular tissue and their associated ducts, blood vessels, nerves and lymphatics, and connective tissue.

The glandular tissue consists of multiple clusters of milk-secreting alveoli surrounded by band-like myoepithelial cells that are sensitive to oxytocin and promote the ejection of milk during suckling.

The cuboidal alveolar cells secrete milk into their associated ducts and finally into some 10–20 lactiferous sinuses underlying and draining into the nipples (Fig. 3.3).

Breast development during pregnancy

Proliferation of the ducts during pregnancy is under the influence of high levels of oestrogen with some contribution from growth hormone and glucocorticoids.

Alveolar growth is stimulated in the oestrogen-primed breast by progesterone but is also influenced by prolactin.

Table 3.1
Postpartum weight loss

Delivery loss	6 kg
Delivery to day 3	Weight constant or may rise
Days 3–10.	Weight loss 0.3 kg/day
Day10–10th week	Further loss 2.15 kg
Net weight gain/ pregnancy	2.25 kg

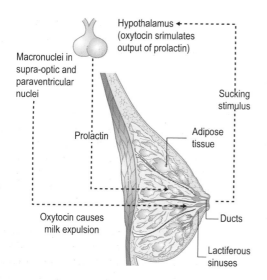

Fig. 3.3 Factors regulating milk production and expulsion.

Secretory activity is initiated during pregnancy and is promoted by prolactin and placental lactogen so that from 3–4 months onwards and for the first 30 hours after delivery, a thick, glossy, protein-rich fluid known as **colostrum** can be expressed from the breast. However, full lactation is inhibited during pregnancy by the high levels of oestrogen and progesterone.

The initiation of lactation

Prolactin is secreted from the anterior pituitary gland and its release is controlled by prolactin inhibitory factors such as dopamine. The hormone acts directly on the cells of the alveoli to stimulate the synthesis of all milk components including casein, lactalbumin and fatty acids. The sudden reduction of progesterone and oestrogen levels following parturition allows prolactin to act in an uninhibited manner and its release is promoted by suckling, with the development of the full flow of milk by day 5 and a further gradual increase over the next 3 weeks. The administration of a dopamine agonist such as bromocriptine inhibits the release of prolactin and abolishes milk production.

Suckling also promotes the release of oxytocin from specialized neurones in the supraoptic and para-ventricular nuclei of the hypothalamus and this in turn results in the milk-ejection reflex as the oxytocin stimulates the myoepithelial cells to contract.

The milk-ejection reflex can also be stimulated by the mother seeing the infant or hearing its cry or just thinking about feeding! It may also be inhibited by catecholamine release or by adverse emotional and environmental factors.

THE UTERUS

During pregnancy, the uterus undergoes a 10-fold increase in weight from around 100 g prepregnant weight to 300–400 g at 20 weeks and 1100 g at term. The uterus consists of bundles of smooth muscle cells separated by thin sheets of connective tissue composed of collagen, elastic fibres and fibroblasts. As with the smooth muscle cells, these structures all undergo hypertrophy during pregnancy.

The smooth muscle cells initially grow by hyperplasia of the cells and later by hypertrophy and elongation of the cells from 50 μm in the non-pregnant state to 200–600 μm at term. The muscle cells are arranged as an innermost longitudinal layer, a middle layer with bundles running in all directions and an outermost layer of both circular and longitudinal fibres that are in part continuous with the ligamentous supports of the uterus (Fig. 3.4).

The myometrium functions as a syncytium so that contractions can pass through the gap junctions linking the cells and produce coordinated waves of contractions.

The uterus is functionally and morphologically divided into three sections: the cervix, the isthmus (later to

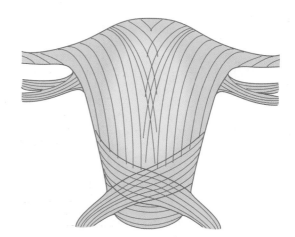

Fig. 3.4 Decussation of muscle fibres in the various layers of the human uterus.

develop into the lower uterine segment and the body of the uterus (corpus uteri).

The cervix

The cervix is predominantly a fibrous organ with only 10% of uterine muscle cells in the substance of the cervix. Eighty per cent of the total protein in the non-pregnant state consists of collagen. The principal function of the cervix is to retain the conceptus (Fig. 3.5).

By the end of pregnancy, the concentration of collagen is reduced to one-third of the amount present in the non-pregnant state.

The characteristic changes in the cervix during pregnancy are:

- Changes in the stroma
- Hypertrophy of the cervical glands producing the appearance of a cervical erosion; an increase in mucous secretory tissue in the cervix during pregnancy leads to a mucous discharge and the development of an antibacterial plug of mucus in the cervix
- A reduction of collagen in the cervix in the third trimester and the accumulation of glycosamino-glycans and water. These changes lead to the

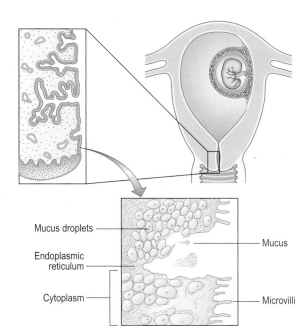

Mucus droplets
Endoplasmic reticulum
Cytoplasm
Mucus
Microvilli

Fig. 3.5 Structure and function of the cervix in pregnancy.

characteristic changes of cervical ripening. An alteration in ground structure also allows stretching and dilatation of the cervix in labour.

The isthmus

The isthmus of the uterus is the junctional zone between the cervix and the body of the uterus. It joins the muscle fibres of the corpus to the dense connective tissue of the cervix both functionally and structurally. By the 28th week of gestation, regular contractions produce some stretching and thinning of the isthmus, resulting in the early formation of the lower uterine segment.

The lower segment is fully formed during labour and is a thin, relatively inert part of the uterus. It contributes little to the expulsive efforts of the uterus and becomes in effect an extension of the birth canal. Because of its relatively avascularity and quiescence in the puerperium, it is the site of choice for the incision for a caesarean delivery.

The corpus uteri

The uterus must adapt to meet the needs of the growing fetus both in terms of physical size and in vascular adaptation to supply the nutrients required. The uterus changes throughout pregnancy to meet these requirements as follows.

- There is a change in the size, shape, position and consistency. In the latter months of pregnancy, the enlargement occurs predominantly in the uterine fundus so that the round ligaments tend to emerge from a relatively caudal point in the uterus. The shape of the uterus changes from a pear-shaped structure in early pregnancy to a more globular and ovoid shape in the second and third trimesters. The cavity expands from some 4 ml in the non-pregnant state to 4000 ml at full term. To retain the pregnancy, the myometrium must remain relatively quiescent until the onset of labour.
- All the vessels supplying the uterus undergo massive hypertrophy. The uterine arteries dilate so that the diameters are 1.5 times those seen in the non-pregnant state. The arcuate arteries that supply the placental bed become 10 times larger and the spiral arterioles reach 30 times the pre-pregnancy diameter. Uterine blood flow increases from 50 ml/min at 10 weeks gestation to 500–600 ml/min at term.

In the non-pregnant uterus, blood flow is almost entirely through the uterine arteries but in pregnancy up to 20–30% is contributed through the ovarian vessels. A small contribution is made by the superior vesical arteries.

The uterine and radial arteries are subject to regulation by the autonomic nervous system and by direct effects from vasodilator and vasoconstrictor humoral agents.

The final vessels delivering blood to the intervillous space (Fig. 3.6) are the spiral arterioles; there are a total of 100–150 supplying this space. Two or three spiral arterioles arise from each radial artery and each placental cotyledon is provided with one or two.

In the first 10 weeks of normal pregnancy, extravillous cytotrophoblast invades the decidua and the walls of the spiral arterioles, producing destruction of the smooth muscle in the wall of the vessels, which then become inert channels unresponsive to humoral and neurological control. From 10–16 weeks, a further wave of invasion of villous trophoblast occurs and extends down the luminal portion of the decidual portion of the vessel and from 16–24 weeks this invasion extends to involve the myometrial portion of the spiral arterioles. The net effect of these changes is to turn the spiral arterioles into flaccid sinusoidal channels.

Failure of this process, particularly in the myometrial portion of the vessels, is a feature of pre-eclampsia and intrauterine growth restriction and this means that this portion of the vessels remains sensitive to vasoactive stimuli with a consequent reduction in blood flow.

Uterine contractility

Myometrial growth is almost entirely due to muscle hypertrophy, although some hyperplasia may occur during early pregnancy. The stimulus for myometrial growth and development is derived from the direct effects of the growing conceptus and from the effects of oestrogens and progesterone produced initially by the ovary but later predominantly by the placenta.

The pregnant myometrium has a much greater compliance than non-pregnant myometrium in response to distension. Thus, although the uterus becomes distended by the growing conceptus, intrauterine pressure does not increase, although the uterus does maintain the capacity to develop maximal active tension. This capacity may depend on some changes in contractile proteins but is predominantly due to changes in connective tissue.

The continuation of successful pregnancy depends on the fact that the myometrium remains quiescent until the fetus is mature and capable of sustaining extrauterine life. Progesterone appears to be the major hormone responsible. It achieves this effect by increasing the resting membrane potential of the myometrial cells while at the same time impairing the conduction of electrical activity and limiting muscle activity to small clumps of cells. Progesterone antagonists such as mifepristone can induce labour.

The uterus has both afferent and efferent nerve supplies, although it can function normally in a denervated state. The main sensory fibres from the cervix arise from S1 and S2 whereas those from the body of the uterus arise from the dorsal nerve routes on T11 and T12. There is an afferent pathway from the cervix to the hypothalamus so that stretching of the cervix and upper vagina stimulates the release of oxytocin. This is known as *Ferguson's reflex*. The cervical and uterine vessels are well supplied by adrenergic nerves whereas cholinergic nerves are confined to the blood vessels of the cervix.

The development of myometrial activity

Uterine activity occurs throughout pregnancy and is measurable as early as 7 weeks gestation, with contractions that are frequent but of low intensity. As preg-

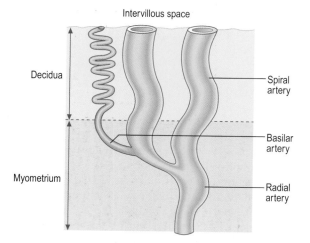

Fig. 3.6 Vascular structure in the uteroplacental bed.

Intervillous space

Decidua

Spiral artery

Basilar artery

Myometrium

Radial artery

nancy advances into the second trimester, contractions increase in intensity but remain of relatively low frequency; in the third trimester they increase in both frequency and intensity, leading up to the first stage of labour. Contractions during pregnancy are usually painless and are felt as 'tightenings' known as *Braxton Hicks contractions*. However, these contractions may sometimes be sufficiently powerful to produce discomfort. They do not produce cervical dilatation, which occurs with the onset of labour.

Once labour has begun, the contractions in the late first stage may reach pressures up to 100 mmHg and occur every 2–3 minutes (Fig. 3.7).

THE VAGINA

The vagina is lined by stratified squamous epithelium, which becomes markedly hypertrophic during pregnancy. The musculature in the vaginal wall also becomes hypertrophic and the connective tissue, as in the cervix, shows a reduction in collagen and an increase in water and glycosaminoglycans. The rich venous vascular network in the vaginal walls becomes engorged and gives rise to a slightly bluish appearance.

The three layers of superficial, intermediate and basal cells change their relative proportions so that the intermediate cells predominate and can be seen in the cell population of normal vaginal secretions.

Epithelial cells generally multiply and enlarge and become filled with vacuoles rich in glycogen. High oestrogen levels stimulate glycogen synthesis and deposition and, as these epithelial cells are shed into the vagina, lactobacilli known as Döderlein's bacilli break down the glycogen in these cells to produce lactic acid. The vaginal pH falls in pregnancy to 3.5–4.0 and this acid environment serves to keep the vagina clear of bacterial infection.

At the same time, yeast infections may thrive in this environment and thus *Candida* infections are common in pregnancy.

CHANGES IN THE SKIN

The characteristic feature of skin changes in pregnancy is the appearance of pigmentation on the face, known as *chloasma*, the areola of the nipples and the linea alba of the anterior abdominal wall, giving rise to the *linea nigra*. These changes are due to increased secretion of pituitary melanocyte-stimulating hormone (MSH).

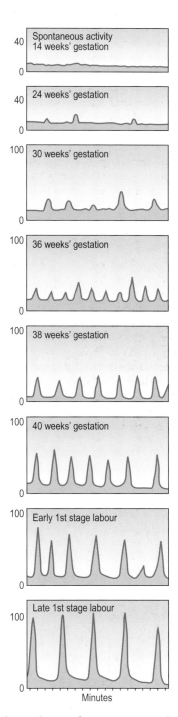

Fig. 3.7 The evolution of uterine activity during pregnancy.

The development of stretch marks or *striae gravidarum* varies greatly in different races and different women. In the first pregnancy, these marks often have a distinctly purplish colour; in subsequent pregnancies the scars become silvery in appearance. Although they predominantly occur in the lines of stress of the abdominal wall, they also occur on the lateral aspects of the thighs and breasts. Striae gravidarum are the product of the disruption of collagen fibres in the subcuticular zone and are related more to the increased production of adrenocortical hormones in pregnancy than to the stress and tension in the skin folds associated with the expansion of the abdominal cavity (see Fig. 6.6).

THE CARDIOVASCULAR SYSTEM

Major changes occur in the cardiovascular system in pregnancy, the most significant taking place by 12–16 weeks gestation. Although the longer-term needs of pregnancy are met by these changes, they tend to occur well before the full impact of the biological demands of pregnancy is felt.

Cardiac position and size

With increasing enlargement of the uterus, the diaphragm is pushed upwards and the heart is correspondingly displaced: the apex of the heart is displaced upwards and laterally. Radiologically, the upper left cardiac border is straightened, with increased prominence of the pulmonary conus.

The heart enlarges by 70–80 ml, some 12%, between early and late pregnancy; this enlargement is due to a small increase in wall thickness but predominantly to increased venous filling. The increase in ventricular volume results in dilatation of the valve rings and hence an increase in regurgitant flow velocities.

Myocardial contractility is increased during pregnancy, as indicated by shortening of the pre-ejection period, and this is associated with lengthening of the myocardial muscle fibres.

Cardiac output

A number of techniques have been used to study cardiac output in pregnancy, ranging from dye dilution techniques to cardiac catheterization. There is general agreement that the major rise in cardiac output occurs in the first 14 weeks of pregnancy, with an increase of 1.5 litres

from 4.5 to 6.0 l/min. This increase occurs under standardized conditions of posture and time. During labour, a further increase of 2 l/min may occur, with an average increase in labour of 0.6 l/min. Pulsed Doppler ultrasound has allowed the study of cardiac output in labour and, after delivery, cardiac output remains elevated for 24 hours and then gradually declines to the non-pregnant levels by 2 weeks post-partum.

Cardiac output commonly falls in late pregnancy when the woman lies supine, as the enlarged uterus can seriously impede venous return through compression of the inferior vena cava. There is also a small decline in output from 34 weeks gestation to term.

Twin pregnancies are associated with a 15% greater increase throughout pregnancy.

 Pregnancy imposes a 40% increase in cardiac output and is likely to precipitate heart failure in women with heart disease.

The increase in cardiac output is achieved by an increase in both heart rate and stroke volume. Heart rate is increased in pregnancy by about 15 beats/min with, typically, an increase from 70 to 85 beats/min and this contributes to, although it is not essential for, the increase in cardiac output.

Stroke volume

Stroke volume increases from about 64 to 71 ml and plays an important role in the increase in cardiac output. Indeed, women who have an artificial pacemaker and thus a fixed heart rate compensate well in pregnancy on the basis of increased stroke volume alone.

Arterial blood pressure

Blood pressure changes occur during the menstrual cycle. Systolic blood pressure increases during the luteal phase of the cycle and reaches its peak at the onset of menstruation, whereas diastolic pressure is 5% lower during the luteal phase than in the follicular phase of the cycle.

In normal pregnancy, there is a fall of some 10 mmHg in mean arterial pressure; 80% of this fall occurs in the first 8 weeks of pregnancy. Thereafter, a small additional fall occurs, until arterial pressure reaches its nadir by 24 weeks gestation.

Posture has a significant effect on blood pressure in pregnancy and is lowest with the woman lying supine on her left side. The pressure falls in a similar way whether the pressure is recorded sitting, lying supine or in the left lateral supine position, but the levels are significantly different (Fig. 3.8).

Mothers attending for antenatal visits must have their blood pressure recorded in the same position at each visit if the pressures are to be comparable. Also, special care must be taken to use an appropriate cuff size for the measurement of brachial pressures.

Profound falls in pressure may occur in late pregnancy when the mother lies on her back. This phenomenon is described as the *supine hypotension syndrome*. It results from the restriction of venous return from the lower limbs due to compression of the inferior vena cava but it must be remembered that aortic compression also occurs and that this will result in conspicuous differences between brachial and femoral blood pressures in pregnancy. When a woman turns from a supine to a lateral position in late pregnancy, the blood pressure may fall by 15%, although some of this fall can be accounted for by the raising of the right arm above the level of the heart.

Central venous pressure and pressure in the upper arms remain constant in pregnancy but pressure from the uterus and the fetal presenting part in late pregnancy result in a marked increase in femoral venous pressure.

One factor that may cause discrepancies in the measurement of diastolic pressure in pregnancy is the widening of the gap between the fourth Korotkoff sound and the fifth sound as the fifth Korotkoff sound may be difficult to define. Although most published studies of blood pressure are based on the use of Korotkoff fourth sound, there is now a move towards using the fifth sound where it is clear and only using the fourth sound where the point of disappearance is unclear.

Peripheral resistance

Peripheral resistance is calculated from the mean arterial pressure divided by cardiac output and, as the cardiac output rises during pregnancy and the blood pressure falls, it follows that peripheral resistance must fall; it is estimated that it falls to almost 50% of the non-pregnant values. In the non-pregnant normotensive female, values are around 1700 dyn/s/cm, whereas in mid-trimester these fall to 980 dyn/s/cm and they rise slowly again towards term, to 1200–1300 dyn/s/cm in late pregnancy.

The fall in total peripheral resistance is associated with the expansion of the vascular space in the uteroplacental bed and the renal vasculature in particular, but there is abundant evidence that blood flow to the skin is also greatly increased in pregnancy as the result of vasodilatation. The mechanism by which these changes are achieved remains uncertain but the balance between vasodilatation and vasoconstriction in pregnancy is a critical determinant of blood pressure and lies at the heart of the pathogenesis of pre-eclampsia.

RESPIRATORY FUNCTION

Alterations to the configuration of the thorax occur during pregnancy. The level of the diaphragm rises and the intercostal angle increases from 68° in early pregnancy to 103° in late pregnancy. Although there is upward pressure on the diaphragm in late pregnancy, the costal changes occur well before there is any possibility that they could be attributed to mechanical pressure. Nevertheless, breathing in pregnancy is more diaphragmatic than costal, with greater excursion of the diaphragm than in the non-pregnant state.

Vital capacity is a measure of the maximum amount of gas that can be expired after maximum inspiration. Studies are equally divided between reporting an

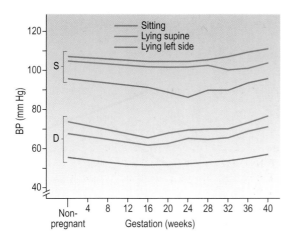

Fig. 3.8 The effect of posture on blood pressure during pregnancy.

apparent increase in vital capacity and a decrease, and the likelihood is that there is no consistent change. There does appear to be a relationship with body weight and there is evidence that vital capacity is reduced by obesity.

Respiratory rate and tidal volume

Respiratory rate remains constant during pregnancy at 14–15 per minute, whereas tidal volume increases from about 500 ml in the non-pregnant state to about 700 ml in late pregnancy (Fig. 3.9). Thus there is about a 40% increase during pregnancy and, consequently, the minute ventilation, which is the product of tidal volume and respiratory rate, also increases by 40%, from about 7.5 to 10.5 l/min.

As the result of this increase in minute ventilation and the effect of progesterone increasing the level of carbonic anhydrase B in red cells, arterial P_{CO_2} falls in pregnancy. At the same time, there is a fall in plasma bicarbonate concentration and the arterial pH therefore remains constant.

Inspiratory capacity, which is a measure of tidal volume plus inspiratory reserve volume, increases progressively during pregnancy by an order of 300 ml and residual volume decreases by about 300 ml.

Forced expiratory volume in 1 second (FEV₁) and *peak expiratory flow* (PFR) remain constant in pregnancy and women with asthma do not appear to be affected by pregnancy.

In general terms, respiratory diseases and in particular obstructive airway diseases have far less implications for the mother's health than cardiac disorders, with the exception of those conditions, such as severe kyphoscoliosis where the lung space is severely restricted.

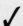 Pregnancy does not generally impose any increased risk on women with respiratory disease.

CHANGES IN BLOOD

Blood volume is a measurement of plasma volume and total red cell mass. The indices are under separate control mechanisms.

Plasma volume increases in pregnancy to a peak between 32 and 34 weeks from a non-pregnant level of 2600 ml by an additional 1250 ml in a first pregnancy and 1500 ml in subsequent pregnancies. Where measurements of plasma volume are made by dye dilution techniques in the supine position, there is an apparent fall in plasma volume in late pregnancy that is probably due to poor mixing of dye because of obstructed venous return from the legs.

Multiple pregnancies are associated with a significantly higher increase in plasma volume and pregnancies exhibiting impaired fetal growth are associated with a poor increase in plasma volume (Fig. 3.10).

Red cell mass is a measurement of the total volume of red cells in the circulation and is much more difficult to measure. However, the evidence available suggests that

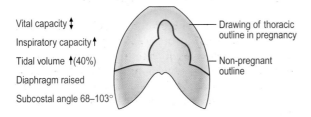

Vital capacity $\updownarrow$
Inspiratory capacity $\uparrow$
Tidal volume $\uparrow$(40%)
Diaphragm raised
Subcostal angle 68–103°

Drawing of thoracic outline in pregnancy
Non-pregnant outline

Fig. 3.9 Changes in respiratory function in pregnancy.

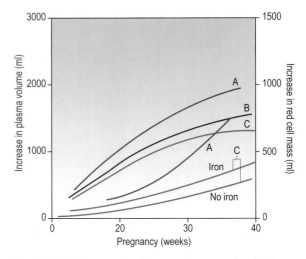

Fig. 3.10 Changes in plasma volume and red cell mass in (A) twins, (B) healthy multigravidae and (C) healthy primigravidae.

there is a steady increase in pregnancy and the increase appears to be linear throughout pregnancy.

The figure for non-pregnant women is around 1400 ml and this increases by some 240 ml in the pregnant woman who does not take iron supplements. However, this figure is substantially greater in multiple pregnancies and where iron supplementation is given.

Haemoglobin concentration, haematocrit and red cell count decline during pregnancy because of the discrepancy between the expansion of plasma volume and the red cell mass. At the same time, in normal pregnancy the mean corpuscular haemoglobin concentration remains constant.

The white cells

The total white cell count rises during pregnancy. This increase is mainly due to an increase in neutrophil polymorphonuclear leukocytes that reaches its peak at the 30th week of gestation (Fig. 3.11). A further massive neutrophilia occurs during labour and immediately after delivery, with a fourfold increase in the number of polymorphs.

There is also an increase in the metabolic activity of granulocytes during pregnancy, which may result from the action of oestrogens. This can be seen in the normal menstrual cycle, where the neutrophil count rises with the oestrogen peak in mid-cycle.

It is important to remember to consider white cell counts in labour and immediately post-delivery in the light of these observations and not to interpret the results as an indication of infection.

 A massive neutrophilia is normal during labour and the immediate puerperium and cannot be assumed to be due to infection.

Eosinophils, basophils and monocytes appear to remain relatively constant during pregnancy but there is a profound fall in eosinophils during labour and they are virtually absent at delivery.

The lymphocyte count remains constant and the numbers of T and B cells do not alter. However, lymphocyte function and cell-mediated immunity in particular are depressed, possibly by the increase in concentrations of glycoproteins coating the surface of the lymphocytes, reducing the response to stimuli.

Although this suppression has advantages in preventing the rejection of the conceptus, it has the disadvantage that it lowers resistance to viral and bacterial infections as well as parasitic diseases such as malaria. There is, however, no evidence of suppression of humoral immunity or the production of immunoglobulins.

Platelets

Longitudinal studies on platelet counts during pregnancy show a significant fall and, at the same time, after 28 weeks gestation there is a substantial increase in mean platelet volume. The fall in platelet numbers may be a dilutional effect but the increase in platelet volume suggests that there is increased destruction of platelets in pregnancy with an increase in the number of larger and younger platelets in the circulation (Fig. 3.12).

Clotting factors in pregnancy

There are major changes in the coagulation system in pregnancy, with an increased tendency towards clotting. In a situation where haemorrhage from the uterine vascular bed may be sudden, profuse and life-threatening, the increase in coagulability may play a life-saving role. On the other hand, it increases the risk of thrombotic disease.

Many clotting factors remain constant in pregnancy but there are notable and important exceptions.

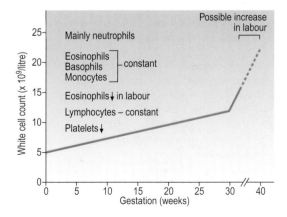

Fig. 3.11 Pregnancy is associated with an increased white cell count; the increase occurs predominantly in polymorphonuclear leukocytes.

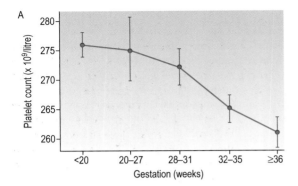

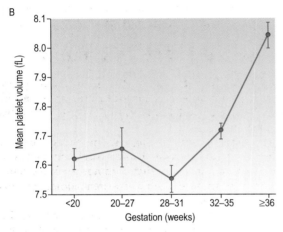

Fig. 3.12 Platelet count and platelet volume in normal pregnancy. (With permission from James et al. 1994 High risk pregnancy: management options. Baillière Tindall, London.)

Factors VII, VIII, VIII:C, X and IX (Christmas factor) all increase during pregnancy, whereas factors II and V tend to remain constant. Factor XI falls to 60–70% of the non-pregnant values and concentrations of factor XIII fall by 50%.

Plasma fibrinogen levels increase from non-pregnant values of 2.5–4.0 g/l to levels as high as 6.0 g/l in late pregnancy and there is an increase in the concentration of high-molecular-weight fibrin/fibrinogen complexes during normal pregnancy.

On the other hand, there is a reduction in plasma fibrinolytic activity and the rapid return to normal non-pregnant levels of activity within 1 hour of delivery suggests that this inhibition is mediated through the placenta.

Common screening tests for the coagulation system

- **Bleeding time** is a measure of the length of time a skin wound continues to bleed and is an in-vivo test of platelet vascular interaction. The normal range is 7–10 minutes.
- The **platelet count** is a valuable screening test for assessing acute obstetric haemostatic failure, particularly disorders such as disseminated intravascular coagulation.
- The **activated partial thromboplastin time** is the test used to monitor therapeutic heparin levels and normally lies between 35 and 45 seconds, but must always be assessed against a normal control.
- **Prothrombin time** measures the clotting time after the addition of thromboplastin. It is the test used to monitor the dosage of warfarin and usually lies between 10 and 14 seconds.
- **Fibrinogen estimation** is important in the presence of severe consumptive coagulopathy, which may occur following severe placental abruption or in cases of severe pre-eclampsia. The normal value in late pregnancy lies between 4.0 and 6.0 g/l.
- **Fibrinogen/fibrin degradation products (FDP)** are present in low concentrations in healthy subjects but high levels can be detected in the presence of severe disseminated intravascular coagulation. Values in the presence of this disorder may exceed 40 µg/l.

 There is an increased tendency to clotting in pregnancy and the puerperium.

Changes in osmolality

Plasma osmolality falls abruptly during the first 8 weeks in pregnancy and this change is associated with a resetting of the osmoreceptor system to preserve the new low level of osmolality. The ability to excrete a water load is significantly affected by posture, the upright posture being more antidiuretic than in non-pregnant subjects.

Nutrients in blood

Maternal carbohydrate metabolism

Carbohydrate metabolism in pregnancy is of the utmost importance to the development of the fetus, as glucose provided by the mother across the placenta is the major substrate for fetal growth and nutrition.

Glucose metabolism in both mother and fetus is regulated by insulin and, at the same time as it moves glucose into the cells, insulin reduces the level of circulating amino acids and free fatty acids.

Maternal levels of glucose determine blood glucose levels in the fetus but levels run at a value some 20% lower than in the maternal circulation.

Maternal fasting blood glucose levels fall, reaching their nadir by 12 weeks at about 0.5–1 mmol/l lower than non-pregnant values. At the same time, plasma insulin levels increase.

Pregnant women exhibit insulin resistance and, for any given glucose challenge, will produce extra insulin, which does not reduce the blood glucose levels as quickly as the response in the non-pregnant female. The implications of these observations on the management of women with diabetes will be discussed in the section on diabetes in pregnancy.

Changes in plasma proteins

The total protein concentration falls by about 1 g/dl during the first trimester from 7 to 6 g/dl. This fall is largely due to the fall in albumin concentration and is associated with a corresponding fall in colloid osmotic pressure. The fall is insufficient to affect drug-carrying capacity.

The globulins show a rise of about 10% in concentration during pregnancy, from about 0.2 to 0.3 g/dl, although there are marked differences in the globulin fractions.

Lipoproteins are classified according to their density into four groups: very-low-density, intermediate-density, low-density and high-density lipoprotein. Alpha-lipoprotein generally lies in the high-density fraction and beta-lipoproteins in the low-density fraction. Within the very-low-density and intermediate-density lipoprotein fractions, three to fourfold increases in triglyceride, cholesterol and phospholipid concentrations occur.

Amino acids

With the exception of alanine and glutamic acid, amino acid levels in plasma decrease below non-pregnant values.

Lipids

Pregnancy is a hyperlipidaemic state and most lipids increase in concentration during pregnancy. The total lipid concentration rises from about 600 to 1000 mg per 100 ml of serum. The main increases occur in triglycerides, cholesterol, and free fatty acids. However, levels of free fatty acids are particularly unstable in pregnancy and may be affected by fasting, exertion, emotional stress and smoking. The levels are consistently elevated above non-pregnant and early pregnancy values in late pregnancy.

Levels of fat-soluble vitamins rise in pregnancy whereas levels of water-soluble vitamins tend to fall.

IMMUNOLOGY OF PREGNANCY

Pregnancy defies the laws of transplant immunology. The fetus constitutes an allograft that, according to the laws that protect 'self' from 'non-self', should be rejected by the mother.

The mother continues to respond to and destroy other foreign antigens and confers passive immunity to the newborn but the mother does not reject the fetus. The mechanism by which this apparent anomaly occurs remains uncertain.

The intimate contact between a large area of syncytiotrophoblast and the maternal circulation implies that trophoblast plays a primary role in immunologically protecting the fetus.

The fetus expresses paternal antigens and these are capable of stimulating the production of maternal antibodies. In addition, pregnancy may induce blocking antibodies but these do not appear to be vital to the continuation of pregnancy. The placenta is not an impermeable immunological barrier, as is shown by the presence of maternal antibodies in the fetus.

Furthermore, the uterus is not an immunologically privileged site, because other tissues implanted in the uterus are rejected.

Cell-surface antigens

The major histocompatability complex for cell-surface antigens is encoded on chromosome 6. These antigens are central to transplant and cytotoxic responses. They are absent on trophoblast, which cannot therefore elicit allogeneic responses. Fetal stem cells and Hofbauer cells are able to bind maternal immunoglobulin and may therefore act as a filter.

In addition, the fetus has a less well-defined local immunoregulatory capacity, signalling the maternal immune system not to attack via special HLA-like surface antigens expressed by elements of the cytotrophoblast.

Decidual response

The endometrium undergoes the process of decidualization in response to implantation of the embryo. The decidua contains all the common immunological cell types, such as lymphocytes and macrophages, but it also contains additional cell types such as large granular lymphocytes.

Conventional natural killer (NK) cells are also found in the decidua, where they may downgrade antifetal activity.

Lymphoid cells do not appear to be activated and may act as suppressor cells by inhibiting the action of lymphokines essential for cytotoxic and NK action.

In summary, the fetus appears to avoid attack by the maternal immune system by a combination of having a relatively non-immunogenic interface with the maternal circulation, filtering out harmful antibodies in the placenta and a locally mediated manipulation of the maternal immune response.

Changes in the lymphatic system and the thymus gland

There is evidence that the thymus undergoes involution during pregnancy, both in humans and in various animal species. The involution appears to be caused by the exodus of lymphocytes from the thymic cortex and data from rats and mice suggests that this phenomenon may be due to the action of progesterone.

There is also some evidence that the spleen enlarges during pregnancy in humans; this may be due to the accelerated production of immunoglobulin-producing cells.

The lymph nodes in the para-aortic chain that drain the uterus may increase in size, although the germinal centres of these nodes may shrink.

The number of circulating T-cells remains constant while the number of B-lymphocytes appears to increase.

Maternal humeral responses are generally enhanced in pregnancy, with increased antibody synthesis in the IgG fraction.

Overall, there is however some diminution in maternal immunocompetence, although this is not sufficient to account for the suppression of fetal rejection.

RENAL FUNCTION IN PREGNANCY

In line with many other organs during pregnancy, the kidneys undergo changes in both size and function. The kidneys enlarge as the result of expansion of vascular volume and renal parenchymal volume. While the microscopic appearances of the kidney do not change, parenchymal volume increases by 70% by the third trimester. Renal enlargement during pregnancy is a physiological phenomenon and must not be interpreted as indicative of pathological changes in the kidney.

Renal blood flow increases by 30–50% in the first trimester and remains elevated throughout pregnancy. At the same time, glomerular filtration rate (GFR) increases by 50% by 16 weeks gestation and then shows some decline from 26 to 36 weeks gestation (Fig. 3.13). Effective renal plasma flow increases by 50–80% by mid-pregnancy. These changes are apparent soon after conception and are fully developed by the end of the first trimester. The increase in glomerular filtration rate is not associated with an increased production of creatinine or urea and plasma levels of these solutes therefore decline.

> **!** Glycosuria is a feature of normal pregnancy.

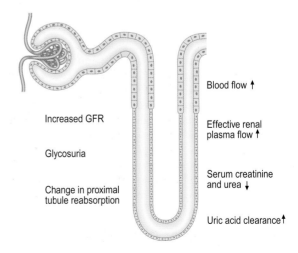

Increased GFR

Glycosuria

Change in proximal tubule reabsorption

Blood flow ↑

Effective renal plasma flow ↑

Serum creatinine and urea ↓

Uric acid clearance ↑

Fig. 3.13 Changes in renal function in pregnancy. GFR, glomerular filtration rate.

The 24-hour creatinine clearance has increased by 25% 4 weeks after the last menstrual period and by 45% at 9 weeks. In the third trimester, there is a decrease, towards non-pregnant values before delivery. Creatinine clearance provides a simple and valuable indicator of GFR but gives values that are significantly less than those obtained by infusion tests of inulin or endogenous creatinine and must therefore be interpreted with caution.

Associated with the increase in the glomerular filtration rate, the filtered load of sodium increases by 5000–10 000 mmol/day. Tubular reabsorption increases in parallel with the glomerular filtration rate, with the retention of 3–5 mmol of sodium per day into the fetal and maternal stores. The total net sodium gain amounts to 950 mmol; this increased load is mainly stored in the maternal compartment.

A similar change occurs with potassium ions, with a net gain of approximately 350 mmol.

Renal tubular function

Renal tubular function also undergoes significant change during pregnancy. Uric acid clearance increases from between 6 and 12 ml/min up to 12–20 ml/min, resulting in a reduction in serum uric acid levels. While uric acid is freely filtered through the glomerulus, most is reabsorbed. Serum uric acid concentration falls by 25%. The normal values in pregnancy range from 148 to 298 μmol/l, with an upper limit of 327 μmol/l.

As the pregnancy progresses, the filtered load increases while excretion remains constant and serum levels therefore begin to return towards non-pregnant values in late pregnancy.

Glucose excretion increases during pregnancy and glycosuria is therefore a feature of normal pregnancy and is unrelated to blood glucose levels. The glycosuria of pregnancy is intermittent and may be the result of increased glomerular filtration or a change in the pattern of tubular reabsorption. Present evidence suggests that the most likely cause is that tubular reabsorption is less complete during pregnancy, resulting in the escape of more glucose into the urine.

The excretion of other sugars, such as lactose, fructose, xylose and fucose, are also increased during pregnancy.

The renin–angiotensin system

The renin–angiotensin system shows an early and persistent increase in activity and it now appears that it plays a role in a far wider range of activities than was originally thought.

Renin is a proteolytic enzyme that exists in an active and inactive form (prorenin). Active renin acts on a substrate of alpha-2-globulin, produced in the liver, to create a decapeptide, angiotensin I. Under the action of angiotensin-converting enzyme (ACE), produced predominantly in the lungs but also in the placenta, angiotensin I is converted to the octapeptide angiotensin II (AII). This peptide is a potent vasoconstrictor that elevates blood pressure and also acts on the adrenal cortex to produce aldosterone, which in turn promotes the retention of sodium and water.

What has now become apparent is that the activities of this system are much wider and more fundamental than originally proposed and that the system plays a fundamental role in the process of growth and development of the fetus.

Renin and prorenin are produced in a number of sites other than the kidney; these include the brain, the genital tract and in particular the chorion, decidua, uterus and ovary.

In the general circulation, up to 70% of total renin is in the form of prorenin. Both plasma renin activity and prorenin levels exhibit a 2.5-fold increase in the first trimester and remain elevated throughout pregnancy, although there is some fall in levels as pregnancy progresses. High concentration of prorenin, up to 40 times the plasma level, can be found in amniotic fluid. The renin substrate increases gradually throughout pregnancy and this increase seems to be mediated by oestrogen stimulation. At the same time, levels of angiotensin II in the plasma also increase, by a similar amount and in a similar pattern to plasma renin activity.

With all this increase in activity of the system, the effect on blood pressure is offset by a parallel reduction in vascular sensitivity to angiotensin II, a change that is probably mediated by the downregulation of the vascular receptors to AII. The loss of sensitivity to AII in normal pregnancy is altered in pre-eclampsia, where sensitivity increases even before the onset of hypertension.

Recent studies on AT1 and AT2 receptor subtypes now suggest that the important role of the renin–angiotensin system in the uterus and placenta may be in the regulation of fetal and placental growth. AT1 receptors promote angiogenesis and vasoconstriction and AT2 receptors promote apoptosis. Evidence is now available to show intense activity of AT1 receptors throughout pregnancy over the site of implantation of the conceptus and, to a lesser extent, on the syncytiotrophoblast, where they may play an important role in angiogenesis and cell growth.

Other changes in the urinary system

Apart from the functional changes in the kidney, various anatomical changes occur in the urinary tract (Fig. 3.14).

There is marked dilatation of the calyces, renal pelves and ureters. The changes occur in the first trimester and it is likely that they are due to the influence of progesterone rather than the effect of back-pressure.

However, the ureteric dilatation terminates as the ureter crosses the pelvic brim, suggesting that there may be some effect from back pressure as the uterus enlarges in later pregnancy. Furthermore, these changes are invariably more pronounced on the right side, an observation that is not compatible with hormonal effects alone.

Despite the changes seen in the collecting system, the ureters do not exhibit actual hypotonicity and hypomotility and there is hypertrophy of the ureteral smooth muscle and hyperplasia of the connective tissue. Vesicoureteric reflux occurs sporadically and the combination

of reflux and ureteric dilatation is associated with a high incidence of urinary stasis and an increased tendency to urinary tract infection.

THE ALIMENTARY SYSTEM

Heartburn is a common disorder of pregnancy and this has generally been ascribed to reflux oesophagitis. However, it is known that reflux also occurs in women without any symptoms of heartburn. With increased intra-abdominal pressure, there is commonly displacement of the lower oesophageal sphincter through the diaphragm but this is not necessarily the cause of heartburn. The predominant factors appear to be a decreased sphincter response to raised intra-abdominal pressure.

Gastric secretion is reduced in pregnancy and gastric motility is low. As a consequence, gastric emptying is delayed.

Reduced motility also occurs in both the small bowel and the large bowel and there is also evidence that absorption of water and sodium is increased in the colon. This may account for the increased tendency to constipation that characterizes pregnancy.

ENDOCRINE CHANGES

Massive production of sex steroids by the placenta tends to dominate the endocrine picture but there are also significant changes in all the maternal endocrine organs during pregnancy. It is important to be aware of these changes so that they are not interpreted as indicating abnormal function.

The pituitary gland

Anterior pituitary

The pituitary gland enlarges during pregnancy: the weight is estimated to increase by 30% in primigravid women and 50% in multiparous women. The weight increase is largely due to changes in the anterior lobe, which produces six hormones: three glycoproteins – luteinizing hormone (LH), follicular stimulating hormone (FSH) and thyroid stimulating hormone (TSH) – and three polypeptide and peptide hormones – growth hormone, prolactin and adrenocorticotrophic hormone (ACTH).

Prolactin is the only pituitary hormone that exhibits a progressive rise in plasma concentrations during preg-

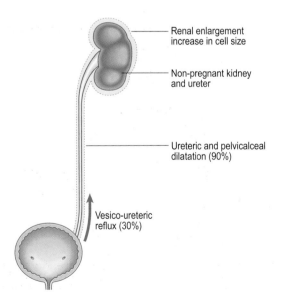

Fig. 3.14 Changes in the urinary tract include renal enlargement and ureteric dilatation.

Renal enlargement increase in cell size

Non-pregnant kidney and ureter

Ureteric and pelvicalceal dilatation (90%)

Vesico-ureteric reflux (30%)

nancy. The increases in oestrogen levels during pregnancy stimulate the number and secretory activity of the lactotrophs and thereby increase prolactin synthesis, with a surge at the time of delivery and a subsequent fall with the disappearance of placental oestrogens. Levels of prolactin remain raised above basal levels in women who continue to breast-feed.

Gonadotrophin secretion is inhibited, as is the secretion of growth hormone. Corticotrophin-releasing hormone (CRH) and ACTH show increased plasma levels but these hormones are also produced in the placenta. Thyrotrophin levels remain constant in pregnancy.

Posterior pituitary

The posterior pituitary is derived from a downgrowth of neural tissue that forms the floor of the third ventricle. It consists of glial cells and nerve terminals, where the bodies all lie in the hypothalamic nuclei.

The posterior pituitary releases vasopressin and oxytocin.

The secretion of vasopressin plays a role in regulating plasma osmolality. In the third trimester, measurable basal levels of vasopressin can be detected. Renal response to vasopressin may increase during pregnancy.

Oxytocin stimulates uterine contractions as well as having an important role to play in breast-feeding. It is present in low concentrations in both men and women. Oxytocin levels are not raised in labour but there is an upregulation of oxytocin receptors in the uterus, so there is enhanced sensitivity to oxytocin. This appears to be related to the oestrogen:progesterone ratio, as oestrogen upregulates binding sites and progesterone downregulates them. In addition, dilatation of the cervix stimulates the release of oxytocin, thus reinforcing uterine activity.

Oxytocin also plays an important role in lactation as it is released following stimulation of the nipples. It then acts on the myoepithelial cells surrounding the breast alveoli, causing these cells to contract and resulting in ejection of milk.

Thyroid function

The thyroid gland enlarges in up to 70% of pregnant women and was relied on by the ancient Egyptians as a sign of pregnancy. The percentage varies according to the level of iodine intake in the population. In the USA,

where there is a higher iodine content in the diet because of the wider usage of iodized salt, no significant difference occurs in the prevalence of goitre.

In normal pregnancy, there is increased urinary excretion of iodine and transfer of iodothyronines to the fetus. This in turn results in a fall of plasma inorganic iodide levels in the mother. At the same time, the thyroid gland triples its uptake of iodide from the blood, creating a relative iodine deficiency that is probably responsible for a compensatory follicular enlargement of the gland.

Thyroid-binding globulin (TBG) is doubled by the end of the first trimester and remains elevated throughout pregnancy (Fig. 3.15).

As a result of the increase in TBG, total triiodothyronine (T_3) and thyroxine (T_4) increase in pregnancy, although free T_3 and T_4 rise in early pregnancy and then fall to remain in the non-pregnant range. TSH may increase slightly but tends to remain within the normal range. T_3, T_4 and TSH do not cross the placental barrier and there is therefore no direct relationship between maternal and fetal thyroid function. However, iodine and antithyroid drugs do cross the placenta, as does the long-acting thyroid stimulator (LATS). Hence,

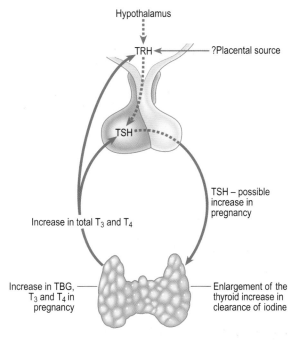

Fig. 3.15 Thyroid function in pregnancy.

the fetus may be affected by the level of iodine intake and by the presence of autoimmune disease in the mother.

The adrenal gland

The adrenal glands remain constant in size but exhibit changes in function. Plasma levels of ACTH rise in pregnancy but remain within the normal non-pregnant range. Some of the increase in ACTH may be the result of placental production.

Total plasma cortisol increases from 3 months to term. Much of this cortisol is bound to cortisol binding globulin (CBG) or to albumin and only 10% is present in the free state. CBG increases throughout pregnancy to reach twice non-pregnant levels. Mean unbound cortisol levels increase during pregnancy, with the loss of diurnal variation.

Plasma levels of CRH increase greatly in the third trimester of pregnancy.

Plasma aldosterone rises progressively throughout pregnancy, probably as compensation for the natriuretic effects of progesterone, and there is also a substantial increase in the weak mineralocorticoid deoxycorticosterone that is apparent by 8 weeks gestation and may reflect production by the fetoplacental unit.

An oestrogen-induced increase in the production of sex-hormone-binding globulin (SHBG) results in an increase in total testosterone levels.

The function of the adrenal medulla remains unchanged so that levels of catecholamines remain as in the non-pregnant state. However, there are often massive increases in both adrenaline (epinephrine) and noradrenaline (norepinephrine) during labour as the result of stress and muscle activity.

ESSENTIAL INFORMATION

Initiation of lactation

- Sudden fall in oestrogen and progesterone levels at delivery
- Release of inhibition of prolactin action on alveolar cells – milk production
- Prolactin production increased by nipple stimulation
- Milk ejection reflex stimulated by suckling and release of oxytocin
- Milk production inhibited by dopamine agonist and catecholamines
- Full milk flow occurs by day 5

Changes in the cervix

- Increased vascularity
- Reduction in collagen
- Accumulation of glycosaminoglycans and water
- Hypertrophy of cervical glands
- Increased mucus secretions

Vascular changes in the pregnant uterus

- Hypertrophy of the uterine vessels
- Uterine blood flow from 50–500 ml/min 10 weeks to term
- Trophoblast invasion of spiral arterioles up to 24 weeks
- 100–150 spiral arterioles supply intervillous space
- One spiral arteriole per placental cotyledon

Uterine contractility

- Suppressed by progesterone
- Increased resting membrane potential
- Impaired conduction
- Contractions by 7 weeks – frequent low intensity
- Late pregnancy – stronger and more frequent
- In labour, contractions produce cervical dilatation

Changes in the skin

- Increased secretion of pituitary MSH
- Facial pigmentation – chloasma
- Pigmentation of the areola of the nipples
- Linea nigra on lower anterior abdominal wall
- Striae gravidarum

Cardiac output

- 40% increase in the first trimester
- Further increase of up to 2 litres/min in labour
- 15% increment with twin pregnancy
- Heart rate increased by 15 beats/min
- Stroke volume increases from 64 to 71 ml

Nutrients in blood

- Glucose is the major substrate for the fetus
- Albumin falls throughout pregnancy
- Globulin rises by 10%
- Amino acids decrease except alanine and glutamic acid
- Pregnancy is a hyperlipidaemic state

- Free fatty acids are elevated
- Fat-soluble vitamins increase in concentration

Immunological responses

- The uterus is not immunologically a privileged site
- Trophoblast does not elicit allogeneic responses
- Fetus has a non-immunogenic interface with maternal circulation
- Maternal immune response is locally manipulated
- Thymus involutes in pregnancy
- Lymph nodes draining the uterus enlarge

Endocrine changes

- Pituitary gland enlarges
- Increased secretion of prolactin
- Placenta produces CRH and ACTH
- Growth hormone, LH and FSH levels are suppressed
- Thyroid function increases
- Aldosterone and deoxycorticosterone levels increase in pregnancy

4
Placental and fetal growth and development

EARLY PLACENTAL DEVELOPMENT

After fertilization and egg cleavage, the *morula* is transformed into a *blastocyst* by the formation of a fluid-filled cavity within the ball of cells.

The outer layer of the blastocyst consists of primitive cytotrophoblast and, by day 7, the blastocyst penetrates the endometrium as a result of trophoblastic invasion (Fig. 4.1). The outer layer of trophoblast becomes a syncytium. In response to contact with the syncytiotrophoblast, the endometrial stromal cells become large and pale, a process known as the *decidual reaction*. Some endometrial cells are phagocytosed by the trophoblastic cells.

The nature and function of the decidual reaction remain uncertain but it seems likely that the decidual cells both limit the invasion of trophoblastic cells and serve an initial nutritional function for the developing placenta.

During development of the placenta, cords of cytotrophoblast or *Langhans cells* grow down to the basal layers of decidua and penetrate some of the endometrial venules and capillaries. The formation of lacunae filled with maternal blood presages the development of the intervillous space.

The invading cords of trophoblast form the primary villi, which later branch to form secondary villi and, subsequently, free-floating tertiary villi.

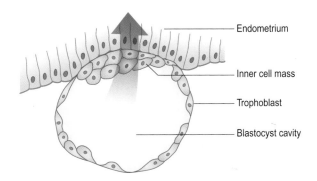

— Endometrium

— Inner cell mass

— Trophoblast

— Blastocyst cavity

Fig. 4.1 Implantation of the blastocyst.

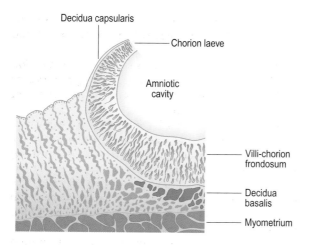

Fig. 4.2 Development of early placentation. The chorion frondosum forms the placental villi. The chorion laeve forms the chorionic portion of the fetal membranes.

The central core of these villi is penetrated by a column of mesoblastic cells that become the capillary network of the villi. The body stalk attaching the developing fetus to the placenta forms the umbilical vessels, which advance into the villi to join the villous capillaries and establish the placental circulation.

Although trophoblastic cells surround the original blastocyst, the area that develops into the placenta becomes thickened and extensively branched and is known as the *chorion frondosum*. However, in the area that subsequently expands to form the outer layer of the fetal membranes or *chorion laeve*, the villi become atrophic and the surface becomes smooth (Fig. 4.2). The decidua underlying the placenta is known as the *decidua basalis* and the decidua between the membranes and the myometrium as the *decidua capsularis*.

FURTHER PLACENTAL DEVELOPMENT

By 6 weeks after ovulation, the trophoblast has invaded some 40–60 spiral arterioles. Blood from the maternal vasculature pushes the free-floating secondary and tertiary capillaries into a tent-shaped *maternal cotyledon*. The tents are held down to the basal plate of the decidua by anchoring villi, and the blood from arterioles spurts towards the chorionic plate and then returns to drain through maternal veins in the basal plate. There are eventually about 12 large maternal cotyledons and 40–50 smaller ones (Fig. 4.3).

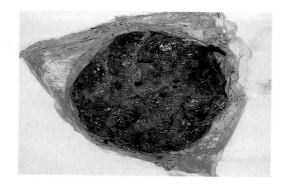

Fig. 4.3 Maternal surface of the full-term placenta showing maternal cotyledons.

The villus

Despite the arrangement of villi into maternal cotyledons, the functional unit of the placenta remains the *stem villus* or *fetal cotyledon*. The end unit of the stem villus, sometimes known as the terminal or chorionic villus is shown in Figure 4.4. There are initially about 200 stem villi arising from the chorion frondosum. About 150 of these structures are compressed at the periphery of the maternal cotyledons and become relatively functionless, leaving a dozen or so large

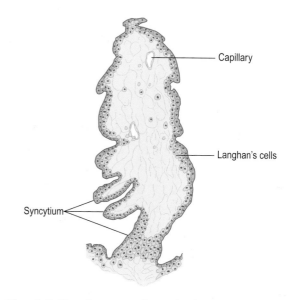

Fig. 4.4 The chorionic villus is the functional unit of the placenta.

cotyledons and 40–50 smaller ones as the active units of placental function.

The estimated total surface area of the chorionic villi in the mature placenta is approximately 11 m^2. The surface area of the fetal side of the placenta and of the villi is enlarged by the presence of numerous microvilli. The core of the villus consists of a stroma of closely packed spindle-shaped fibroblasts and branching capillaries. The stroma also contains phagocytic cells known as *Hofbauer cells*. In early pregnancy, the villi are covered by an outer layer of syncytiotrophoblast and an inner layer of cytotrophoblast. As pregnancy advances, the cytotrophoblast disappears until only a thin layer of syncytiotrophoblast remains. The formation of clusters of syncytial cells, known as *syncytial knots*, and the reappearance of cytotrophoblast in late pregnancy are probably the result of hypoxia. There is evidence that the rate of apoptosis of syncytial cells accelerates towards term and is particularly increased where there is evidence of fetal growth impairment.

STRUCTURE OF THE UMBILICAL CORD

The umbilical cord contains two arteries and one vein (Fig. 4.5). The two arteries carry deoxygenated blood from the fetus to the placenta and the oxygenated blood returns to the fetus via the umbilical vein. Absence of one artery occurs in about 1 in 200 deliveries and is associated with a 10–15% incidence of cardiovascular anomalies. The vessels are surrounded by a hydrophilic mucopolysaccharide known as *Wharton's jelly* and

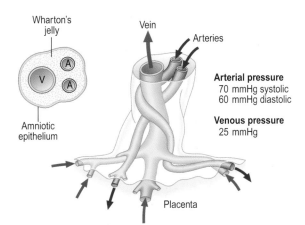

Fig. 4.5 Vascular structure of the umbilical cord. The vein carries oxygenated blood and the two arteries carry deoxygenated blood.

the outer layer covering the cord consists of amniotic epithelium. The cord length varies between 30 and 90 cm.

The vessels grow in a helical shape. This configuration has the functional advantage of protecting the patency of the vessels by absorbing torsion without the risk of kinking or snarling of the vessels.

The few measurements that have been made in situ of blood pressures in the cord vessels indicate that the arterial pressure in late pregnancy is around 70 mmHg systolic and 60 mmHg diastolic, with a relatively low pulse pressure and a venous pressure that is exceptionally high, at approximately 25 mmHg. This high venous pressure tends to preserve the integrity of the venous flow and indicates that the pressure within the villus capillaries must be in excess of the cord venous pressures.

> ! The high capillary pressures imply that, at the point of proximity, the fetal pressures exceed the pressures in the choriodecidual space, so that any disruption of the villus surface means that fetal blood cells enter the maternal circulation and only rarely do maternal cells enter the fetal vascular space.

The cord vessels often contain a false knot consisting of a refolding of the arteries; occasionally, blood flow is threatened by a true knot, although such formations are often seen without any apparent detrimental effects on the fetus.

In the full-term fetus, the blood flow in the cord is approximately 350 ml/min.

UTEROPLACENTAL BLOOD FLOW

Trophoblastic cells invade the spiral arterioles within the first 10 weeks of pregnancy and destroy some of the smooth muscle in the wall of the vessels which then become flaccid dilated vessels. Maternal blood enters the intervillous space and, during maternal systole, blood spurts from the arteries towards the chorionic plate of the placenta and returns to the venous openings in the placental bed. The intervillous space is characterized by low pressures, with a mean pressure estimated at 10 mmHg and high flow. Assessments of uterine blood flow at term indicate values of 500–750 ml/min (Fig. 4.6).

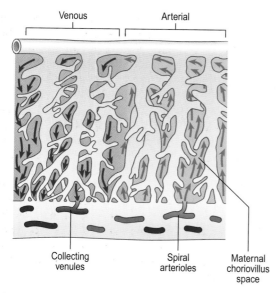

Fig. 4.6 Blood from the spiral arterioles spurts towards the chorionic plate and returns to the collecting venules.

Factors that regulate fetoplacental and uterine blood flow

The fetoplacental circulation is effected by the fetal heart and aorta, the umbilical vessels and the vessels of the chorionic villi, so factors that affect these structures may affect the fetal circulation. Such factors as oedema of the cord, intramural thrombosis and calcification within the large fetal vessels or acute events such as acute cord compression or obstruction of the umbilical cord may have immediate and lethal consequences for the fetus. However, the more common factors that influence the welfare of the fetus arise in the uteroplacental circulation. Access to these factors by the use of Doppler ultrasound has greatly improved our understanding of the control mechanisms of uterine blood flow.

The regulation of uterine blood flow is of critical importance to the welfare of the fetus. The utero-placental blood flow includes the uterine arteries and their branches down to the spiral arterioles, the intervillous blood flow and the related venous return.

Impairment of uterine blood flow leads to fetal growth impairment and under severe circumstances to fetal death. Factors that influence uteroplacental blood flow acutely include maternal haemorrhage, tonic or abnormally powerful and prolonged uterine contractions

and substances such as noradrenaline (norepinephrine) and adrenaline (epinephrine). Angiotensin II increases uterine blood flow at physiological levels, as it has a direct effect on the placental release of vasodilator prostaglandins, but in high concentrations, it produces vasoconstriction.

At the simplest level, acute fetal asphyxia can be produced by the effect of the mother lying in the supine position in late pregnancy, causing compression of the maternal inferior vena cava and hence a sudden reduction in blood flow through the uteroplacental bed.

In terms of chronic pathology, the main causes of impaired uteroplacental circulation are inadequate trophoblast invasion and acute atherosis affecting the spiral arterioles, resulting in placental ischaemia, advanced maturation and placental infarction.

PLACENTAL TRANSFER

The placenta plays an essential role in growth and development in the fetus and in regulating maternal adaptation to pregnancy. The placenta is an organ of fetal nutrition, excretion and respiration, and of hormone synthesis.

Transfer of materials across the placental membrane is governed by molecular weight, solubility and the ionic charge of the substrate involved. Actual transfer is

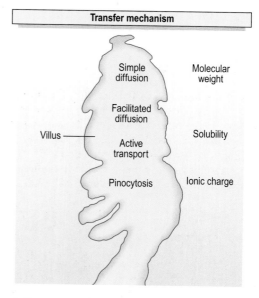

Fig. 4.7 Factors which determine transfer of materials and gases across the placenta.

achieved by simple diffusion, facilitated diffusion, active transport and pinocytosis (Fig. 4.7).

Simple diffusion

Transfer between maternal and fetal blood is regulated by the trophoblast and it must be remembered that the layer separating fetal from maternal blood in the chorionic villus is not a simple semipermeable membrane but a metabolically active cellular layer. However, with regard to some substances, it does behave like a semipermeable membrane and substances pass by simple diffusion.

Although there are some exceptions, small molecules generally cross the placenta in this way and movement is determined by chemical or electrochemical gradients. The quantity of solute transferred is described by the Fick diffusion equation:

$$\frac{Q}{t} = \frac{KA(C^1 - C^2)}{L}$$

where Q/t is the quantity transferred per unit of time, K is a diffusion constant for the particular substance, A is the total surface area available, C^1 and C^2 indicate the difference in concentrations of solute and L represents the thickness of the membrane.

This method is applicable particularly to transfer of gases, although the gradient of oxygen, for example, is exaggerated by the fact that oxygen is extracted by the villous trophoblast.

Facilitated diffusion

Some compounds are transported across the placenta at rates that are considerably enhanced above the rate that would be anticipated by simple diffusion. Transport always occurs in favour of the gradient but at an accelerated rate. This mechanism pertains to glucose transport and can only be explained by the active involvement of enzyme processes and specific transport systems.

Active transport

Transfer against a chemical gradient occurs with some compounds and must involve an active transport system that is energy-dependent. This process occurs with amino acids and water-soluble vitamins and can be demonstrated by the presence of higher concentra-

tions of the compound in the fetal blood as compared with maternal blood. Such transfer mechanisms can be inhibited by cell poisons and are stereo-specific.

Pinocytosis

Transfer of high-molecular-weight compounds is known to occur even where such transfer would be impossible through the villus membrane because of the molecular size. Under these circumstances, microdroplets are engulfed into the cytoplasm of the trophoblast and then extruded into the fetal circulation. This process applies to the transfer of globulins, phospholipids and lipoproteins and is of particular importance in the transfer of immunologically active material. The major source of materials for protein synthesis, which also accounts for some 10% of energy supplies, is amino acids transferred by active transport.

Transport of intact cells

Fetal red cells are commonly seen in the maternal circulation, particularly following delivery. This transfer occurs through fractures in the integrity of the trophoblastic membrane and may also therefore occur at the time of abortion or following placental abruption. Although some maternal cells can be found in the fetal circulation, this is much less common. As previously mentioned, the pressure gradient favours movement from the relatively high pressure of the fetal capillaries to the low pressure environment of the intervillous space.

Water and electrolyte transfer

Water passes easily across the placenta and a single pass allows equilibrium. The net water gain to the fetus in late pregnancy is approximately 20–25 ml. The driving forces for movement of water across the placenta include hydrostatic pressure, colloid osmotic pressure and solute osmotic pressure.

Sodium

The concentration of sodium is higher in the venous plasma of the fetus than in the maternal venous plasma. It therefore seems that the placenta actively regulates sodium transfer, probably through the action of Na/K ATPase on the fetal surface of the villus trophoblast.

Potassium

The transfer of potassium is also controlled at the cell membrane level but the mechanism remains obscure. Fetal plasma potassium levels are significantly higher than maternal plasma levels. In particular, fetal plasma levels become significantly raised in the presence of fetal hypoxia and fetal acidosis with an exaggerated gradient if the acid–base balance remains normal. There is evidence for a carrier-mediated transfer at the maternal surface of the placenta and the transfer of placental potassium may also be modulated by intracellular Ca^{2+}.

Calcium

Calcium is actively transported across the placenta and there are higher concentrations in fetal plasma than in maternal plasma.

PLACENTAL FUNCTION

The placenta has three major functions:

- Gaseous exchange
- Fetal nutrition and removal of waste products
- Endocrine function.

Gaseous exchange

As the transfer of gases occurs by simple diffusion, the major determinants of gaseous exchange are the efficiency and flow of the fetal and maternal circulation, the surface area of the placenta that is available for transfer and the thickness of the placental membrane.

Oxygen transfer

The average oxygen saturation of maternal blood entering the intervillous space is 90–100% at a Po_2 of 90–100 mmHg and these high levels of oxygen favour transfer to the fetal circulation. After the placenta itself has utilized some of this oxygen, the remainder is available to the fetal circulation. Fetal haemoglobin has a higher affinity for oxygen than does adult haemoglobin and haemoglobin concentration is higher in the fetus. All of these factors favour the rapid uptake of oxygen by the fetus at Po_2 levels as low as 30–40 mmHg. The extent to which haemoglobin can be saturated by oxygen is affected by hydrogen ion concentration. The

increase that occurs in deoxygenated blood arriving in the placental circulation from the fetus favours the release of maternal oxygen in the fetoplacental bed. The oxygen dissociation curve is shifted to the right by the increase in H^+ ion concentration, Pco_2 and temperature and this is known as the *Bohr effect* (Fig. 4.8). Oxygen is predominantly transported in the form of oxyhaemoglobin as there is little free oxygen in solution.

Carbon dioxide transfer

Carbon dioxide is readily soluble in blood and transfers rapidly across the placenta. The partial pressure difference is about 5 mmHg. Transport of carbon dioxide may occur in solution as either bicarbonate or carbonic acid. It is also transported as carbaminohaemoglobin. The binding of CO_2 to haemoglobin is affected by factors that influence oxygen release. Thus, an increase in carbaminohaemoglobin results in the release of oxygen. This is known as the *Haldane effect*.

Acid–base balance

Factors involved in the regulation of acid–base balance such as H^+ ions, lactic acid and bicarbonate ions also move across the placenta. As a consequence, acidosis associated with starvation and dehydration in the mother may also result in acidosis in the fetus. However, the fetus may become acidotic as the result of

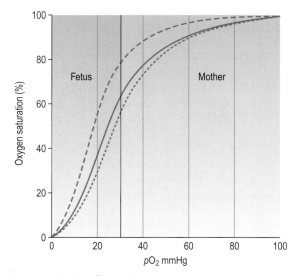

Fig. 4.8 Bohr effect

oxygen deprivation in the presence of normal maternal acid–base balance.

Fetal nutrition and removal of waste products

Carbohydrate metabolism

Glucose transferred from the maternal circulation provides the major substrate for oxidative metabolism in the fetus and placenta and provides 90% of the energy requirements of the fetus. Facilitated diffusion ensures that there is rapid transfer of glucose across the placenta. In late pregnancy, the fetus retains some 10 g/kg body weight and any excess glucose is stored as glycogen or fat. Glycogen is stored in the liver, muscle, the placenta and the heart whereas fat is deposited around the heart and behind the scapulae.

Animal studies have shown that the transfer of sugars is selective. Generally, glucose and the monosaccharides cross the placenta readily whereas it is virtually impermeable to disaccharides such as sucrose, maltose and lactose. The placenta is also impermeable to the sugar alcohols such as sorbitol, mannitol, deleitol and meso-inositol.

In the fasting normal pregnant woman, blood glucose achieves a concentration of approximately 4.0 mmol/l in the maternal venous circulation and 3.3 mmol/l in the fetal cord venous blood. Infusion of glucose into the maternal circulation results in a parallel increase in both maternal and fetal blood until the fetal levels reach 10.6 mmol/l, when no further increase occurs regardless of the values in the maternal circulation.

The hormones that are important in glucose homeostasis – insulin, glucagon, human placental lactogen and growth hormone – do not cross the placenta and maternal glucose levels appear to be the major regulatory factor in fetal glucose metabolism. The placenta itself utilizes glucose and may retain as much as half of the glucose transferred to the fetoplacental unit.

In mid-pregnancy, approximately 70% of this glucose is metabolized by glycolysis, 10% via the pentose phosphate pathway, and the remainder is stored by glycogen and lipid synthesis. By full term, the rate of placental glucose utilization has fallen by 30%.

Glycogen storage in the fetal liver increases steadily throughout pregnancy and by full term is twice as high as the storage in the maternal liver. A rapid fall to adult levels occurs within the first few hours of life.

Fetal glycogen reserves are particularly important in providing an energy source in the asphyxiated fetus when anaerobic glycolysis is activated.

Fat metabolism

Fats are insoluble in water and are therefore transported in blood either as free fatty acids bound to albumin or as lipoproteins consisting of triglyceride attached to other lipids or proteins and packaged in chylomicra.

The fetus needs fatty acids for cell membrane construction and for deposition in adipose tissue. This is particularly important as a source of energy in the immediate neonatal period.

There is evidence that free fatty acids cross the placenta and that this transfer is not selective. Essential fatty acids are also transferred from the maternal circulation and there is evidence to suggest that the placenta has the ability to convert linoleic acid to arachidonic acid. Starvation of the mother increases mobilization of triglycerides in the fetus.

Protein metabolism

Fetal proteins are synthesized by the fetus from free amino acids transported across the placenta against a concentration gradient. The concentration of free amino acids in fetal blood is higher than in the maternal circulation.

The placenta takes no part in the synthesis of fetal proteins, although it does synthesize some protein hormones that are transferred into the maternal circulation – chorionic gonadotrophin and human placental lactogen. By full term, the human fetus has accumulated some 500 g of protein.

Immunoglobulins are synthesized by fetal lymphoid tissue and IgM first appears in the fetal circulation by 20 weeks gestation, followed by IgA and finally IgG.

IgG is the only gamma-globulin to be transferred across the placenta and this appears to be selective for IgG. There is no evidence of placental transfer of growth-promoting hormones.

Urea and ammonia

Urea concentration is higher in the fetus than in the mother by a margin of about 0.5 mmol/l and the rate of clearance across the placenta is approximately 0.54 mg/min/kg fetal weight at term.

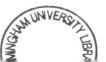

Ammonia transfers readily across the placenta and there is evidence that maternal ammonia provides a source of fetal nitrogen.

Placental hormone production

The placenta plays a major role as an endocrine organ and is responsible for the production of both protein and steroid hormones. The fetus is also involved in many of the processes of hormone production and in this capacity the conceptus functions as a unit involving both fetus and placenta.

Protein hormones

Chorionic gonadotrophin

Human chorionic gonadotrophin (hCG) is produced by trophoblast and has a structure that is chemically very similar to that of luteinizing hormone. It is a glycoprotein with two non-identical α and β subunits and reaches a peak in maternal urine and blood between 10 and 12 weeks gestation. A small sub-peak occurs between 32 and 36 weeks. The β subunit of hCG can be detected in maternal plasma within 7 days of conception.

The only known function of the hormone appears to be the maintenance of the corpus luteum of pregnancy, which is responsible for the production of progesterone until such time as this production is taken over by the placenta.

The hormone is measured by agglutination inhibition techniques using coated red cells or latex particles and this forms the basis for the standard modern pregnancy test. This will be positive in urine by 2 weeks after the period is missed in 97% of pregnant women.

Human placental lactogen

Human placental lactogen (hPL), or chorionic somato-mammotrophin, is a peptide hormone with a molecular weight of 22,000 that is chemically similar to growth hormone. It is produced by syncytiotrophoblast and plasma hPL levels rise steadily throughout pregnancy. The function of the hormone remains uncertain although it does appear to reduce blood glucose levels and to increase levels of free fatty acids and insulin.

Plasma hPL levels have been extensively used in the assessment of placental function as the levels are low in the presence of placental failure. In the last 2 weeks of gestation the levels in the serum fall in normal pregnancy. However, the use of these measurements as placental function tests has largely fallen into disfavour because of their low discriminant function. The hormone is measured by immunoassay.

Steroid hormones

Progesterone

The placenta becomes the major source of progesterone by the 17th week of gestation and the biosynthesis of progesterone is mainly dependent on the supply of maternal cholesterol. In maternal plasma, 90% of progesterone is bound to protein and is metabolized in the liver and the kidneys. Some 10–15% of progesterone is excreted in the urine as pregnanediol. The placenta produces about 350 mg of progesterone per day by full term and plasma progesterone levels increase throughout pregnancy to achieve values around 150 mg/ml by full term. The measurement of urinary pregnanediol or plasma progesterone has been used in the past as a method of assessing placental function but has not proved to be particularly useful because of the wide scatter of values in normal pregnancies.

Oestrogens

Over 20 different oestrogens have been identified in the urine of pregnant women but the major oestrogens are oestrone, oestradiol-17β and oestriol. The largest increase in urinary oestrogen excretion occurs in the oestriol fraction. Whereas oestrone excretion increases 100-fold, urinary oestriol increases 1000-fold.

The ovary makes only a minimal contribution to this increase as the placenta is the major source of oestrogens in pregnancy. The substrate for oestriol production comes from the fetal adrenal gland. Dehydroepiandrosterone (DHEA) synthesized in the fetal adrenal cortex passes to the fetal liver where it is 16-hydoxylated. Conjugation of these precursors with phosphoadenosyl phosphosulphate aids solubility and active sulphatase activity in the placenta results in the release of free oestriol.

Oestradiol and oestrone are directly synthesized by the syncytiotrophoblast. Urinary and plasma oestriol levels increase progressively throughout pregnancy until 38 weeks gestation, when some decrease occurs.

The use of oestriol measurements has now largely been replaced by the use of various forms of ultrasound assessment.

Corticosteroids

There is little evidence that the placenta produces corticosteroids. In the presence of Addison's disease or following adrenalectomy, 17-hydoxycorticosteroids and aldosterone disappear from the maternal urine. In normal pregnancy, there is a substantial increase in cortisol production and this is at least in part due to the raised levels of transcortin in the blood, so that the capacity for binding cortisol increases substantially.

Corticotrophin-releasing hormone

A progressive increase in the levels of corticotrophin-releasing hormone (CRH) in maternal plasma has been noted in the final two trimesters of pregnancy. Any biological effects of CRH are diminished by the presence of a high affinity CRH-binding protein (CRH-BP) in maternal plasma, although the concentrations of CRH-BP fall in the last 4–5 weeks of pregnancy and, as a consequence, free levels of CRH appear to rise.

FETAL DEVELOPMENT

Growth

Up to 10 weeks gestation, a massive increase in cell numbers occurs in the developing embryo but the actual gain in weight is small. Thereafter a rapid increase in weight occurs, until the full-term fetus reaches a final weight of around 3.5 kg.

Protein accumulation occurs in the fetus throughout pregnancy. However, the situation is very different as far as fetal adipose tissue is concerned. Free fatty acids are stored in brown fat around the neck, behind the scapulae and the sternum and around the kidneys. White fat forms the subcutaneous fat covering the body of the full-term fetus. Fat stores in the fetus between 24–28 weeks gestation make up only 1% of the body weight whereas by 35 weeks they make up 15%.

The rate of fetal growth diminishes towards term. Actual fetal size is determined by a variety of factors, including the efficiency of the placenta, the adequacy of the uteroplacental blood flow and inherent genetic and racial factors in the fetus.

Fetal birthweight is determined by gestational age, race, maternal height and weight and parity. Thus, the projected normal birthweight for an infant is determined by a combination of all of these factors (Fig. 4.9). The normal growth curve therefore varies in each infant and can only be determined by taking into

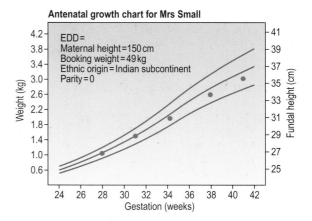

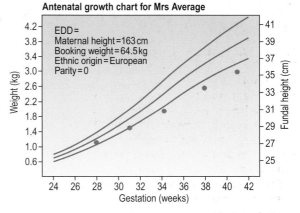

Fig. 4.9 Fetal weight and gestational age plotted on the basis of parity, maternal height and weight and ethnic group. (Courtesy of J. Gardosi.)

account the history of each individual mother. From all these factors, a nomogram for growth can be calculated.

The characteristic appearance of the fetus at 12 weeks gestation is shown in Figure 4.10. The skin is translucent and there is virtually no subcutaneous fat so that the blood vessels in the skin are easily seen, but even at this stage the fetus reacts to stimuli. The upper limbs have already reached their final relative length and the external genitals are distinguishable externally but remain undifferentiated.

By 16 weeks gestation (Fig. 4.11), the crown–rump length is 122 mm and the lower limbs have achieved their final relative length. The external genitalia can now be differentiated.

By 24 weeks gestation (Fig. 4.12), the crown–rump length is 210 mm. The eyelids are separated, the skin is

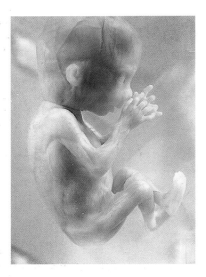

Fig. 4.10 At 12 weeks gestation, the fetus reacts to stimuli. The upper limbs reach their final relative length and the sex of the fetus is distinguishable externally.

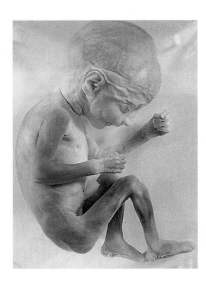

Fig. 4.12 At 24 weeks gestation, the fetal lungs start to secrete surfactant. The eyelids are separated and fine hair covers the body.

The cardiovascular system

The heart develops initially as a single tube and, by 4–5 weeks gestation, a heartbeat is present at a rate of 65 beats/minute. The definitive circulation has developed by 11 weeks gestation and the heart rate increases to around 140 beats/minute. In the mature fetal circulation, about 40% of the venous return entering the right atrium flows directly into the left atrium through the foramen ovale (Fig. 4.13). Blood pumped from the right atrium into the right ventricle is expelled into the pulmonary artery, where it passes either into the aorta via the ductus arteriosus or into the pulmonary vessels.

In the mature fetus, the fetal cardiac output is estimated to be 200 ml/min/kg body weight. Unlike the adult circulation, fetal cardiac output is entirely dependent on heart rate and not on stroke volume. Autonomic control of the fetal heart rate matures during the third trimester and parasympathetic vagal tonus tends to reduce the basal fetal heart rate.

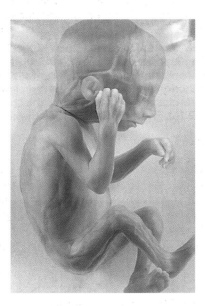

Fig. 4.11 At 16 weeks gestation, the crown–rump length is 122 mm. The lower limbs achieve their final relative length and the eyes face anteriorly.

opaque but wrinkled because of the lack of subcutaneous fat, and there is fine hair covering the body. By 28 weeks, the eyes are open and the scalp is growing hair.

The respiratory system

Fetal respiratory movements can be detected from as early as 12 weeks gestation and, by mid-trimester, a regular respiratory pattern is established. By 34 weeks gestation, respiration occurs at a rate of

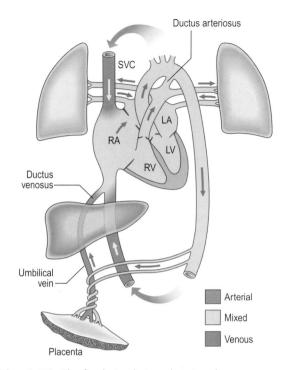

Fig. 4.13 The fetal circulation showing the distribution of arterial, venous and mixed blood.

40–60 movements/min with intervening periods of apnoea. These respiratory movements are shallow, with movement of amniotic fluid only into the bronchioles. There are occasional larger flows of fluid into the bronchial tree but this does not extend into the alveoli because of the high pressure maintained in the developing alveoli from the secretion of alveolar fluid. An exception to this situation may result from episodes of hypoxia, when gasping may lead to the inhalation of amniotic fluid deeper into the alveoli. This fluid may often, under these circumstances, be meconium-stained.

Fetal breathing is stimulated by hypercapnia and by raised maternal glucose levels, as in the postprandial state, whereas hypoxia reduces the number of respiratory movements, as does maternal smoking.

The occurrence of fetal apnoea increases towards term, when breathing movements may be absent for as long as 120 minutes in a normal fetus.

The fetal pulmonary alveoli are lined by two main types of alveolar epithelial cell. Gaseous exchange occurs across the type I cells and the type II cells secrete a surface active phospholipid surfactant that is essential in maintaining the functional patency of the alveoli. The principal surfactants are sphingomyelin and lecithin; production of lecithin reaches functional levels by 32 weeks gestation, although it may begin as early as 24 weeks. In some circumstances, such as in the diabetic pregnancy, the production of surfactant may be delayed and the process can be accelerated by the administration of corticosteroids to the mother.

The measurement of lecithin concentration in the amniotic fluid provides a useful method of assessing functional fetal lung maturity.

The gastrointestinal tract

The development of the fetal gut and gut function proceeds throughout pregnancy and, by 16–20 weeks gestation, mucosal glands appear, heralding the earliest onset of gut function. By 26 weeks gestation, most of the digestive enzymes are present although amylase activity does not appear until the neonatal period. The fetus swallows amniotic fluid and peristaltic gut movement is established by mid-pregnancy. The digestion of cells and protein in amniotic fluid results in the formation of fetal faeces known as *meconium*.

Meconium normally remains in the gut and appears in the amniotic fluid under conditions of fetal stress and asphyxia.

The kidney

Functional renal corpuscles first appear in the juxta-glomerular zone of the renal cortex at 22 weeks gestation and filtration begins at this time. The formation of the kidney is completed by 36 weeks gestation. Glomerular filtration increases towards term as the number of glomeruli increases and fetal blood pressure rises.

In the fetus, only 2% of the cardiac output perfuses the kidney as most of the excretory functions normally served by the kidney are met by the placenta.

The fetal renal tubules are capable of active transport before any glomerular filtrate is received and thus some urine may be produced within the tubules before glomerular filtration starts. The efficiency of tubular reabsorption is low and glucose in the fetal circulation spills into fetal urine at levels as low as 4.2 mmol/l.

Fetal urine makes a significant contribution to amniotic fluid.

The special senses

The external ear can be visualized using ultrasound from 10 weeks onwards. The middle ear and the three ossicles are fully formed by 18 weeks, when they also become ossified; the contents of the inner ear, including the cochlear and the membranous and bony labyrinth, are all fully developed by 24 weeks gestation. The perception of sound by the fetus has to be gauged by behavioural responses and it is generally agreed that the first responses to acoustic stimuli occur at 24 weeks gestation, although some observations have suggest that there may be perception as early as 16 weeks. In view of the developmental timetable of the inner ear, this seems unlikely.

> **!** There is good evidence that the fetus can hear the mother's voice, and indeed sounds delivered internally are much louder than sounds delivered from outside the maternal abdominal wall. Studies with echoplanar functional magnetic resonance imaging have demonstrated temporal lobe vascular changes in the fetus in response to the mother reciting nursery rhymes in late pregnancy. Perhaps mothers should beware what they say to the fetus in late pregnancy!

Visual perception is much more difficult to assess but it seems likely that some perception to light through the maternal abdominal wall does develop in late pregnancy. Certainly, fetal eye movements can be observed during pregnancy and form an important part of the observations made concerning various fetal behavioural states – a subject that is discussed in the chapter on fetal wellbeing.

AMNIOTIC FLUID

Formation

The amniotic sac develops in early pregnancy and has been identified in the human embryo as early as 7 days. The first signs of the development of the amniotic cavity can be seen in the inner cell mass of the blastocyst.

Early in pregnancy, amniotic fluid is probably a dialysate of the fetal and maternal extracellular compartments and therefore is 99% water. It does have a cellular and protein content as well. There is evidence that up to 24 weeks gestation when keratinization of fetal skin begins, significant transfer of water may occur by transudation across the fetal skin. In the second half of pregnancy after the onset of kidney function, fetal urine provides a significant contribution to amniotic fluid volume. Certainly, when the kidneys are missing, as in renal agenesis, the condition is invariably associated with minimal amniotic fluid volume, a condition known as *oligohydramnios*.

The role of the fetus in the regulation of amniotic fluid volume in normal pregnancy is poorly understood but the fetus swallows amniotic fluid, absorbs it in the gut and, in later pregnancy, excretes urine into the amniotic sac (Fig. 4.14).

It must be noted that this is a highly dynamic state, as the total volume of water in the amniotic sac is turned over every 2–3 hours. Any factor that interferes with either formation or removal of amniotic fluid may therefore result in a rapid change in amniotic fluid volume.

Congenital abnormalities that are associated with impaired ability to ingest amniotic fluid are commonly associated with excessive amniotic fluid volume, a condition known as *polyhydramnios*.

In summary, amniotic fluid is formed by the secretion and transudation of fluid through the amnion and fetal skin and from the passage of fetal urine into the amniotic sac. Circulation of amniotic fluid occurs by reabsorption of fluid through the fetal gut, skin and amnion.

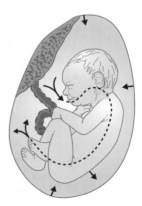

Fig. 4.14 Amniotic fluid secreted into the amniotic sac is swallowed by the fetus, absorbed through the gut and excreted through fetal urine.

Volume

By 8 weeks gestation, 5–10 ml of amniotic fluid has accumulated. Thereafter, the volume increases rapidly in parallel to fetal growth and gestational age up to a maximum volume of 1000 ml at 38 weeks. Subsequently, the volume diminishes so that by 42 weeks, it may fall below 300 ml. The estimation of amniotic fluid volume forms a standard part of the ultrasound assessment of fetal wellbeing.

Clinical significance of amniotic fluid volume

Oligohydramnios

The diminution of amniotic fluid volume is most commonly associated with impaired secretion of fluid and therefore is a sign of the impairment of placental function with the exception of the effect of postmaturity. It may be associated with the preterm rupture of the membranes with chronic loss of amniotic fluid.

Oligohydramnios is commonly associated with intrauterine fetal growth impairment and is therefore an important sign of fetal jeopardy.

It is also associated with congenital abnormalities such as renal agenesis where there is no production of fetal urine.

Oligohydramnios is associated with various structural and functional problems in the fetus. It may be associated with pulmonary hypoplasia and respiratory difficulties at birth. It may also cause physical deformities such as club foot, skull deformities and wry neck. In labour it has been associated with abnormal cord compression during contractions and hence with fetal hypoxia. Amniotic fluid infusions are used in some units to try and avoid these problems but the efficacy of these techniques remains in doubt.

Polyhydramnios

The presence of excessive fluid commonly arises as a chronic condition but may on occasions be acute.

Acute polyhydramnios is a rare condition that tends to arise in the second trimester or the early part of the third trimester and commonly results in the premature onset of labour. The condition is painful for the mother and may cause dyspnoea and vomiting. The uterus becomes acutely distended and it may be necessary to relieve the pressure by amniocentesis. However, this only gives short-term relief and nearly always requires repeated procedures. There is often an underlying congenital abnormality.

Chronic hydramnios may arise in those pregnancies where there is a large placenta, such as occurs in multiple pregnancy or a mother with diabetes. It may also be idiopathic, with no obvious underlying cause, and the fetus may be entirely normal. However, in approximately 30% of all cases, there is a significant congenital anomaly. The distribution of such anomalies is as follows in order of frequency:

- Anencephaly
- Oesophageal atresia
- Duodenal atresia
- Iniencephaly
- Hydrocephaly
- Diaphragmatic hernia.

Hydramnios itself is associated with certain complications and these include:

- Unstable lie
- Cord prolapse or limb prolapse
- Placental abruption if there is sudden release of amniotic fluid
- Postpartum haemorrhage associated with overdistension of the uterus
- Maternal discomfort and dyspnoea.

Clinical value of tests on amniotic fluid

Both the biochemical and cytological components of amniotic fluid can be used for a variety of clinical tests. However, many of the tests previously used have been replaced by ultrasonography and procedures such as cordocentesis and chorionic villus biopsy.

Amniotic fluid contains two distinct types of cell. The first group is derived from the fetus and the second from the amnion. Cells of fetal origin are larger and more likely to be anucleate, whereas those derived from the amnion are smaller, with a prominent nucleolus contained within the vesicular nucleus, and are found in proportionately greater numbers prior to the 32nd week of gestation.

Cells that stain with eosin are most prominent in early gestation and are derived from the amnion. After 38 weeks gestation, numbers of these cells fall to less than 30% of the total cell population.

Basophilic cells increase in number as pregnancy progresses but also tend to decrease after 38 weeks. The presence of large numbers of these cells has been related to the presence of a female fetus; the fetal vagina is thought to be the possible source.

After 38 weeks, a large number of eosinophilic anucleate cells appear. These cells stain orange with Nile blue sulphate and are thought to be derived from maturing sebaceous cells.

These cells have been used in the past as a method of assessing gestational age but this has now been replaced as a method by ultrasound imaging and the assessment of fetal growth.

AMNIOCENTESIS

Amniotic fluid is obtained by the procedure of amniocentesis. This procedure involves inserting a fine-gauge needle under aseptic conditions through the anterior abdominal wall of the mother under local anaesthesia. The procedure, when used for diagnostic testing for congenital abnormalities, is commonly performed at 15–16 weeks gestation but can be performed as early as 12 weeks in some circumstances. The procedure must be performed under ultrasound control in order to identify the best and most accessible pool of amniotic

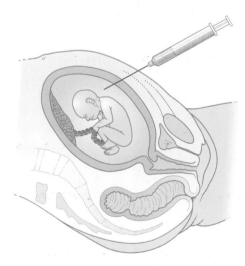

Fig. 4.15 Amniotic fluid is obtained by the procedure of amniocentesis by inserting a needle into the amniotic sac under ultrasound guidance, avoiding the placenta where possible.

fluid and, where possible, to avoid the placenta and the fetus. Up to 10 ml of fluid is withdrawn and the presence of a fetal heart beat is checked both before and after the procedure (Fig. 4.15).

Indications for amniocentesis

Prenatal diagnosis of neural tube defects

Routine screening programmes using serum measurements of α-fetoprotein are discussed elsewhere in more detail but the detection of levels of α-fetoprotein in the mother that are elevated above those appropriate for the gestational age are an indication for detailed ultrasound scanning and occasionally amniocentesis. Elevated levels may be associated with the presence of anencephaly and open neural tube defects. They may also be associated with other abnormalities such as exomphalos, ectopia vesicae and fetal nephrotic syndrome. The high quality of modern ultrasound imaging now means that most of the structural congenital anomalies can be diagnosed by the use of ultrasound alone and thereby reduce the need for diagnostic procedures involving amniocentesis.

Chromosomal abnormalities and sex-linked diseases

The fetal karyotype can be determined by the culture of fetal cells obtained from amniotic fluid. This can reveal chromosome abnormalities such as those found in Down's syndrome, Turner's syndrome and various mosaics. It also allows the determination of fetal sex and hence may be useful in the management of sex-linked disorders such as thalassaemia, haemophilia and Duchenne's muscular dystrophy.

Metabolic disorders

There are a number of rare metabolic disorders, such as Tay–Sachs disease and galactosaemia, that can be diagnosed using fetal cells obtained from amniotic fluid.

Rhesus isoimmunization

A spectrophotometric peak at 450 μm representing unconjugated bilirubin is present in amniotic fluid throughout pregnancy until around 36 weeks gestation when, in normal pregnancy, it disappears. During pregnancies complicated by Rhesus incompatibility, the height of the optical density peak above the baseline slope has been correlated with the severity of fetal anaemia associated with intravascular haemolysis, and this provides a valuable tool in the management of the disease.

Samples can be obtained from 24 weeks onwards depending on the suspected severity of the disease. The height of the peak at 450 μm provides an indication of the severity of the disease and the need for intrauterine fetal transfusion or early delivery. The optical density chart is shown in Figure 4.16.

Estimation of fetal lung maturity

The estimation of lecithin or the lecithin/sphingo-myelin ratio in amniotic fluid has been used to measure functional lung maturity in the fetus after 28 weeks gestation and prior to premature delivery, and where there is a significant risk of the child developing the respiratory distress syndrome. However, it is now routine practice to give the mother corticosteroids under these circumstances. Such is the efficacy of this procedure that it has reduced the need to use the test. Other tests for fetal maturity based on amniotic fluid have now been abandoned in favour of ultrasound techniques.

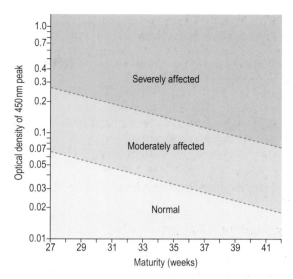

Fig. 4.16 Optical density of amniotic fluid in the prediction of Rhesus isoimmunization.

ESSENTIAL INFORMATION

Early placental development

- Implantation of the blastocyst occurs by day 7
- Formation of placental villi takes place from Langhans cells

Further placental development

- Maternal cotyledons form by 6 weeks after ovulation
- Stem villi remain the functional unit of the placenta

Umbilical cord structure

- Contains two arteries and a vein surrounded by Wharton's jelly and covered in epithelium

Uteroplacental blood flow

- Mean pressure 10 mmHg and flow at term 500–750 ml/min
- Can be impaired by haemorrhage, uterine contractions, adrenaline/noradrenaline
- Impairment leads to fetal growth impairment and possible asphyxia

Placental transfer and function

- Gaseous exchange comes about by simple diffusion
- Oxygen rapidly taken up by the fetal circulation even at low pressure
- Fetal nutrition/excretion

Endocrine function

- hCG – reaches peak between 10 and 12 weeks gestation
- hPL
- Progesterone – placenta produces about 350 mg per day at term
- Oestrogens – placenta major source, 20 different hormones

Fetal development

- Rate of fetal growth increases after 10 weeks and dimishes again towards term
- Heartbeat present at 4–5 weeks
- Cardiac output at term 200 ml/min/kg, entirely dependent on heart rate
- Regular respiratory pattern by mid-trimester
- 40–60 movements/min at 34 weeks
- Principal surfactants sphingomyelin and lecithin
- Production of lecithin reaches functional levels by 32 weeks
- Surfactant production may be delayed by maternal diabetes
- Most digestive enzymes present by 26 weeks
- Fetal kidney completely formed by 36 weeks but most excretory functions performed by the placenta
- Perception of sound begins between 16 and 24 weeks

Amniotic fluid

- Fetal urine major contributor
- Total volume turned over every 2–3 hours
- Oligohydramnios
  - Associated with intrauterine growth impairment and congenital abnormalities, e.g. renal agenesis
  - May cause pulmonary hypoplasia, club foot, skull deformity, wry neck and fetal hypoxia in labour
- Polyhydramnios
  - May be associated with multiple pregancy, diabetes or congenital abnormality
  - May cause unstable lie, cord prolapse, placental abruption, postpartum haemorrhage

Clinical tests

- Amniocentesis may help to detect neural tube defects and chromosome abnormalities
- Amniocentesis also detects fetal sex
- Spectrophotometry can detect fetal anaemia associated with Rhesus isoimmunisation
- Can be used to estimate fetal lung maturity where premature delivery is likely

Perinatal and maternal mortality

Definitions

The definition of perinatal death is linked to the concept of viability and, as the likelihood of survival of a low-birthweight infant has increased progressively over recent decades, UK definitions have been changed. The present legal definitions that apply to England and Wales are as follows:

- **Stillbirth:** a child which has issued forth from its mother after the 24th week of pregnancy and which did not at any time after being completely expelled from its mother breathe or show any signs of life
- **Neonatal death:** death of a liveborn infant within 28 days of birth; an **early neonatal death** is defined as death during the first week of life (0–6 completed days inclusive)
- **Perinatal death:** fetal death after 24 completed weeks gestation and death before 6 completed days.

All perinatal deaths in England, Wales and Northern Ireland must be registered within 5 days of birth or death.

Mortality rates

The current definitions related to mortality rates are as follows:

- **Perinatal mortality rate:** the number of stillbirths and early neonatal deaths (those occurring in the first week of life) per 1000 total births (live births and stillbirths)
- **Stillbirth rate:** the number of stillbirths per 1000 total births
- **Neonatal death rate:** the number of neonatal deaths occurring within the first 28 days of life per 1000 live births.

Incidence

Perinatal mortality rates vary widely – both between different countries and within different regions of the

Table 5.1
International comparison of perinatal mortality rates in 1995 (per 1000 total births)

Country	Rate/1000 births
Somalia	120
Mozambique	105
Bangladesh	85
Nepal	75
China	45
Greece	15
UK	10
USA	10
Germany	5
Sweden	5
Japan	5

same country. For example, in 1995 the highest rate occurred in Somalia and the lowest in Japan (Table 5.1). In western European countries, perinatal mortality has fallen markedly over the last 30 years. However since 1993 these trends have flattened, so that mortality rates demonstrated in the figures for the UK (Fig. 5.1) have remained remarkably constant. The exception is the neonatal death rate, which fell from 4.06 in 1997 to 3.5

in 2001. In 1992, the definition of a stillbirth was changed from a baby born dead after 28 completed weeks to one born dead after 24 completed weeks, so data reported before 1992 cannot be compared with subsequent figures.

The causes for this improvement include:

- Improved antenatal and intrapartum care
- Improved socioeconomic conditions
- Reduction in parity
- An active screening programme for common congenital abnormalities such as Down's syndrome and abnormalities of the central nervous system such as anencephaly and spina bifida.

Factors that are known to affect perinatal mortality in England and Wales include social class, country of birth of the mother, maternal age and parity and marital status. Smoking also has a significant adverse effect on birthweight and perinatal mortality.

Many developing nations in sub-Saharan Africa and Asia do not collect routine statistics, and the data available are collected by governmental and other agencies. Among the poorest countries, in terms of their gross national product, such as Mozambique, Tanzania, Bangladesh and Nepal, the perinatal mortality rate is above 75 per 1000 total births. A comparison of the role of obstetric care in perinatal mortality must take account of the incidence of congenital abnormalities and low birthweight.

Aetiology

The commonest causes of stillbirth (Fig. 5.2) are related to:

- Major congenital abnormalities incompatible with life, such as heart disease, abnormalities of the central nervous system and renal agenesis
- Asphyxia – a final diagnosis of intrauterine asphyxia may represent the end product of a variety of different pathological processes, including:
  - Placental abruption
  - Pre-eclampsia and eclampsia
  - Placental dysfunction associated with intrauterine growth retardation
  - Cord entanglement or prolapse
  - Abnormal uterine activity and cephalopelvic disproportion
- Traumatic cerebral haemorrhage and intracranial damage from difficult labour and delivery

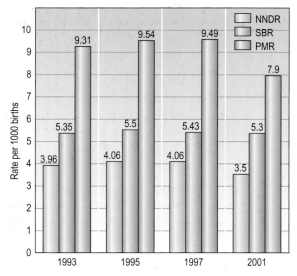

Fig. 5.1 Stillbirth (SBR), neonatal (NNDR) and perinatal (PMR) mortality rates for England, Wales and Northern Ireland. The figures for 2001 (ONS) are for England and Wales.

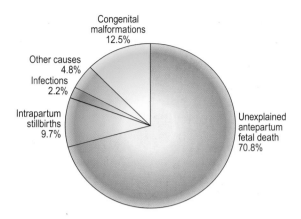

Fig. 5.2 Causes of stillbirths in 1997 in England, Wales and Northern Ireland, using the Wigglesworth classification. Data from the CESDI report 1999.

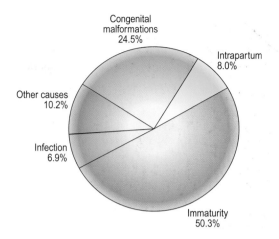

Fig. 5.3 Neonatal deaths in England, Wales and Northern Ireland, using the Wigglesworth classification. Data from the CESDI Report 1999.

- Blood group incompatibility – this is now a rare cause of intrauterine death associated with severe Rhesus isoimmunization and hydrops fetalis.

The data produced by the Confidential Enquiry into Stillbirths and Deaths in Infancy (CESDI) in the UK, shown in Figure 5.2, shows that the commonest reason for stillbirths (70.8%) is listed as 'unexplained antepartum fetal death'. This reflects the difficulty of identifying the cause of antepartum stillbirth, particularly where the stillborn infant is macerated. Only 9.7% of deaths were intrapartum and related to the events of labour.

The common causes of neonatal death (Fig. 5.3) are those related to:

- Major congenital abnormalities incompatible with life
- Prematurity – the most important single factor in causing neonatal death – associated with:
  - Respiratory distress syndrome and hyaline membrane disease
  - Pneumonia
  - Intracranial haemorrhage and cerebral damage sustained during labour and delivery or in the early neonatal period
  - Necrotizing enterocolitis.

The 1997 CESDI data on neonatal deaths show that just over half of all neonatal deaths were associated with immaturity of the infant. Congenital malformations incompatible with life accounted for a further 24.5% of neonatal deaths.

Social factors and perinatal mortality

Maternal age

Maternal age at both extremes is associated with an increase in perinatal mortality. The death rate in the under-16-years age group is twice as high as at any other age. The most recent figures published by the Office of National Statistics in the UK (2001) show that the safest time to have a baby is between the ages of 24 and 29 years.

Parity

There seems to be little doubt that the introduction of the 1967 Abortion Act has been a major factor in the reduction of perinatal mortality. High parity is associated with higher fetal and neonatal losses. The data published in 2001 for England and Wales show that the lowest perinatal mortality rate (6.1/1000 total births) occurs in women having their second child, with women having their third or more having the highest rate (12.0/1000).

Social class

Each country tends to exhibit in microcosm the international differences that are dependent on economic status. The impact of socioeconomic class on perinatal mortality means that women of social classes 4 and 5 have a higher perinatal mortality rate than social classes 1 and 2.

Many countries do not collect routine annual statistics and, in those countries where figures are published, there are often difficulties in interpreting the data because of inaccuracies in the data collection. However, the grosser discrepancies do generally say something about social indices in a country and the quality of medical care.

The figures published for 1995 show a remarkable 24-fold difference between those countries with the highest and lowest perinatal mortality rates (Table 5.1). Although perinatal mortality rates have tended to fall over the last 10 years in most countries, there are still marked differences between countries. The magnitude of these differences is tending to increase.

Smoking has also been shown to affect perinatal mortality, as does substance abuse.

Racial factors

The data published by the Office of National Statistics (ONS) in the UK show that racial factors have a significant bearing on mortality rates. The data published for 2001 based on the country of birth in those women now giving birth in England and Wales is shown in Table 5.2. The differences are quite marked despite the fact that, in general, the standards of maternity services around the UK tend to be at a consistent level. It is, however, likely that there is a bias in the social conditions of the various groups. For example, the low mortality rates seen in those women born in Australia, Canada and New Zealand may be due to the fact that this group of women includes a higher proportion of professional people, as these rates are actually better than those seen in the countries of origin! It is also clear that, to improve mortality rates, more attention will need to be directed towards those groups with the high mortality rates.

The impact of low birthweight on neonatal mortality

Low birthweight is defined as a live birth of less than 2500 g. The rate varies from 4% in Sweden to an estimated 25% in Bangladesh. The overall figure in Britain is 6.7% of all live births. The mortality rate in relation to birthweight is shown in Figure 13.2. The figures shown are national figures and tend to vary substantially in relation to the quality of special intensive care baby units. Figures published in the Health Statistics (ONS) for 2001 show that the neonatal mortality rates for infants with a birthweight of less than 1500 g is 172/1000 live births whereas the rate falls to 13.6/1000 for a birthweight of 1500–1999 g and to 0.9/1000 for a birthweight of 3000–3499 g.

Figures published as a group for birthweights below 1500 g are of limited value because the rates vary greatly with every 50 g of birthweight. Thus, the prognosis is considerably worse for an infant with a birthweight less than 1000 g whereas the rate for infants between 1400 g and 1500 g is similar to that for babies of 1500–2000 g.

MATERNAL MORTALITY

Maternal mortality rate is the number of maternal deaths per million maternities in 1 year. This figure is often expressed as deaths per 100 000 maternities. A maternal death is defined as death occurring within 1 year of delivery. Death may be directly due to pregnancy and childbirth, including abortion, or may sim-

Table 5.2
Perinatal mortality in the UK by country of birth, 2001

Country of birth	Stillbirths	Neonatal deaths	Perinatal mortality
All	5.3	3.5	7.9
England & Wales	5.1	3.4	7.6
Scotland	5.1	3.4	7.6
Australia, Canada, NZ	3.2	3.2	5.9
India	7.7	4.2	10.7
Pakistan	9.3	6.8	14.8
Caribbean	8.7	7.1	15.1

ply occur within a year of childbirth, but be unrelated to the process.

The Tenth Revision of the International Classification of Diseases (ICD10) defines a maternal death as: 'the death of a woman while pregnant or within 42 days of termination of pregnancy, irrespective of the duration and site of the pregnancy, from any cause related to or aggravated by the pregnancy or its management but not from accidental or incidental causes'.

This definition is also divided into two groups:

- **Direct obstetric deaths:** those resulting from obstetric complications of the pregnant state (pregnancy, labour, and the puerperium) from interventions, omissions, or incorrect treatment, or from a chain of events resulting from any of the above
- **Indirect obstetric deaths:** those resulting from previous existing disease or disease that developed during pregnancy and that was not due to obstetric causes but was aggravated by the physiological effects of pregnancy.

The report issued by the World Health Organization (WHO) in 1999 entitled *Reduction of Maternal Mortality* points out that, world-wide, nearly 600 000 women aged between 15 and 49 die each year as the result of complications arising from pregnancy and childbirth. Most of these deaths would be avoidable if adequate antenatal and intrapartum care were available. The deaths are a largely the consequence of poor health and nutrition as well as inadequate care.

This WHO report states that, on a global basis, the five main causes of death are haemorrhage, infections, high blood pressure, obstructed labour and unsafe abortion. Indirect causes include anaemia, malaria, hepatitis, heart disease and HIV/AIDS. The proportional contribution of all these conditions varies from country to country.

In a comparative study of maternal mortality rates in five European countries for mortality rate changes between 1970 and 1998, the European Longitudinal Study of Pregnancy and Childhood draws attention to the large differences in mortality rates within the countries studied in Europe. The data are summarized in Table 5.3.

Part of the explanation for the high death rates in Russia and Ukraine lies in the number of deaths resulting from abortion, which is used as a method of contraception in these countries. In many rural regions of Russia, where contraceptive services are rarely avail-

Table 5.3
Maternal mortality rates in five European countries (deaths/100 000 live births)

Country	1970–86	1998
Czech Republic	15.00	5.52
Russia	68.01	44.03
Slovakia	–	8.64
Ukraine	41.33	27.19
UK	18.03	5.37

able, many women resort to clandestine abortions, with often lethal results. In Russia, 23.8% of all maternal deaths are accounted for by abortions, despite the fact that abortion is legal and available on request. In the UK, abortion contributes only 0.28/100 000 to the total figure for maternal deaths.

Every year, detailed reports of each individual maternal death are recorded and submitted to a National Review Committee. The purpose of these enquiries is to examine, in detail and in an unbiased way, the facts surrounding all maternal deaths with a view to making recommendations concerning the quality of care in order to further reduce the risks to women during childbearing. Some events are so catastrophic and carry such a high risk to the mother that it may not be possible to avoid a fatal outcome. In general, the level of risk to any mother in the UK has been reduced to a near minimal level and stands as a good example of the benefits of a well-organized maternity service.

The system of confidential enquiry into maternal deaths was introduced in England and Wales in 1952, and triennial reports have been published since that time. Ninety nine per cent of all deaths are now documented in the reports. Information gathered by the area or, now, district medical officers, based on reports of all those staff involved in management of the pregnant woman, together with the results of the post-mortem, are passed to regional obstetric assessors and finally to central assessors, who are the Department of Health advisers in obstetrics and gynaecology. Strict confidentiality is maintained throughout this procedure and the name of the patient is removed from the public record. An attempt is made to classify deaths into avoidable and unavoidable groups.

The statistics in Figures 5.4 and 5.5 are based on the triennial reports from the Department of Health in England and Wales. The report for 1997–99 showed a

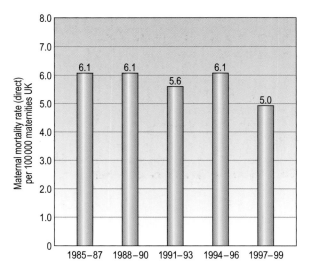

Fig. 5.4 Maternal death rates (direct causes) expressed as deaths/100,000 maternities.

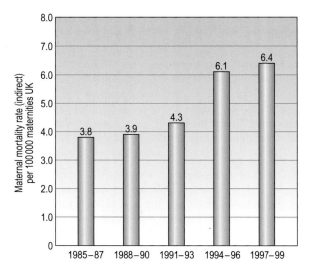

Fig. 5.5 Maternal death rates (indirect causes) expressed as deaths/100,000 maternities.

direct death rate of 61/1 000 000 maternities (Fig. 5.4) and an 'indirect' death rate of 39.4/1 000 000 maternities (Fig. 5.5). The rates in the UK vary according to the region, as with the perinatal mortality rate.

Major causes of maternal death in the UK

The five major direct causes of maternal death in the UK (1997–99), in order of importance, are as follows:

1. Thromboembolism
2. Hypertensive diseases of pregnancy
3. Uterine haemorrhage
4. Amniotic fluid embolism
5. Sepsis, excluding abortion.

The commonest three indirect causes of maternal death in the year following delivery are cardiac disease, psychiatric causes and, in particular, suicides and cancer.

It is important to remember that the ranking order of this list of the causes of death varies from country to country. In the statement of the WHO in their Safe Motherhood Initiative, it was observed that 'the low social status of women in developing counties is an important factor as it limits access to economic resources and basic education'. WHO figures show that some 80% of all maternal deaths are the direct result of complications arising during pregnancy or delivery, or in the first 6 weeks after birth. The remaining 20% arise as the result of pre-existing conditions.

At the same time, only 53% of deliveries in developing countries are attended by health professionals and only 40% take place in a hospital or health centre.

ESSENTIAL INFORMATION

Perinatal mortality

- UK stillbirth rate 2001 5.3/1000
- Neonatal death rate 3.5/1000
- Perinatal mortality rate 7.8/1000

Aetiology

- Stillbirths
  - 70% uncertain
  - 12.5% congenital malformations

History taking and examination in obstetrics

There are many features that are common to history taking in any section of medical practice. However, there are also special subjects that are central to history taking in obstetrics and gynaecology, and knowledge of these factors is essential to good practice in these disciplines.

The term 'obstetrics' relates to the study and management of normal and abnormal pregnancy. The term 'gynaecology' describes the study of diseases of the female genital tract and reproductive system.

There is a continuum between both subjects, so the division is somewhat arbitrary. Complications of early pregnancy such as miscarriage and ectopic pregnancy are generally considered under the title of gynaecology but more properly lie within the remit of obstetrics.

OBSTETRIC HISTORY

The relevant history in obstetrics can be considered under details of the present pregnancy, previous obstetric and gynaecological history, and previous medical and family history.

Present pregnancy

The commonest presenting symptom of pregnancy is the cessation of periods, i.e. the onset of secondary amenorrhoea in a woman previously experiencing regular menstrual cycles. It is important to ascertain the date of the *first day of the last menstrual period (LMP)*. It must be remembered that this information is often inaccurate, simply because many women do not record the days on which they menstruate and, unless the date of the period is associated with some particular event or the woman is actively trying to conceive, the precise dates may not be remembered.

The duration of the menstrual cycle is also important. Ovulation occurs on the 14th day before menstruation but the time interval between menstruation and ovulation – the proliferative phase of the menstrual cycle – may vary substantially.

The length of the menstrual cycle is defined by the time interval between the first day of the period and the first day of the subsequent period. This may vary from

21 to 35 days in normal women, but menstruation usually occurs every 28 days.

It is important to note the method of contraception prior to conception, as hormonal contraception may be associated with a delay in ovulation in the first cycle after discontinuation. In general history taking, the date of onset of menstruation – the *menarche* – should be noted, although this is principally of relevance in the gynaecological history.

The *estimated date of delivery (EDD)* can be calculated if one knows the date of the first day of the last menstrual period and the usual duration of the menstrual cycle (Fig. 6.1). The average duration of human gestation is 269 days from the date of conception and, in a woman with a 28-day cycle, this is 283 days from the first day of the last menstrual period. In a 28-day cycle, the estimated date of delivery can be calculated by subtracting 3 months from the first day of the LMP and adding on 7 days. Some obstetricians prefer to add on 10 days but, in any event, only 40% of women will deliver within 5 days of the EDD and about two-thirds deliver within 10 days. The calculation is therefore at best a guide to women as to the date that delivery is likely to occur.

If the normal menstrual cycle is less than 28 days or greater than 28 days, then an appropriate number of days should be subtracted from or added to the estimated date of delivery. For example, if the normal cycle is 35 days, 7 days should be added to the estimated date of delivery.

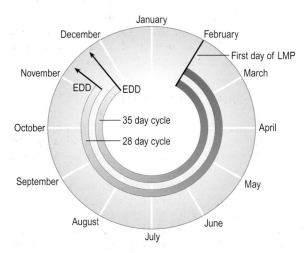

Fig. 6.1 Calculation of the estimated date of delivery.

Symptoms of pregnancy

In addition to a history of amenorrhoea, various symptoms are experienced in early pregnancy.

Nausea and vomiting commonly occur within 2 weeks of missing the first period. Although described as *morning sickness*, vomiting may occur at any time of the day and is often precipitated by the smell or sight of food. Morning sickness commonly occurs in the first 3 months but may persist throughout pregnancy. Occasionally, the vomiting may become severe and persistent, leading to dehydration and electrolyte imbalance; this condition is known as *hyperemesis gravidarum*.

Frequency of micturition occurs in early pregnancy and cannot be explained on the basis of pressure on the bladder from the gravid uterus, as it tends to diminish after the first 12 weeks of pregnancy. Plasma osmolality falls soon after conception and the ability to excrete a water load is altered in early pregnancy. There is an increased diuretic response after water loading when the woman is sitting in the upright position and this response declines by the third trimester. However it may be sufficient to cause urinary frequency in early pregnancy.

Excessive lassitude is a common symptom of early pregnancy and may become apparent even before the first period is missed. Again, it tends to disappear after 12 weeks gestation but is often the most prominent symptom reported.

Breast tenderness and heaviness, which are really an extension of those experienced by many women in the premenstrual phase of the cycle, are common and are particularly common in the month after the first period is missed.

Fetal movements or 'quickening' are not usually noticed until 20 weeks gestation in the woman having her first pregnancy and 18 weeks in the second or subsequent pregnancies. However, many women experience fetal movements earlier than these times and others reach full term without being aware of movements at all.

Occasionally, an abnormal desire for a particular food may occur and this is know as **pica**.

Pseudocyesis

All these symptoms and many of the signs may develop in the absence of pregnancy, giving rise to a condition known as pseudocyesis.

An intense desire for or fear of pregnancy may result in hypothalamic amenorrhoea but, with the present widespread use of ultrasound scanning in early pregnancy, it is unlikely to proceed into late 'pregnancy' unless the woman presents late to a booking clinic.

Biochemical data, in particular a negative pregnancy test, and ultrasound scan information will provide confirmation that pregnancy has not occurred but subsequent sympathetic management and support will be necessary to resolve the underlying anxieties. Menstruation usually returns after the woman is informed of her condition.

Previous obstetric history

The term 'gravidity' is the same as the term 'pregnancy' and a *gravida* is a woman who is pregnant. A *primigravida* is a woman who is pregnant for the first time and a *multigravida* is a woman who has been pregnant on two or more occasions.

The term 'gravidity' must be distinguished from the term 'parity', which describes a woman who has given birth to a potentially viable infant, alive or dead, with a birth weight of 500 g or more and a gestational age in excess of 24 weeks. Thus a *primipara* is a woman who has given birth to one infant or more as a result of one pregnancy. Multiple pregnancies are counted as singleton as far as parity is concerned.

A *multiparous* woman is one who has given birth on two or more occasions to viable infants. A *nulliparous* woman has not given birth to a viable infant. A *grand multipara* has given birth to viable infants on five or more separate occasions.

Thus, a pregnant woman who has given birth to three viable singleton pregnancies and has also had two miscarriages would be described as gravida 5 para 3 – a multigravid multiparous woman.

A *parturient* is a woman in labour and a *puerpera* is a woman who has given birth to a child during the preceding 42 days.

A record should be made of all previous pregnancies, including previous miscarriages, and the duration of gestation in each pregnancy. In particular, it is important to note any previous antenatal complications, details of induction of labour, the duration of labour, the presentation and the method of delivery as well as the birthweight and sex of each infant.

The condition of each infant at birth and the need for care in a special care baby unit should be noted.

Complications of the puerperium such as postpartum haemorrhage, infections of the genital tract and urinary tract, deep vein thrombosis and perineal complications such as breakdown of the perineal wounds may all be relevant to future pregnancies.

PREVIOUS MEDICAL HISTORY

Various medical conditions will have significant bearing on the outcome of a pregnancy, both for the mother and for the baby.

It is important to note a history of diabetes, renal disease, hypertension, cardiac disease, and various endocrine disorders such as thyrotoxicosis and Addison's disease. Infectious diseases such as tuberculosis, HIV, syphilis and hepatitis A or B may have an effect on the outcome of the pregnancy and may cause deterioration in the maternal condition.

FAMILY HISTORY

A wide variety of conditions that are genetically transmitted may have importance in the family history. In practical terms, most women will be aware of any significant family history of the common genetically based diseases and it is not necessary to list all the possibilities to the mother. A general enquiry as to whether there are any known inherited conditions in the family will be sufficient, unless one partner (or both) is adopted and not aware of their family history.

Meticulous attention to the family history and past obstetric history, maternal age and any medical conditions will provide a firm basis for the identification of the risk of congenital abnormalities and fetal and maternal risk. It will also point the way to performing the appropriate tests to screen for these risks.

OBSTETRIC EXAMINATION

At the initial visit to the clinic, a complete physical examination should be performed to identify any physical problems that may be relevant to the antenatal care.

Height is recorded, as it may provide the first indication of a small pelvis. Weight is recorded at the first and all subsequent visits.

Blood pressure is recorded with the patient supine and in the left lateral supine position to avoid compression of the inferior vena cava by the gravid uterus

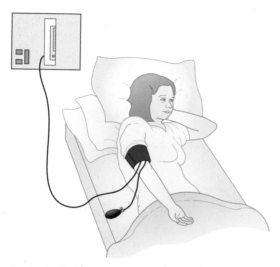

Fig. 6.2 Blood pressure recording standardized in the left lateral position.

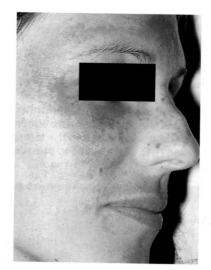

Fig. 6.3 'Chloasma' – facial pigmentation over the forehead and cheeks.

(Fig. 6.2). If blood pressure is to be recorded in the sitting position, then it should be recorded in the same position for all visits and on the same arm. The effect of posture on blood pressure has been noted in Chapter 3. Vena caval compression in late pregnancy may cause symptoms of syncope and nausea and this is associated with postural hypotension, the condition being known as the *supine hypotensive syndrome.*

Although in the past the diastolic pressure has always been taken as Korotkoff fourth sound, where the sound begins to fade, it is now agreed that, where the fifth sound (i.e. the point at which the sound disappears) is clear, this should be used as representing the diastolic pressure. If the point at which the sound disappears cannot be identified because it continues towards zero, then the fourth sound should be used.

Head and neck

Many women develop pigmentation over the forehead and cheeks, particularly where there is frequent exposure to sunlight. This brownish discoloration is known as *chloasma* or 'the mask of pregnancy' (Fig. 6.3). The pigmentation fades after completion of the pregnancy.

The colour of the mucosal surfaces and the conjunctivae should be examined for pallor, as anaemia is a common complication of pregnancy.

The general state of dental hygiene should be noted, as pregnancy is often associated with hypertrophic gingivitis and dental referral may be needed.

Some degree of thyroid enlargement commonly occurs in pregnancy but, unless it is associated with other signs of thyroid disease, it can generally be ignored.

Heart and lungs

A careful examination of the heart should be made to identify any cardiac murmurs. With the hyperdynamic state of the cardiovascular system in normal pregnancy, flow murmurs are common and are of no significance. These are generally soft systolic bruits heard over the

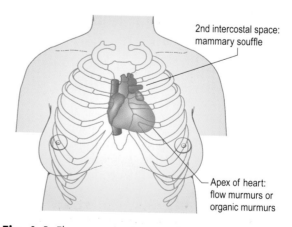

2nd intercostal space: mammary souffle

Apex of heart: flow murmurs or organic murmurs

Fig. 6.4 Flow murmurs in normal pregnancy.

apex of the heart, and occasionally a mammary souffle is heard, arising from the internal mammary vessels and audible in the second intercostal spaces. This will disappear with pressure from the stethoscope (Fig. 6.4).

The presence of all other murmurs should be investigated by a cardiologist, as the early identification of any valvular pathology has implications for the management of the pregnancy.

Gross lung pathology may also affect the outcome of the pregnancy, both for the mother and for the baby, and should therefore be identified as early in the pregnancy as possible.

Breasts

The breasts show characteristic signs characterized by increased vascularity, the development of Montgomery's tubercles and pigmentation of the areolae of the nipples (Fig. 6.5). Although routine breast examination is not indicated, it is important to ask about inversion of nipples, as this may give rise to difficulties during suckling, and to look for any pathology such as breast cysts or solid nodules in women who complain of any breast symptoms.

Abdomen

Examination of the abdomen commonly shows the presence of stretch marks or *striae gravidarum* (Fig. 6.6). The scars are initially purplish in colour and appear in the lines of stress in the skin. These scars may also extend on to the thighs and buttocks and on to the

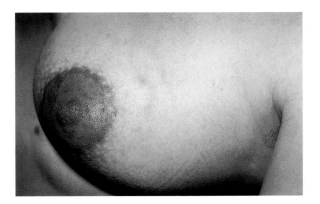

Fig. 6.5 Physiological changes in the breast in early pregnancy. The areola becomes pigmented and Montgomery's tubercles develop.

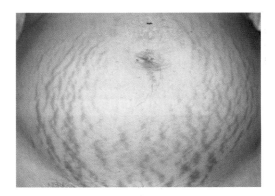

Fig. 6.6 Striae gravidarum on the anterior abdominal wall.

breasts. In subsequent pregnancies, the scars adopt a silvery-white appearance. The linea alba often becomes pigmented and is then known as the *linea nigra*. This pigmentation often persists after the first pregnancy.

Hepatosplenomegaly should be excluded as well as any evidence of renal enlargement. The uterus does not become palpable as an abdominal organ until 12 weeks gestation.

Limbs and skeletal changes

The legs should be examined for oedema and for varicose veins.

They should also be examined for any evidence of shortening of the lower limbs, as this may give problems with gait as the abdomen expands.

In addition, posture also changes in pregnancy as the fetus grows and the maternal abdomen expands, with a tendency to develop some kyphosis and, in particular, to develop an increased lumbar lordosis as the upper part of the trunk is thrown backwards to compensate for the weight of the developing fetus (Fig. 6.7). This often results in the development of backache and sometimes gives rise to sciatic pain.

Pelvic examination

The widespread use of ultrasound has removed the need for routine pelvic examination to confirm pregnancy and gestation at booking. If a routine cervical smear is due at the time of booking, this can usually be deferred until after the puerperium, as interpretation of cervical cytology is more difficult in pregnancy. Clinical assess-

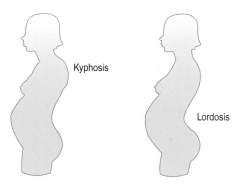

Kyphosis

Lordosis

Fig. 6.7 Postural changes in pregnancy. With enlargement of the gravid uterus, there is an increased lumbar lordosis and a tendency to some degree of kyphosis.

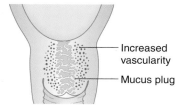

Increased vascularity

Mucus plug

Fig. 6.8 Cervical changes in pregnancy include increased glandular content and a thick mucus plug.

ment of the size and shape of the pelvis may be useful in unusual circumstances such as a previous fractured pelvis but has not be shown to be of value otherwise and is generally no longer carried out as part of the routine antenatal examinations.

Vaginal examination in early pregnancy is indicated in the assessment of bleeding (see Chapter 18). Pelvic examination in later pregnancy is indicated for cervical assessment (Chapter 12), the diagnosis of labour and to confirm ruptured membranes (Chapter 12). Vaginal examination is contraindicated in later pregnancy in cases of antepartum haemorrhage until placenta praevia can be excluded.

The role of vaginal examination in normal labour is discussed in Chapter 12.

The technique of pelvic examination in early pregnancy is the same as that for the non-pregnant woman and is described in Chapter 17 but noting the following.

The vulva should be examined to exclude any abnormal lesions and to assess the perineum in relation to any damage sustained in previous pregnancies. Varicosities of the vulva are common and may become worse during pregnancy.

The vaginal walls become more rugous in pregnancy as the stratified squamous epithelium thickens with an increase in the glycogen content of the epithelial cells.

There is also a marked increase in the vascularity of the paravaginal tissues so that the appearance of the vaginal walls become purplish red. There is an increase in vaginal secretions, with increased vaginal transudation, increased shedding of epithelial cells and some contribution from enhanced production of cervical mucus.

The cervix becomes softened and shows signs of increased vascularity. Enlargement of the cervix is associated with an increase in vascularity as well as oedema of the connective tissues and cellular hyperplasia and hypertrophy. The glandular content of the endocervix increases to occupy half the substance of the cervix and produces a thick plug of viscid cervical mucus that occludes the cervical os (Fig. 6.8).

Assessment of the bony pelvis

Although the shape and size of the bony pelvis are critical to labour, routine antenatal estimation of pelvic size, either clinically or radiologically, has not been shown to be of value in predicting outcome. However, it is important to assess the pelvis and fetus for possible disproportion when managing cases of poor progress in labour. Clinical pelvimetry may be of value where there has been previous trauma or abnormal development of the bony pelvis, although in these cases more precise information about the dimensions is usually obtained by imaging.

In a normal female or *gynaecoid* pelvis, because the sacrum is evenly curved, maximum space for the fetal head is provided in the pelvic mid-cavity. The sacrum should feel evenly curved.

If the sacrum feels flat, then the pelvis may contract towards the pelvic outlet, as in the *android* or male-like pelvis, and may lead to impaction of the fetal head as it descends through the pelvis.

The bony pelvis consists of the sacrum, the coccyx and two innominate bones. The pelvic area above the iliopectineal line is known as the *false pelvis* and the area below the pelvic brim is the *true pelvis*. The latter is the important section in relation to childbearing and parturition. Thus, the wall of the true pelvis is formed by the sacrum posteriorly, the ischial bones and the sacrosciatic notches and ligaments laterally, and anter-

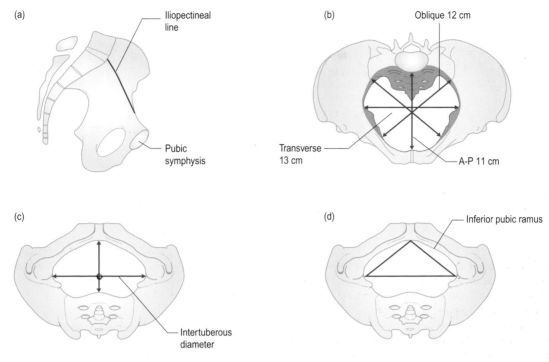

Fig. 6.9 (a) Inlet of the true pelvis is bounded by the sacral promontory, iliopectineal lines, pubic rami and pubic symphysis. (b) Dimensions of the inlet of the true pelvis. (c) Pelvic outlet bounded by the inferior pubic rami and the ischial tuberosities and the sacrosciatic ligaments. (d) the inferior pubic rami should form an angle of 90°.

iorly by the pubic rami, the obturator fossae and membranes, the ascending rami of the ischial bones and the pubic rami (Fig. 6.9). The shape and the dimensions of the true pelvis are best understood by consideration of the four planes of the pelvis.

Plane of the pelvic inlet

The plane of the pelvic inlet or pelvic brim is bounded posteriorly by the sacral promontory, laterally by the iliopectineal lines and anteriorly by the superior pubic rami and upper margin of the pubic symphysis. The plane is almost circular in the normal gynaecoid pelvis but is slightly larger transversely than anteroposteriorly.

The true conjugate or anteroposterior diameter of the pelvic inlet is the distance between the midpoint of the sacral promontory and the superior border of the pubic symphysis anteriorly (Fig. 6.10). The diameter measures approximately 11 cm. The shortest distance and the one of greatest clinical significance is the obstetric conjugate diameter. This is the distance between the midpoint of

the sacral promontory and the nearest point on the posterior surface of the pubic symphysis.

It is not possible to measure either of these diameters by clinical examination; the only diameter at the pelvic inlet that is amenable to clinical assessment is the distance from the inferior margin of the pubic symphysis to the midpoint of the sacral promontory. This is known as the diagonal conjugate diameter and is approximately 1.5 cm greater than the obstetric diameter. In practical terms it is not usually possible to reach the sacral promontory on clinical examination and the highest point that can be palpated is the second or third piece of the sacrum. If the sacral promontory is easily palpable, the pelvic inlet is contracted (Fig. 6.11b).

Plane of greatest pelvic dimensions

The plane of greatest pelvic dimensions has little clinical significance and has an anteroposterior and transverse diameter of approximately 12.7 cm. The anteroposterior diameter extends from the midpoint of

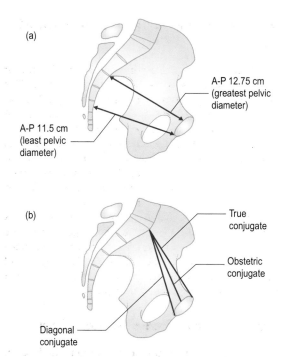

(a)

A-P 12.75 cm
(greatest pelvic
diameter)

A-P 11.5 cm
(least pelvic
diameter)

(b)

True
conjugate

Obstetric
conjugate

Diagonal
conjugate

Fig. 6.10 (a) Anteroposterior diameters of the mid-cavity and pelvic outlet. (b) Conjugate diameters of the pelvic inlet.

the posterior aspect of the pubic symphysis to the junction of the second and third pieces of the sacrum. The transverse diameter passes laterally through the middle of the acetabuli.

The only indication of the shape of the pelvis at this level is the curvature of the sacrum and the shape of the sacrosciatic notch, which should subtend an angle of 90°. This normally allows the admission of two fingers along the sacrospinous ligaments, which extend from the ischial spines to the lateral aspects of the second and third pieces of the sacrum.

Plane of least pelvic dimensions

The plane of least pelvic dimensions represents the level at which impaction of the fetal head is most likely to occur. The anteroposterior diameter extends from the inferior margin of the pubic symphysis and transects the line drawn between the ischial spines. Both the transverse (interspinous) and the anteroposterior diameter can be assessed clinically and the interspinous diameter is the narrowest space in the pelvis (10 cm). The ischial spines should be palpated to see if they are prominent and also to make an estimate of the interspinous diameter (Fig. 6.11a).

Outlet of the pelvis

The outlet of the pelvis consists of two triangular planes. Anteriorly, the triangle is bounded by the area under the pubic arch and this should normally subtend an angle of 90°. The transverse diameter is the distance between the ischial tuberosities, the intertuberous diameter, which is normally not less than 11 cm. The posterior triangle is formed anteriorly by the intertuberous diameter and posterolaterally by the tip of the sacrum and the sacrosciatic ligaments.

Clinically, the intertuberous diameter can be assessed by placing the knuckles of the clenched fist between the ischial tuberosities. The subpubic angle can be assessed

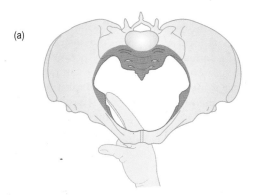

(a)

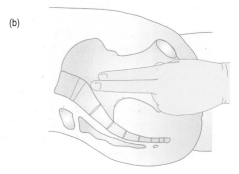

(b)

Fig. 6.11 (a) Clinical assessment of the ischial spines at the plane of least pelvic dimensions. (b) Assessment of the pelvic inlet.

by placing the index fingers of both hands along the inferior pubic rami or by inserting two fingers of the examining hand under the pubic arch.

Obstetrical examination at subsequent routine visits

At all subsequent antenatal visits, the blood pressure should be recorded and the urine tested for glucose, protein and ketone bodies. Maternal weight should be measured at each visit and should increase by an average of approximately 0.5 kg per week after the 16th week of gestation.

Rapid and excessive weight gain is nearly always associated with excessive fluid retention and static weight or weight loss may indicate the failure of normal fetal growth. Excessive weight gain is often associated with signs of oedema and this is most readily apparent in the face, the hands, where it may become difficult to remove rings, on the anterior abdominal wall and over the lower legs and ankles. Oedema over the sacral pad is rare in pregnancy.

ABDOMINAL PALPATION

Palpation of the uterine fundus

The estimation of gestational age is the first step in examination of the abdomen in the pregnant woman. There are several methods employed to assess the size of the fetus.

The ulnar border of the left hand is placed on the uterine fundus. The uterus first becomes palpable suprapubically at 12 weeks gestation and by 24 weeks gestation it has reached the level of the umbilicus. At 36 weeks gestation the uterine fundus is palpable at the level of the xiphisternum and then tends to remain at this level until term, or to fall slightly as the presenting part enters the pelvic brim.

All methods of clinical assessment of gestational age are subject to considerable inaccuracies, particularly in the early assessment related to the position of the umbilicus, and the fundal height will be affected by the presence of multiple fetuses, excessive amniotic fluid or, at the other extreme, the presence of a small fetus or oligohydramnios.

Direct measurement of the girth or the symphysial–fundal height provides a more reliable method of assessing fetal growth and gestational age.

Measurement of symphysial–fundal height

The distance between the uterine fundus and the top of the pubic symphysis is measured in centimetres. The mean fundal height measures approximately 20 cm at 20 weeks and increases by 1 cm/week so that at 36 weeks the fundal height will be 36 cm (Fig 6.12).

Using two standard deviations from the mean, it is possible to describe the 10th and 90th centile values. Using this technique on a serial basis, approximately 75% of all small-for-dates infants can be detected and the maximum accuracy of detection occurs at 32–33 weeks gestation. The accuracy is considerably reduced as a random observation after 36 weeks gestation. The predictive value is also lower at approximately 65% for large-for-dates infants. The technique is simple and easily applicable and is particularly useful where other more precise techniques are not available.

Measurement of abdominal girth

Measurement of girth provides another method of assessment. The measurement of girth is made at the level of the maternal umbilicus. Assuming that the average non-pregnant girth is 60 cm, no significant increase will occur until 24 weeks gestation. Thereafter the girth should increase by 2.5 cm weekly so that at full term the girth will be 100 cm.

If the non-pregnant girth is greater or smaller than 60 cm, then an appropriate allowance must be made. Thus, a woman with a normal 65 cm girth would have a measurement of 95 cm at 36 weeks gestation.

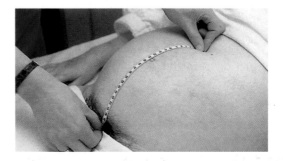

Fig. 6.12 Measurement of symphysial–fundal height.

PALPATION OF FETAL PARTS

Fetal parts are not usually palpable before 24 weeks gestation. When palpating the fetus, it must be remembered that the presence of amniotic fluid necessitates the use of 'dipping' movements with flexion of the fingers at the metacarpophalangeal joints. The purpose of palpation is to describe the relationship of the fetus to the maternal trunk and pelvis (Fig. 6.13).

Lie

The term 'lie' describes the relationship of the long axis of the fetus to the long axis of the uterus (Fig. 6.14). Facing the feet of the mother, the examiner's left hand is placed along the left side of the maternal abdomen and the right hand on the right lateral aspect of the uterus. Systematic palpation towards the midline with the left

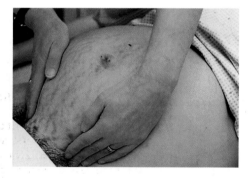

Fig. 6.13 Palpation of the presenting part and the fetal back.

and then the right hand will reveal either the firm resistance of the fetal back or the irregular features of the fetal limbs.

If the lie is *longitudinal*, the head or breech will be palpable over or in the pelvic inlet. If the lie is *oblique*, the long axis of the fetus lies at an angle of 45° to the long axis of the uterus and the presenting part will be palpable in the iliac fossa. In a *transverse* lie, the fetus lies at right angles to the mother and the poles of the fetus are palpable in the flanks.

Having ascertained the lie and the location of the fetal back, it is now important to feel for the head and breech by firm pressure with alternate hands. The head is hard, round and discrete. It can be 'bounced' between the examining hands and is described as being 'ballotable'. The buttocks are softer and more diffuse and the breech is not ballotable. The head should be sought in the lower abdomen or in the uterine fundus. Facing the mother's feet, firm pressure is applied over the presenting part. If the head is presenting, note is made as to whether it is easily palpable or whether it is necessary to apply deep pressure.

The normal attitude of the fetus is one of flexion (Fig. 6.15) but on occasions, as with the 'flying fetus', it may exhibit an attitude of extension.

Presentation

In a longitudinal lie, the presenting part may be the head (*cephalic*) or the breech (*podalic*). In a transverse lie, the presenting part is the shoulder.

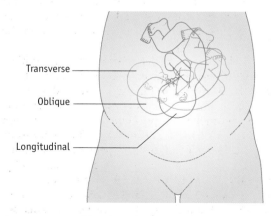

Fig. 6.14 Fetal lie describes the relationship of the long axis of the fetus to the long axis of the uterus.

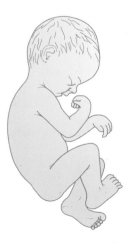

Fig. 6.15 The normal attitude of the fetus is one of flexion.

Depending on the degree of flexion or deflexion, various parts of the head will present to the pelvic inlet. Where the head is well flexed, the presentation is the *vertex* – the area that lies between the anterior and posterior fontanelles. If the head is completely extended, the face presents to the pelvic inlet (*face presentation*) and if it lies between these two attitudes, the brow presents (*brow presentation*). The brow is the area between the base of the nose and the anterior fontanelle. The diameter of presentation for the vertex is the suboccipitobregmatic diameter (Table 6.1,

Fig. 6.16). If the head is deflexed, the occipitofrontal diameter presents. With a brow presentation, the verticomental diameter presents to the pelvic inlet. Presentation and position can be accurately determined only by vaginal examination when the cervix has dilated and the suture lines and fontanelles can be palpated. This situation only really pertains when the mother is well established in labour.

Position

The position of the fetus is a description of the relationship of the denominator to the inlet of the maternal pelvis. It must not be confused with the presentation, although it provides a further description of the relationship of the presenting part to the maternal pelvis and is of particular importance during parturition. The denominators for the various presentations are as follows:

Table 6.1
Diameters of presentation

Presenting part	Diameter	size (cm)
Vertex	Suboccipitobregmatic	9.5
Brow	Verticomental	13.5
Face	Submentobregmatic	9.5
Deflexed vertex	Occipitofrontal	11.7

Presentation	Denominator
Vertex	Occiput
Face	Chin (mentum)
Breech	Sacrum

Thus, in a vertex presentation, six different positions are described (Fig. 6.17).

Viewed from below the pelvis, these include right and left occipitotransverse positions as well as left and right anterior and posterior positions. Except in the advanced second stage, it is very rare for the head to be identified in a direct anterior or posterior position.

With a face presentation, the prefix *mento-* is included and with a breech presentation the prefix is *sacro-*. No such description is given to a brow presentation, as there is no mechanism of vaginal delivery unless the presentation is corrected.

The position can be determined from abdominal palpation by palpating the anterior shoulder of the fetus. If this is near the midline and easily palpable, the position is anterior. If it is not easily palpable and the limbs are prominent, the position is probably posterior.

However, the position of the presenting part can be most accurately determined by palpating the suture lines and fontanelles or the breech presentation through the dilated cervix once labour has started.

The degree of flexion of the head can also be determined. On abdominal palpation, a deflexed or extended head tends to feel large and the nuchal groove between the occiput and the fetal back is easily identified.

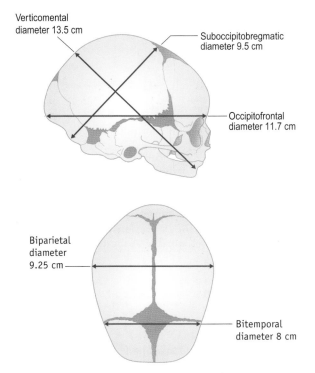

Fig. 6.16 Diameters of presentation of the mature fetal skull.

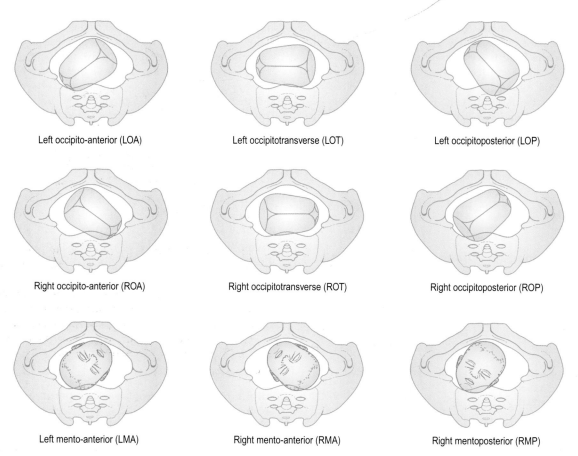

Left occipito-anterior (LOA)   Left occipitotransverse (LOT)   Left occipitoposterior (LOP)

Right occipito-anterior (ROA)   Right occipitotransverse (ROT)   Right occipitoposterior (ROP)

Left mento-anterior (LMA)   Right mento-anterior (RMA)   Right mentoposterior (RMP)

Fig. 6.17 Positions of the head in vertex and face presentations viewed from below.

Station and engagement

The station of the head is described in fifths above the pelvic brim (Fig. 6.18). The head is *engaged* when the greatest transverse diameter (the biparietal diameter) has passed through the inlet of the true pelvis. The head that is engaged is usually fixed and only two-fifths palpable. It is usually difficult to feel abdominally.

> **!** A small head may still be mobile even though it is engaged. A large head may be fixed in the pelvic brim and yet not be engaged. At the simplest level, a head that is easily palpable abdominally is not engaged, whereas a head that is presenting and is deeply engaged is difficult to palpate.

Where it is difficult to locate the head, this may either be because the head is under the maternal rib cage, as with a breech presentation, or because it is a case of anencephaly.

Under these circumstances, a vaginal examination should be performed, as the leading part of the engaged head will be palpable at the level of the ischial spines.

Auscultation

Auscultation of the fetal heart rate is a routine part of the obstetric examination and is usually performed with a Pinard fetal stethoscope (Fig. 6.19). The bell of the instrument is placed over the anterior fetal shoulder or in the midline where there is a posterior position. It is now standard practice to use a hand-held Doppler

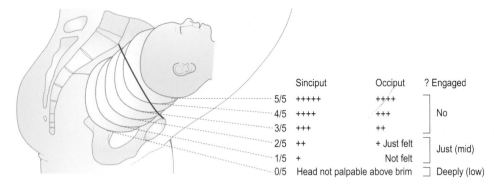

		Sinciput	Occiput	? Engaged
	5/5	+++++	++++	No
	4/5	++++	+++	
	3/5	+++	++	
	2/5	++	+ Just felt	Just (mid)
	1/5	+	Not felt	
	0/5	Head not palpable above brim		Deeply (low)

Fig. 6.18 Stations of the fetal head.

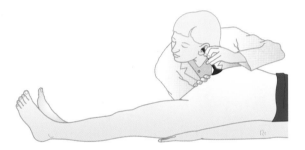

Fig. 6.19 Auscultation of the fetal heart.

ultrasound device that will produce an electronic signal to enable the heartbeat to be recognized and counted.

With the Pinard's stethoscope, the low frequency sound is best heard in late pregnancy below the level of the umbilicus but with a breech presentation, the sound is best heard at the level of the umbilicus. The rate and rhythm of the heart beat should be recorded.

ESSENTIAL INFORMATION

Obstetric history present pregnancy

- Date of LMP
- Length of menstrual cycle
- EDD – subtract 3 months/ add 7 days
- Contraceptive history

Symptoms of pregnancy

- Nausea and vomiting
- Frequency of micturition
- Excessive lassitude
- Breast tenderness

Previous obstetric history

- Previous miscarriages
- Previous viable pregnancies
- Stillbirths or neonatal deaths
- Method of delivery
- Gestational age and sex of infants
- Previous antenatal or postnatal complications

Previous medical history

- Diabetes
- Cardiac disease
- Hypertension
- Renal disease
- Infectious disease such as HIV, Hepatitis B or C

Obstetric examination

- General examination including CVS
- Flow murmurs are common
- Examine breasts and nipples if clinically indicated

Abdominal palpation

- Palpate fundus
- Measure symphysial–fundal height
- Feel for presenting part
- Determine lie
- Assess station of presenting part
- Determine position of presenting part
- Auscultation of fetal heart

7 Normal pregnancy and antenatal care

The concept that the general wellbeing and reproductive performance of a woman might be improved by antenatal supervision is surprisingly recent and was first introduced in Edinburgh in 1911. In many societies, antenatal care is not available or, for social or religious reasons, is not used when it is available. Unfortunately, it is often least available in those communities where the need is greatest and where antenatal disorders, particularly those linked to malnutrition, are most common.

The basic aims of antenatal care are:

- To ensure optimal health of the mother throughout pregnancy and in the puerperium
- To detect and treat disorders arising during pregnancy that relate to the welfare of both the mother and the fetus and to ensure that the pregnancy results in a healthy mother and a healthy infant.

The ways by which these objectives are achieved will vary according to the initial health and history of the mother and are a combination of screening tests, educational and emotional support and monitoring of fetal growth and maternal health throughout the pregnancy.

The frequency of antenatal visits was first established by a group of providers of antenatal care as long ago as 1929 and this protocol advised that antenatal visits should occur monthly from 8 weeks gestation until 28 weeks and then every 2 weeks until 36 weeks and thereafter weekly until the time of delivery.

In modern antenatal care, the timing of visits, particularly in the first 28 weeks of pregnancy, is now more closely geared to attendance for screening tests. Nevertheless, in the last 4 weeks of pregnancy, weekly visits are advised as it is not possible to anticipate those cases where hypertension and pre-eclampsia will develop.

Antenatal care is provided through a variety of different mechanisms and may be provided by general practitioners, midwives and obstetricians, often in a pattern of shared care. Pregnancies that are considered to be high risk should receive a high proportion of their care by obstetricians or specialists in fetomaternal medicine.

ROUTINE CLINICAL EXAMINATIONS

The details of antenatal history and routine clinical examinations have been discussed in Chapter 6 and will not be discussed again in this chapter. However, certain observations should be stressed at the first visit and it is preferable that these observations should be made within the first 10 weeks of pregnancy. The measurement of maternal height and weight is important and has value in prediction of pregnancy outcomes. Women with a low body mass index (BMI) – less than 20 where BMI is estimated as weight (kg) divided by height (m)^2 – are at increased risk of fetal growth restriction and perinatal mortality. Poor weight gain during pregnancy may also be associated with intrauterine growth impairment and thus regular checks on maternal weight throughout pregnancy, as well as the measurement of blood pressure (BP) and urinary testing for proteinuria, haematuria and glycosuria, are all part of good antenatal care.

The initial measurement of blood pressure should be taken as soon as possible as this may provide evidence that, if there is hypertension, it is likely to have predated the pregnancy.

ROUTINE SCREENING TESTS

Beginning at the first visit, a number of screening tests are introduced. Some will be repeated later in the pregnancy. The omission of these tests will generally now be considered to be evidence of substandard practice so they have medicolegal importance as well as clinical relevance.

Haematological investigations

Anaemia is a common disorder in pregnancy and in most communities will be due to iron deficiency, either because of the depletion of iron stores or because of reduced iron intake. Over 90% of pathological anaemia in pregnancy is due to iron deficiency. However, it may also be macrocytic and due to folate deficiency or may be related to various parasitic infections.

Haemoglobin concentration and a complete blood picture should therefore be performed at the first visit and repeated at 28 and 36 weeks gestation. Women who

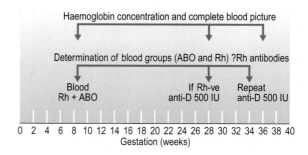

Fig. 7.1 Schedules for routine tests of haemoglobin estimation and detection and administration of Rhesus antibodies.

have deficient iron intakes should be given oral supplements of iron from early in pregnancy. Screening for haemoglobinopathies should be routinely offered to those racial groups where conditions such as thalassaemia and sickle cell disease are common.

Blood groups

Blood group should be determined in all pregnant women and screening for red cell antibodies should be undertaken in early pregnancies. In Rhesus-negative women, screening for Rh antibodies should be performed at the first visit (preferably in the first trimester) and then repeated at least at 28 and 34 weeks gestation. Now that anti-D antibodies are readily available, it has become standard practice to give 500 IU at 28 and 34 weeks gestation (Fig. 7.1). This will prevent maternal immunization by a Rhesus-positive fetus in all but 1–1.5% Rhesus-negative women, in whom the infusion of cells from the fetus overwhelms the dose of antibody administered. ABO antibodies may also cause problems in the fetus but there is no method available to counter this problem.

Infection screening

Rubella

All females in the UK are offered rubella vaccination between the ages of 11 and 14. By the time they present for their first confinement, 22% of nulliparous women will still be found to be non-immune, as well as 1.2% of multiparous women. Around 50% of non-immune women will have been previously vaccinated. All seronegative women should be offered immunization in the immediate puerperium. Vaccination is performed with a live attenuated rubella virus with vaccines such as Almevax and involves a single dose of 0.5 ml injected subcutaneously. Although there is no evidence to suggest any significant abnormality rate in women who have conceived immediately before or following rubella vaccination, it is generally recommended that pregnancy should be avoided for 2 months after vaccination. Non-immune women should be advised to avoid contact with infected individuals and any clinically suspected infection should be investigated with paired sera, preferably with the original sample taken at the time of booking.

Syphilis

Routine screening for syphilis is recommended practice. Despite the fact that the condition is relatively rare in the UK, with 200–300 new cases being detected annually, the condition is treatable and has major neonatal sequelae if left untreated. Various tests are available.

Non-specific tests. The *Wasserman reaction* is a complement-fixation test that was the first successful serological test described for use in clinical practice. The test is dependent on the presence of treponemal antibodies in the serum, which unite with a colloidal suspension of lipoids to produce visible flocculation. A similar flocculation test that is widely used is the *Venereal Disease Research Laboratory test (VDRL)*, which employs a cardiolipin antigen. The difficulty with these tests is that they may give a false-positive reaction in association with malaria or viral pneumonia, or in autoimmune conditions such as lupus erythematosus, haemolytic anaemias, Hashimoto's disease or rheumatoid arthritis.

Specific tests. Where there is doubt about the diagnosis, specific tests should be employed. The *Treponema pallidum immobilization test (TPI)* is the most specific test available and is based on the fact that the serum from syphilitic patients contains an antibody that, in the presence of complement, immobilizes virulent treponemes. Positive tests are also found in patients with yaws and other treponemal diseases. Other tests include the *fluorescent treponemal antibody tests (FTA)* and the *Treponema pallidum haemagglutination test (TPHA)*. In the TPHA, the antigen consists of a suspension of Turkey red blood cells in formalin and tannin that have been sensitized by contact with virulent treponemes. Positive tests are characterized by agglutination of the sensitized cells on contact with affected serum. The test is easy to perform and is highly specific. The VDRL usually becomes nega-

tive within 6 months of treatment, whereas the TPHA remains positive for many years. The VDRL, therefore assumes the most important role in monitoring treatment.

Hepatitis B

There is a case for universal screening for hepatitis B in pregnancy. Passive and active vaccination is recommended for at-risk infants, although often the completion of full vaccination, which involves a course of three injections, is not achieved. Full vaccination protects infants from hepatitis B infection in 90% of cases.

Human immunodeficiency virus

The basis of tests for the detection of human immunodeficiency virus (HIV) is the detection of HIV antibodies. The virus can be isolated and grown but this is difficult. As the virus has a predilection for the T-helper subset of lymphocytes, there is an altered T-helper/T-suppressor ratio. All these tests can be normal, even in the presence of infection. The most important confounding variable is that HIV antibodies may be absent in the incubation phase.

Seropositive mothers always have seropositive babies but this may not indicate the acquired immune deficiency syndrome (AIDS) in the baby. However, anywhere between 30% and 50% of babies will have AIDS if active management programmes are not used. While screening is obviously important in high-risk populations such as intravenous drug users, a sexual partner who is a drug user or bisexual, or haemophiliacs, there is now a strong case for routine screening of all women. The change in philosophy to an opt-out policy has now arisen because there is compelling evidence that mother-to-child transmission rates can be reduced from more than 30% to less than 5% by strategies including caesarean section, avoidance of breastfeeding and antiretroviral therapy.

Screening for fetal anomalies

Structural fetal anomalies account for some 20–25% of all perinatal deaths and for about 15% of all deaths in the first year of life. There is therefore a strong case to be made for early detection and termination of pregnancy where this is appropriate. The frequency of the major structural anomalies is shown in Table 7.1. It has to be remembered that these figures vary in different

Table 7.1
Structural anomalies

Type of anomaly	Frequency (per 1000)
Cardiovascular	8
Craniospinal	2–4
Renal tract	1
Gastrointestinal	1

countries and under different environmental circumstances. Congenital anomalies are one of the markers of socio-economic deprivation.

These anomalies are generally detectable by ultrasound scanning and this will be discussed in the chapter on congenital abnormalities.

Neural tube defects

In 1972, Brock and Sutcliffe described an increased concentration of α-fetoprotein in amniotic fluid in the presence of neural tube defects. This is also reflected in serum values, so that serum α-fetoprotein testing is offered as a routine test in the UK. The likelihood of a major neural tube defect is increased where there is a previous history of an affected child. The risk of a subsequent abnormal child is 1 in 20 and increases to 1 in 10 after two affected children and 1 in 5 after three affected children. Ingestion by the mother of folic acid supplements, preferably starting pre-pregnancy, significantly reduces the recurrence rate. Using a cut-off point of 2.5 multiples of the median, 79% of fetuses with spina bifida and 88% of anencephalic fetuses will be detected, with 3% of unaffected fetuses falling into this range.

Total population screening is now undertaken on serum measurements but emphasis is placed on the value of these measurements in screening for neural tube defects as well as for Down's syndrome.

Blood samples are taken between 15 and 19 weeks gestation. It is critical to have an accurate assessment of gestational age using ultrasound if these values are to have any value. The combination of raised values of serum α-fetoprotein and a detailed ultrasound examination will identify 95% of neural tube defects. If there is any doubt about the diagnosis, a sample of amniotic fluid should be collected by amniocentesis and tested for α-fetoprotein and acetyl cholinesterase (Fig. 7.2).

Some difficulty may arise in detecting or confirming a closed neural tube defect as, if the spinal defect is covered by skin, detection may be difficult and the levels of alpha-fetoprotein in amniotic fluid may be within the normal range. This is not such a problem, as covered lesions are associated with a good functional prognosis.

Down's syndrome

Screening for Down's syndrome has become routine in most antenatal services but not in all countries. As the logical consequence of such a programme is to offer termination of pregnancy where there is evidence of Down's syndrome, such a screening programme is not relevant if termination is not an option. Screening is by the use of biochemical and ultrasound tests. It is important that women understand that these are screening tests and therefore have their limitations. They will not detect every case and high-risk results do not necessarily mean that the baby is affected. Despite the increased incidence of Down's syndrome in mothers over 35 years, screening on the basis of age alone is not generally recommended and it is now common practice to offer screening to all women. Routine amniocentesis for the over-35s is not recommended as the pick-up rate is one abnormality for every 125 tests and one chromosomally normal pregnancy is lost for every chromosomally abnormal fetus detected.

Biochemical tests are based on the use of maternal serum alpha-fetoprotein (levels are reduced in the presence of all autosomal trisomy pregnancies), human chorionic gonadotrophin (either free beta or intact hCG) where levels are raised and, in some centres, measurement of low serum unconjugated oestriol levels. This is known as the triple test.

The test is normally performed at 15–20 weeks gestation and is critically gestational-age-dependent for its interpretation. This means that determination of gestational age by ultrasound is an essential ingredient of this type of screening programme. In screening a general population, approximately 70% of cases of Down's syndrome should be detected and 20% of women over 35 can expect to fall into a high-risk category.

The other major modality for screening for Down's syndrome is the use of ultrasound measurement of nuchal translucency, a measurement of fluid behind the fetal neck.

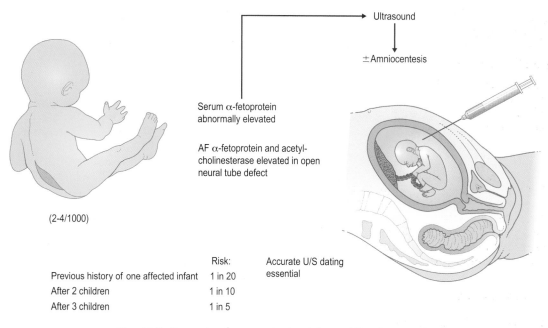

Ultrasound

±Amniocentesis

Serum α-fetoprotein
abnormally elevated

AF α-fetoprotein and acetylcholinesterase elevated in open
neural tube defect

(2–4/1000)

Accurate U/S dating
essential

	Risk:
Previous history of one affected infant	1 in 20
After 2 children	1 in 10
After 3 children	1 in 5

Fig. 7.2 Screening for neural tube defects. AF, α-fetoprotein.

It is now standard practice to use a combination of these measurements for screening purposes. It is also important to note that, in addition to the detection of trisomy 21, other trisomies such as 18 and 13 also have lowered α-fetoprotein values. Furthermore, other causes for low maternal α-fetoprotein levels are fetal death, hydatidiform mole, diabetes, obesity and wrong dates.

Some centres also include the measurement of pregnancy-associated plasma protein A (PAPP-A) and the combination of ultrasound screening, free beta-hCG and PAPP-A can produce a detection rate of 86% for Down's syndrome.

Amniocentesis

Where tests indicate a significant risk of abnormality, amniocentesis should be performed between 15 and 17 weeks gestation. Between 10 and 15 ml of amniotic fluid is aspirated transabdominally using a spinal needle under ultrasound guidance. The procedure carries a 0.5–1% risk of causing a miscarriage. Fetal cells are harvested by centrifugation and the cells are then cultured for up to 3 weeks to obtain the karyotype.

There is a failure rate in the culture process of 2–5%, which may necessitate repeating the procedure if there is a significant risk.

Chorion villus sampling

Fetal cells can also be obtained by obtaining a sample of chorionic villi either transcervically or transabdominally. The advantage of this technique is that it is carried out before 12 weeks gestation and the karyotype can be obtained within 2–3 days. This allows for an early decision to be made and for termination to be performed within the first 14 weeks. The disadvantage is a slightly higher rate of pregnancy loss.

Screening for gestational diabetes

Gestational diabetes is associated with an increased incidence of intra-uterine fetal death. Screening programmes follow one of two pathways:

- **Selection by history:**
  - History of a pregnancy complicated by gestational diabetes or impaired glucose tolerance

- First-degree relative with diabetes
- Previous unexplained stillbirth
- Previous macrosomic infant with a birthweight in excess of 4 kg
- Maternal BMI > 35
- Repeated episodes of glycosuria.

Under these circumstances, if the fasting blood glucose level is less than 4.5 mmol/l, then a full glucose tolerance test (GTT) is unnecessary but, if this not the case, a full GTT should be performed using either a 75 g or 100 g loading dose of glucose. The test should be performed at the booking visit and again at 28 weeks gestation if there is any doubt about the diagnosis. There is an argument that says that the test will give more reliable results at 28 weeks. The desirability of the early GTT is in part determined by the initial fasting blood glucose level.

- **Universal screening:** The screening of all women at booking, with a further test at 28 weeks, will identify more women with impaired glucose tolerance or diabetes with a sensitivity of about 78% and specificity of 90%. A modified GTT involving a loading dose of 50 g and a 1 hour blood glucose is considered positive if the blood glucose exceeds 7.7 mmol/l.

Most units prefer to screen at-risk populations because of the practical difficulties and costs of screening the whole population, particularly in large maternity hospitals.

Screening for urinary tract infection

Screening for asymptomatic bacteriuria is now used as a routine procedure and is of proven benefit. The presence of pathogenic organisms in excess of 10 000 organisms/ml indicates significant bacteruria. As the incidence of ascending urinary tract infection including acute pyelonephritis is increased in pregnancy and is associated with increased pregnancy loss and maternal morbidity, early treatment of asymptomatic bacteruria reduces the incidence of such infections and thus improves maternal health.

FOLLOW-UP VISITS

Although the pattern of antenatal care will vary with circumstances and with the normality or otherwise of the pregnancy, a general pattern of visits will partly revolve around the demands of the screening proce-

dures and the obstetric and medical history of the mother. The measurement of blood pressure and urinalysis are performed at all visits and the measurement of symphysis/fundal height should be recorded, even accepting that this observation has a limited capacity to detect fetal growth retardation. Serial ultrasound measurements will have a greater detection rate if performed at every visit but this is not practicable for all women who are not considered to be at high risk. A suggested regime for antenatal visits is listed in Table 7.2.

In general, where pregnancies have been accurately dated by early ultrasound so that the gestational age is secure, induction of labour after 41 weeks reduces section rates, operative vaginal deliveries, the incidence of meconium staining, macrosomia and the risk of fetal and neonatal deaths.

ANTENATAL EDUCATION

An important and integral part of antenatal care is the education of the mother and her partner about pregnancy, childbirth and the care of the infant. This process should start before pregnancy and as part of school education and should continue throughout pregnancy and the puerperium. There are various ways by which this can be achieved but, commonly, the needs are met by regular antenatal classes during the course of the pregnancy. It is preferable that those staff who are involved in general antenatal care and delivery should be part of the team that deliver the woman so that the processes of care and education are seen as one entity.

Dietary advice

There can be no doubt about the importance of diet in pregnancy. At one extreme, gross malnutrition is known to result in intrauterine growth retardation, anaemia, prematurity and fetal malformation. Lesser degrees of malnutrition may also be associated with an increased incidence of fetal malformations, particularly neural tube defects, and it is therefore important to provide guidance on diet and to ensure that a diet of appropriate quality and quantity is maintained throughout pregnancy and the puerperium.

Where there is a history of a previous neural tube defect, the mother should be advised to take a folic acid supplement of 5 mg/day starting before conception and continuing for at least 12 weeks into the pregnancy. In fact, mothers are usually advised to continue the supplements throughout pregnancy.

Table 7.2
Visits for antenatal care (from Kean 2001)

8–12 weeks	Initial visit, confirmation of pregnancy, search for risk factors in maternal history. Cervical smear where indicated, advice on general health, smoking and diet. Discuss screening procedures
11–14 weeks	Dating scan and scan for multiple pregnancies ± nuchal translucency. Confirm booking arrangements. Offer dietary supplements of iron and folic acid if any evidence of anaemia
16 weeks	Alpha-fetoprotein/serum screen for Down's syndrome offered
18 weeks	Check all blood results. Offer routine ultrasound anomaly scan
24 weeks	BP, urinalysis. Fundal height and maternal weight
28 weeks	BP, urinalysis, fetal activity, full blood count and antibody screen. Administer 500 IU anti-D if Rh-negative
32 weeks	BP, urinalysis, fundal height, maternal weight, fetal activity and fetal growth scan where pattern of fetal growth is in doubt
34 weeks	Routine checks, also second dose of anti-D 500 IU for Rh-negative women
36 weeks	BP, urinalysis, fundal height, maternal weight, determine presentation, full blood count and antibody screen where indicated
40 weeks	BP, urinalysis, fundal height presentation, maternal wellbeing
41 weeks	Routine checks, assessment by pelvic examination as to the state of the cervix for induction of labour

Clearly, there will be substantial variation in the nature of the diet depending on racial group and actual physical size but there are general principles that can be laid down as advice to meet the needs of the mother and of the developing fetus.

Routine supplementation with iron and vitamins should not be necessary during pregnancy, but where there is evidence of dietary deficiency, iron and vitamin supplements should be given from the first trimester onwards.

One of the authors worked in the north-west of England in the 1960s. At that time, nutritional anaemias were so common in pregnancy, as a result of both iron deficiency and megaloblastic anaemia due to folic acid deficiency, that it was routine practice to encourage women to take both iron and folate supplements from the first visit. Such a practice is no longer necessary as the general availability of good, cheap food makes the likelihood of nutritional deficiencies as high in women with nutritional fads as in women from deprived socioeconomic circumstances.

Energy intake

A total energy intake of 2000–2500 kcal/day is necessary during the last two trimesters of pregnancy because of the demands of both maternal and fetal metabolism. This requirement may increase to 3000 kcal in the puerperium in lactating women.

Protein

First-class protein is expensive in most countries, with some notable exceptions such as Argentina and Australia, and is therefore likely to be deficient in industrialized nations. However, it is also likely to be deficient in the diet because of particular choice in those who choose to avoid meat and meat products. Animal protein is obtained from meat, poultry, fish, eggs and cheese. Vegetable protein occurs in nuts, lentils, beans and peas. An average of 60–80 g daily is desirable. The source can be either animal or vegetable.

Fats

Although fats are generally regarded with suspicion in the diet, they provide an important component of a balanced diet. Essential fatty acids may play an important part in cellular growth and in preventing the development of hypertension during pregnancy. Fats are also an important source of energy and a source of fat-soluble vitamins, including vitamins A, D and K.

Animal fats are found in meat, eggs and dairy products and contain a high percentage of saturated fats. Vegetable fats, on the other hand, are important because they contain unsaturated fats such as linoleic and linolenic acids.

Carbohydrates

Carbohydrates are the primary source of energy for both mother and fetus and are therefore an essential dietary component during pregnancy. Although excessive carbohydrate consumption can result in excessive weight gain and fat accumulation, a balanced dietary intake of carbohydrate is an essential component of the diet during pregnancy. In particular, it should be remembered that there is a close correlation between maternal and fetal blood glucose levels and that glucose is the major source of energy for the fetus.

Mineral and vitamins

The requirements for iron, calcium, iodine and various trace elements such as magnesium and zinc are all increased in pregnancy. These elements are found in lean meat, various stone fruits, beans and peas, dairy produce and seafood.

Vitamins A and B are found in kidney, liver and dark green vegetables. Vitamin B2 is found in whole grain and cereals, and Vitamin B5 in fish, lean meat, poultry and nuts.

Ascorbic acid is essential for fetal growth and maternal health and is found in citrus fruits, brussel sprouts and broccoli. Vitamin D and folic acid are also important. Vitamin D deficiency in pregnancy is now very rare. However, in those women who cover themselves completely for religious reasons or for protection against skin cancers, there is a risk of vitamin D deficiency. Folic acid deficiency is still relatively common and is associated with the development of megaloblastic anaemia in pregnancy. Green vegetables, nuts and yeast are all rich sources of folic acid and are now readily available in the UK throughout the year in supermarkets so there is no need for these deficiencies to arise, as the cost of green vegetables is not high.

Where deficiencies do arise, this is generally because of dietary choice rather than from economic pressures. This situation can be overcome by giving folic acid supplements. In some urban environs, folate deficiency tends to be part of a pattern of malnutrition and should be anticipated in early pregnancy so that supplements of iron and folic acid can be given.

A general protocol for diet in pregnancy is given in Table 7.3.

Table 7.3
General advice on foodstuffs recommended in pregnancy (quantity per day unless otherwise stated)

Foodstuff		Quantity
Dairy	Milk	600–1000 ml
	Butter	150 g
	Cheese	1 serving
Meat	Chicken, pork or beef	2 servings
	Liver	Once a week or more
	Fish	Once or twice a week
Vegetables	Potato	1–2 servings
	Other	1–2 servings
	Salads	Freely
Fruit	Citrus	1 serving
	Other	2–3
Cereals	Wheat, maize, rice, pasta	4 servings

1 serving = half a cup

Exercise in pregnancy

Pregnant women should be encouraged to undertake reasonable activity during pregnancy. This will be limited with advancing gestation by the physical restrictions imposed by the changes in abdominal size and by the balance restrictions imposed on the mother, but during early pregnancy, there is no need to limit sporting activities beyond the common sense limits of avoiding excessive exertion and fatigue. There may be exceptions to this situation in women with a history of previous pregnancy losses. Swimming is a useful form of exercise, particularly in late pregnancy, when the water tends to support the enlarged maternal abdomen.

Coitus in pregnancy

There are no contraindications to coitus in normal pregnancies at any stage of gestation other than the physical difficulties imposed by changes in abdominal size. It is, however, sensible to avoid coitus where there is evidence of threatened miscarriage or a previous history of recurrent miscarriage. Because of the risk of introducing infection, it is also advisable to avoid coitus where there is evidence of premature rupture of the membranes and also where there is a history of antepartum haemorrhage.

SOCIAL HABITS

Smoking in pregnancy

Smoking has an adverse effect on fetal growth and development and is therefore generally contraindicated in pregnancy. The mechanisms for these effects are as follows (Fig. 7.3).

- **The effect of carbon monoxide on the fetus.** Carbon monoxide has an affinity for haemoglobin 200 times greater than oxygen. Fresh air contains up to 0.5 ppm of carbon monoxide but in cigarette smoke, values as high as 60 000 ppm may be detected. Carbon monoxide shifts the oxygen dissociation curve to the left in both fetal and maternal haemoglobin. Maternal carbon monoxide saturation may rise to 8% in the mother and 7% in the fetus, so that there is specific interference with oxygen transfer.
- **The effect of nicotine on the uteroplacental vasculature as a vasoconstrictor.** Animal studies on

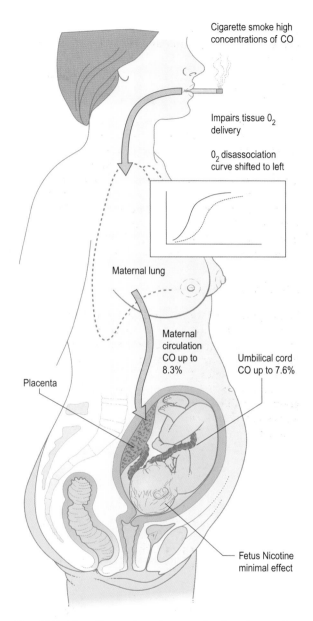

Fig. 7.3 The effects of smoking on the fetoplacental unit.

the effect of infusions of nicotine on cardiac output have shown that high-dose infusions produce a fall in cardiac output and utero-placental blood flow. However, at levels up to five times greater than those seen in smokers there are no measurable effects and it is therefore unlikely that nicotine exerts any adverse effects by reducing uteroplacental blood flow.

- **The effect of smoking on placental structure.** The placenta seems to be spared any significant damage as a result of smoking in pregnancy. However, some changes are seen in the placental morphology. The trophoblastic basement membrane shows irregular thickening and some of the fetal capillaries show reduced calibre. These changes are not consistent or gross and are not associated with any gross reduction in placental size. The morphological changes have not been demonstrated in those women subjected to passive smoking.
- **The effect on perinatal mortality.** Smoking during pregnancy reduces the birthweight of the infant and also reduces the crown–heel length. Perinatal mortality is increased as a direct effect of smoking and this risk has been quantified at 20% for those women who smoke up to 20 cigarettes per day and 35% in excess of one packet per day. Mothers should be advised to stop smoking during pregnancy.

> **!** Paradoxically, there is a considerable volume of evidence to show that women who smoke in pregnancy have a substantially reduced chance of developing pre-eclampsia. However, if they do develop pre-eclampsia, there is a significantly increased risk of perinatal loss.

Alcohol intake in pregnancy

Excessive alcohol intake (in excess of eight standard drinks a day) is associated with a specific syndrome known as the *fetal alcohol syndrome*. Features in the infant include growth retardation, various structural defects and, in particular, facial defects, multiple joint anomalies and cardiac defects. However, these problems arise in women who consume 80 g of alcohol per day and who will almost inevitably have an unsatisfactory dietary intake as well. This is equivalent to an intake of 8 units per day, where 1 unit is equivalent to one glass of wine or half a pint of beer or lager. Although there is some evidence to suggest that even as little as 4 units per day has some effect on fetal growth, there is no evidence to show that a consumption of 20 g a day has any detrimental effect on the fetus or the mother.

In the USA, it is common to see notices in restaurants or bars advising that pregnant women should avoid all alcohol intake and that the proprietors take no responsibility for the outcome should they purchase any alcohol. In reality, the responsibility lies with the woman to adopt a reasonable approach to her alcohol intake. There is no evidence that the occasional social glass of wine or beer has any detrimental effect.

Substance abuse

The common forms of drug abuse that occur during pregnancy are from heroin, cocaine and marijuana. All of these drugs have adverse effects on both the mother and the fetus but many of the adverse effects are related to life style and malnutrition.

Heroin addiction is associated with an increased incidence of intrauterine growth restriction, perinatal deaths and preterm labour. Furthermore, about 50% of infants exposed to heroin will suffer from neonatal withdrawal manifestations. The mother should be screened for HIV, syphilis, Chlamydia and gonorrhoea and should be referred to a drug dependence unit for withdrawal of heroin and replacement with methadone.

Cocaine usage may induce cardiac arrhythmias and central nervous system damage in mothers as well as placental abruptions, fetal growth retardation and preterm labour. Management of cocaine addiction is directed at withdrawing the drug.

Marijuana has no apparent adverse effect on pregnancy although the active ingredient of 9-tetrahydrocannabinol has been shown to have teratogenic effects in animal studies.

BREAST CARE

Breastfeeding should be encouraged in all women unless there are specific contraindications that would have adverse fetal or maternal consequences. Previous damage to the breasts or grossly inverted nipples may make breast feeding difficult or impossible. There are also drugs that are concentrated in breast milk and may be hazardous for the infant, in which case breastfeeding is contraindicated. These drugs are listed in the British National Formulary and the list is updated every 6 months. In some maternal infections, such as HIV, breastfeeding is contraindicated. However, these circumstances are uncommon and, in most circumstances, the mother should be advised of the benefits to her child of breast milk. Not all women find breastfeeding acceptable, even when it is not contraindicated, and it must be remembered that, while breastfeeding is highly

8 Antenatal disorders

HYPERTENSION IN PREGNANCY

Hypertension remains the commonest complication of pregnancy in the UK. The incidence varies substantially in different countries and is influenced by a number of factors such as parity, ethnic group and dietary intake. In the UK, the condition occurs in 10–15% of all pregnancies but only 2–3% of the population will develop both hypertension and proteinuria. While most episodes of hypertension are specifically related to the pregnancy and will resolve when the pregnancy is completed, some women will conceive who suffer from other forms of hypertension such as essential hypertension or renal disease. These diseases may influence the outcome of the pregnancy and the progress of the disease may be influenced by the pregnancy.

In its mildest form, hypertension alone arising in late pregnancy appears to be of minimal risk to mother or child.

In its most severe form, the condition is associated with convulsions, proteinuria, severe hypertension and oedema and may result in cerebral haemorrhage, renal and hepatic failure as well as disseminated intravascular coagulopathy. This may lead to fetal and maternal death.

The association between convulsions and pregnancy was described in ancient Greek and Egyptian writings. The first description of eclampsia, with the occurrence of convulsions, hypertension and proteinuria, was given by Vasquez in 1897.

Classification

Numerous attempts have been made to classify hypertension in pregnancy and this is a subject of ongoing debate. Any classification should be simple and related to factors that can be clearly defined. There are many biochemical and functional changes that are manifest when hypertension arises in pregnancy. Not all of these changes can be measured in those environments where the diseases are most prevalent. On this basis, most classifications are based on the signs of hypertension, proteinuria and oedema. The classification introduced by the American College of Obstetrics and Gynecology in the 1970s remains the basis for most subsequent classifications and is based on the different outcomes associated with different types of hypertension. The definitions included in this classification are as follows.

Hypertension is defined as a systolic pressure of at least 140 mmHg or a diastolic pressure of at least 90 mmHg on two or more occasions after 20 weeks gestation. In the past, diastolic pressure was taken at the fourth Korotkoff sound but, over the last 5 years, this has been changed and the recommendation is now that it should be taken at the fifth sound. This clearly affects earlier observations on prevalence and will lead to occasional difficulty where there is no fifth sound – in these circumstances, it may still be necessary to use the fourth sound. The definition also includes reference to a rise in systolic pressure of at least 30 mmHg or a rise in diastolic pressure of at least 15 mmHg. However, it is unlikely that this addition to the classification does more than complicate the definition as maternal and fetal risks do not increase if the blood pressure remains less than 140/90 mmHg.

Proteinuria is defined as the presence of urinary protein in concentrations greater than 0.3 g/l in a 24 hour collection or in concentrations greater than 1 g/l on a random sample on two or more occasions at least 6 hours apart.

Oedema is defined as the development of pitting oedema or a weight gain in excess of 2.3 kg in a week. Oedema occurs in the limbs, particularly in the feet and ankles and in the fingers, or in the abdominal wall and face (Fig. 8.1). It is not seen as a lumbar pad and can usually be demonstrated in the pretibial area. Because ankle oedema is very common in otherwise uncomplicated pregnancies, this is the least useful component of any classification and has been dropped from many classifications.

The various types of hypertension are classified as follows:

1. Gestational hypertension
2. Pre-eclampsia
3. Eclampsia
4. Superimposed pre-eclampsia/eclampsia on pre-existent forms of hypertension
5. Chronic hypertensive diseases
6. Unclassified hypertensive disease.

Gestational hypertension, sometimes known as *pregnancy-induced hypertension*, is defined as the develop-

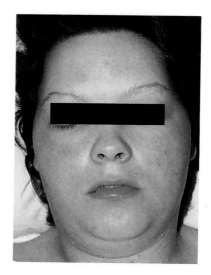

Fig. 8.1 Facial oedema in severe pre-eclampsia.

ment of hypertension alone after 20 weeks of pregnancy or within the first 24 hours postpartum in a previously normotensive woman. The blood pressure usually returns to normal within 10 days after delivery.

Pre-eclampsia is the development of hypertension and proteinuria after the 20th week of gestation. It is predominantly a disorder of primigravidae.

Eclampsia is defined as pre-eclampsia with the development of convulsions. These normally occur antenatally or up to 48 hours after delivery but may occasionally occur up to a week after delivery. However, fits occurring for the first time more than 48 hours after delivery are less likely to be due to eclampsia and a careful search should be made to exclude other causes.

Chronic hypertensive disease is the presence of hypertension that has been present before pregnancy and may be due to various pathological causes.

Superimposed pre-eclampsia or eclampsia is the development of pre-eclampsia in a woman with chronic hypertensive disease or renal disease.

Unclassified hypertension includes those cases of hypertension arising in pregnancy on a random basis where there is insufficient information for classification.

> ! The critical factor that changes the prognosis for the mother and infant is the development of proteinuria. Those women who develop hypertension alone tend to have normal fetal growth with a good prognosis for the infant whereas those that develop proteinuria as well have small placentas and intrauterine growth retardation, with a poor fetal prognosis. From a management point of view, the final diagnosis can only be made after the pregnancy has been completed so the assumption must be made that any woman who develops hypertension must be considered to be at risk.

Pathogenesis and pathology of pre-eclampsia and eclampsia

The exact nature of the pathogenesis of pre-eclampsia remains uncertain. Nearly every major system in the body is affected by the advanced manifestations of the condition and therefore every system that is studied appears to show changes without necessarily doing more than manifesting secondary effects.

However, the pathophysiology of the condition, as outlined in Figure 8.2, is characterized by the effects of:

.• Arteriolar vasoconstriction – particularly in the vascular bed of the uterus and placenta and in the kidney
• Disseminated intravascular coagulation.

Blood pressure is determined by cardiac output, blood volume and peripheral vascular resistance. Both cardiac output and blood volume increase substantially in normal pregnancy but blood pressure actually falls in the mid-trimester. Thus, the most important regulatory factor is the loss of peripheral resistance that occurs in pregnancy. Without this effect, all pregnant women would presumably become hypertensive!

As sympathetic tone appears to remain unchanged, peripheral resistance is determined by the balance between humoral vasodilators and vasoconstrictors. There is a specific loss of sensitivity to angiotensin II, which is associated with locally active vasodilator prostaglandins. Thus, factors that increase the activity of the renin–angiotensin system or reduce the activity of tissue prostaglandins will result in raising of the blood pressure.

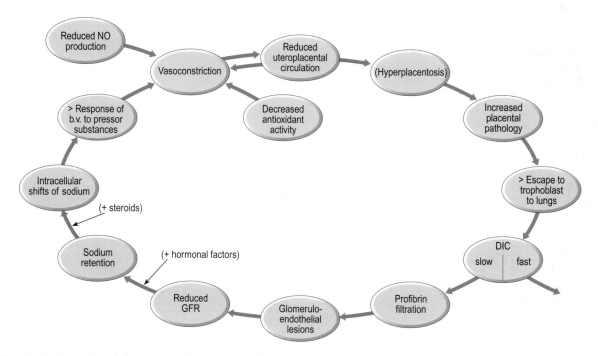

Fig. 8.2 The cycle of changes involved in the pathogenesis of pre-eclampsia. b.v., blood vessels; GFR, glomerular filtration rate; DIC, disseminated intravascular coagulation.

The reduced sensitivity to infused angiotensin II is associated with downregulation of vascular and platelet AII receptors and there is evidence that platelet AII receptors are increased in pre-eclamptic women.

Current evidence also suggests that pre-eclampsia is a disease of endothelial dysfunction. Nitric oxide (NO) or endothelial-derived relaxing factor (EDRF) is a potent vasodilator. In pre-eclampsia, NO synthesis is reduced, possibly by the inhibition of NO synthetase activity.

A further area of consideration is the damaging effect of lipid peroxides on the endothelium. Normally, the production of antioxidants limits these effects but, in pre-eclampsia, antioxidant activity is decreased and endothelial damage occurs.

Once vasoconstriction occurs in the placental bed, it results in placental damage and the release of tropho-blastic material into the peripheral circulation. This trophoblast is rich in thromboplastins, which precipitate disseminated intravascular coagulation. This process gives rise to the pathological lesions in the kidney, liver and placental bed. The renal lesion results in sodium and water retention, with most of this fluid accumulated in the extracellular space. In fact, the intravascular space is reduced in severe pre-eclampsia as plasma volume diminishes. At the same time, increased sodium retention results in increased vascular sensitivity and therefore promotes further vasoconstriction and tissue damage in a vicious circle of events that may ultimately result in cerebral haemorrhage, acute cardiac failure and pulmonary oedema, acute renal failure with tubular or cortical necrosis and hepatic failure with periportal necrosis.

The placenta becomes grossly infarcted and this results in intrauterine growth retardation and sometimes fetal death. There are many factors that may precipitate this sequence of events, including immunological and dietary factors and the existence of underlying chronic renal disease or essential hypertension.

Why do some women develop pre-eclampsia and others do not? Is there a genetic predisposition in some women? The answer to this question is almost certainly yes. Longitudinal studies in the USA, Iceland and Scotland have shown that the daughters of women who have suffered from pre-eclampsia or eclampsia have themselves a 1/4 chance of developing the disease, a risk that is 2.5 times higher than in the daughters-in-law of such women. The data suggests that a single recessive maternal gene is associated with pre-eclampsia. However, the data could also support a hypothetical model of dominant inheritance with partial penetrance.

Although various gene loci have been proposed, there are further long-term studies ongoing to try and identify the correct candidate gene. It is in fact unlikely that there is a single pre-eclampsia gene; it is probable that there are interactions between several genes with external environmental factors enhancing this predisposition.

The renal lesion

The renal lesion is, histologically, the most specific feature of pre-eclampsia (Fig. 8.3). The features are:

- Swelling and proliferation of endothelial cells to such a point that the capillary vessels are obstructed
- Hypertrophy and hyperplasia of the intercapillary or mesangial cells
- Fibrillary material (profibrin) deposition on the basement membrane and between and within the endothelial cells.

The characteristic appearance is therefore one of increased capillary cellularity and reduced vascularity. The lesion is found in 71% of primigravid women who develop pre-eclampsia but in only 29% of multiparous women. There is a much higher incidence of women with chronic renal disease in multiparous women.

The glomerular lesion is always associated with proteinuria and with reduced glomerular filtration. Tubular changes result in impaired uric acid secretion, leading to hyperuricaemia.

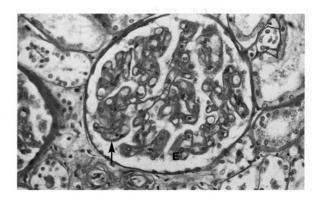

Fig. 8.3 Renal changes in pre-eclampsia include endothelial swelling (E), apparent avascularity of the glomerulus and fibrin deposition (arrow) under the basement membrane.

Placental pathology

Placental infarcts occur in normal pregnancy but are considerably more extensive in pre-eclampsia. The characteristic features in the placenta (Fig. 8.4) include:

- Increased syncytial knots or sprouts
- Increased loss of syncytium
- Proliferation of cytotrophoblast
- Thickening of the trophoblastic basement membrane
- Villous necrosis.

In the uteroplacental bed, the normal invasion of extravillous cytotrophoblast along the luminal surface of the spiral arterioles does not occur beyond the deciduomyometrial junction and there is apparent constriction of the vessels between the radial artery and the decidual portion (Fig. 8.5). These changes result in reduced uteroplacental blood flow.

Disseminated intravascular coagulation (DIC)

In severe pre-eclampsia and eclampsia, thrombosis can be seen in the capillary bed of many organs. Multiple platelet and fibrin thrombi can be identified in the brain. Similar changes are seen in the periportal zones of the liver and in the spleen and the adrenal cortex. In some cases, thrombocytopenia may occur but in only 10% of eclamptic women does the platelet count fall below 100 000/ml. There is an increase in fibrin deposi-

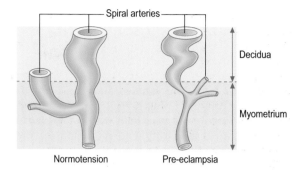

Fig. 8.5 Trophoblast invasion of the spiral arterioles results in dilatation of these vessels. This process is defective in pre-eclampsia.

tion and in circulating fibrin degradation products as a result of increased fibrin production and impaired fibrinolysis. There seems to be little doubt that, while these changes are not the cause of pre-eclampsia, they do play an important role in the pathology of the disease.

Immunological aspects of pregnancy hypertension

It has been postulated that pre-eclampsia may be due to an abnormality of the fetomaternal host response. There is a lower incidence of pre-eclampsia in consanguineous marriages and an increased incidence of hypertension in first pregnancies of second marriages.

Indices of cell-mediated immune response have also been shown to be altered in severe pre-eclampsia. However, there are many other factors that operate independently from any potential immunological factors, such as race, climatic conditions and the genetic or familial factors.

The HELLP syndrome

A severe manifestation of pre-eclampsia occurs in a variant known as the HELLP syndrome. In this syndrome, there is a triad of manifestations that include haemolysis (H), raised liver enzymes (EL) and a low platelet count (LP). The thrombocytopenia is often severe and may result in haemorrhage into the brain and the liver. The syndrome demands intervention and termination of the pregnancy as soon as the acute manifestations are controlled.

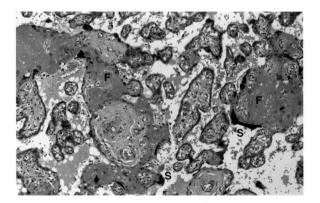

Fig. 8.4 Placental changes in pre-eclampsia include an increase in syncytial knots, proliferation of cytotrophoblast and thickening of trophoblastic basement membrane.

Management of gestational hypertension and pre-eclampsia

The object of management is to prevent the development of eclampsia and to minimize the risks of the condition to both the mother and the fetus. The achievement of these objectives depends on careful scrutiny of the condition of both the mother and the fetus and timely intervention to terminate the pregnancy when the risks of continuation outweigh the risks of intervention.

Bed rest

A rise in blood pressure is usually the first sign to be noted at the antenatal visit. Blood pressure should be recorded in a constant position at each visit, as it is posture-dependent. The most comfortable position is seated, with a cuff of an appropriate size applied to the right upper arm. If the pressure is elevated, the measurement should be repeated after a short period of rest. If the blood pressure remains elevated, then continuing close observation is essential. This may be achieved by hospital admission or by careful scrutiny at home by a visiting midwife or doctor. The woman should be advised to rest. This may not be possible at home if she has other children or a family dependent on her efforts; under these circumstances, hospital admission is preferable. On the other hand, some women develop 'white coat' hypertension and therefore may be better managed at home. However, there is evidence from home monitoring projects that women who are prone to white coat hypertension also become hypertensive in response to other forms of stress and may be better managed away from home.

Bed rest improves renal blood flow and uteroplacental flow and commonly results in a diuresis and improvement in the blood pressure.

The development of proteinuria is an absolute indication for hospital admission as this change constitutes the dividing line between minimal risk and significant risk to both mother and baby.

If the hypertension persists or worsens, treatment with antihypertensive drugs should be considered.

Diuretics and sedation

Although there is fluid retention associated with pre-eclampsia, the retention of fluid is extracellular and blood volume actually falls. In general, diuretics will make this situation worse. There are occasions when diuretics have a role to play:

- The symptomatic relief of oedema
- In some cases of essential hypertension treated with diuretics before the pregnancy
- In the immediate postpartum period where there is oliguria, the use of osmotic diuretics such as mannitol may promote the return of urinary flow.

Sedation has little part to play in the management of pre-eclampsia although, in the more severe forms, drugs such as diazepam have been used to reduce cerebral excitability and to minimize the risk of convulsions. A dose of 10–20 mg given 6-hourly should achieve this objective. However, this drug has the disadvantage that, on a long term basis, diazepam and its metabolite, desmethyl diazepam, are transferred across the placenta and may cause hypothermia and hypotonia in the fetus – a condition known as the *floppy baby syndrome*. Diazepam has now been largely replaced by magnesium sulphate but it may on occasions still be used to prevent or control convulsions.

Antihypertensive drug therapy

In the presence of an acute hypertensive crisis, controlling the blood pressure is essential but, in the case of mild gestational hypertension and moderate pre-eclampsia, their role is more contentious. There is convincing evidence that the treatment of mild or moderate chronic hypertension in pregnancy reduces the risk of developing severe hypertension and the need for hospital admission.

In women with gestational hypertension, treatment with antihypertensive drugs should be confined to those women who fail to respond to conservative management with bed rest, where the gestational age is less than 34 weeks and where there is a clear advantage from the point of view of fetal welfare to prolong the pregnancy. There is some evidence that early treatment reduces the risk of progression to proteinuric hypertension. Management is based on the principle of minimizing both maternal and fetal morbidity and mortality. Where the blood pressure stays above 160/100, antihypertensive treatment is essential as there is a risk of maternal cerebral haemorrhage.

The drugs most commonly used are:

- Methyldopa
- Hydralazine

- Beta-blockers such as atenolol, oxyprenolol, metoprolol
- Combined alpha- and beta-blockers such as labetalol
- Calcium channel blockers such as nifedipine
- Selective serotonin receptor blockers such as ketanserin.

Where acute control is required, an intravenous bolus of hydralazine 5 mg or labetalol 20 mg should be administered

Maternal investigations

The most important investigations for monitoring the mother are, first, the 4-hourly measurement of blood pressure until such time that the blood pressure has returned to normal. Second, routine urine checks for proteinuria. Initially, screening is done with dipsticks but, once proteinuria is established, 24-hour urine samples should be collected. Values in excess of 0.3 g/l over 24 hours are abnormal. Third, excessive maternal weight gain should be noted, although it is a poor predictor of maternal outcome. Weight loss or failure to gain weight may indicate placental failure and fetal growth retardation.

Laboratory investigations

- Full blood count with particular reference to platelet count
- Tests for renal function and liver function
- Uric acid measurements – a useful indicator of progression in the disease
- Clotting studies where there is severe pre-eclampsia
- Catecholamine measurements in the presence of severe hypertension, particularly where there is no proteinuria.

Fetoplacental investigations

Pre-eclampsia is an important cause of fetal growth retardation and prenatal death and it is therefore essential to monitor fetal wellbeing using the following methods:

- **Biophysical profile:** Ultrasound assessment of fetal wellbeing has replaced all previous methods of assessment with the exception of fetal cardiotocography. A biophysical profile involves ultrasound assessment of fetal breathing movements, gross body movements, fetal tone, reactive fetal heart

Case study

Mrs F was pregnant with her first child after a long history of subfertility. She had been admitted to hospital before her pregnancy for tubal evaluation by dye laparoscopy but at no time then or subsequently during her pregnancy had she shown any evidence of hypertension. At 32 weeks gestation, she was admitted to hospital at 10 pm with acute headache and severe hypertension, with a blood pressure reading of 220/140. There was no proteinuria and no hyper-reflexia. There was no evidence of fetal growth retardation. Despite initial attempts to control her blood pressure with hydralazine and labetalol, her hypertension remained severe and uncontrollable and she went into high-output cardiac failure and died at 7 o'clock the following morning. Autopsy revealed a large phaeochromocytoma in the right adrenal gland.

This is an extremely rare form of hypertension in pregnancy. It has an appalling prognosis unless it is detected early. In this case it presented late. All other antenatal recordings of blood pressure had been normal. Although it would not have helped in this case, where hypertension is severe and presents antenatally it is always worth checking urinary catecholamines.

rate and quantitative amniotic fluid volume measurement.
- **Serial ultrasound measurements of growth:** Assessment of fetal biparietal diameter, head circumference and abdominal girth performed on a bi-weekly basis.
- **Doppler flow studies:** The use of serial measurements of umbilical Doppler analysis may give an estimate of umbilical blood flow but, more importantly, makes it possible to assess vascular resistance and hence an assessment of impairment of uteroplacental function. An increase in the ratio of flow in systole to that in diastole and the absent flow in diastole or, on occasions, reversal of flow indicate increasing vascular resistance and increasing fetal compromise.
- **Antenatal cardiotocography:** Used in conjunction with Doppler assessment, the measurement of fetal

heart rate in relation to uterine activity provides a useful, but by no means infallible indication of fetal wellbeing. The presence of episodes of fetal bradycardia and the loss of baseline variability may indicate fetal hypoxia.

A summary of the various management strategies is shown in Figure 8.6. This flow diagram shows the various pathways of progression and their management. Mild hypertension may get better with conservative management or it may progress rapidly to the severe forms of pre-eclampsia and ultimately eclampsia.

Prevention of pre-eclampsia

There is no doubt that careful management and anticipation can largely prevent the occurrence of eclampsia, but preventing pre-eclampsia is much more difficult.

The use of a variety of dietary supplements such as calcium or essential fatty acids has been tried without notable success. Low dose aspirin acts as an inhibitor of cyclooxygenase activity and of platelet aggregation. It also inhibits thromboxane synthesis. On this basis, several large trials have been undertaken on the use of low-dose aspirin for the prevention of pre-eclampsia, but generally the trials have been disappointing. However, there is a case for the use of low-dose aspirin – 60 mg daily taken after the 16th week of pregnancy and

continued to term – is indicated where there is a history of severe early-onset disease. In these women, a thrombophilia screen should be undertaken, as there is an incidence of underlying thrombotic tendencies that may also benefit from anticoagulant therapy.

Symptoms of pre-eclampsia and eclampsia

Pre-eclampsia is commonly an asymptomatic condition. However, there are symptoms that must not be overlooked and these include frontal headache, blurring of vision and epigastric pain. Of these symptoms, the most important is the development of abdominal pain – either during pregnancy or in the immediate puerperium (Fig. 8.7).

> **!** The occurrence of epigastric pain is commonly misdiagnosed or overlooked as a feature of severe pre-eclampsia and impending eclampsia. Presenting often in the late second trimester, an erroneous diagnosis of indigestion or heartburn is made and, unless the blood pressure is recorded and the urine checked for protein, the significance of the pain is overlooked until the woman presents with fitting.

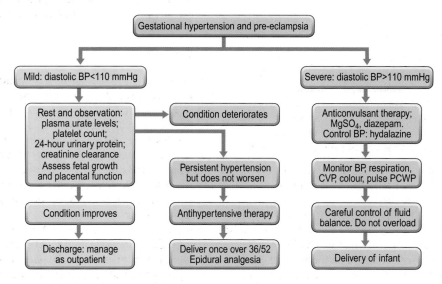

Fig. 8.6 Flow diagram of the management of gestational hypertension and pre-eclampsia. BP, blood pressure; CVP, central venous pressure; PCWP, pulmonary capillary wedge pressure.

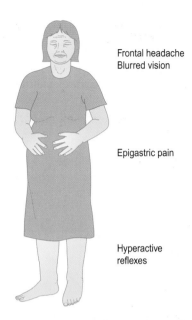

Frontal headache
Blurred vision

Epigastric pain

Hyperactive
reflexes

Fig. 8.7 Presenting signs of impending eclampsia.

Induction of labour

The decision as to when a pregnancy should be terminated is determined by:

- The maturity of the fetus
- The severity of the pre-eclampsia and in particular the development of persistent proteinuria – eclampsia is an absolute indication for delivery
- The presence of additional complications such as placental abruption where the risk to the fetus becomes greater than the risk of premature delivery.

If the decision has been made to proceed to delivery, the choice will rest with either the induction of labour or delivery by caesarian section.

If the cervix is unripe and unsuitable for surgical induction, it can often be ripened by the introduction of prostaglandin E_2 into the posterior fornix. This comes in the form of a gel or tablet. If the Bishop score is less than 5, an initial dose of 2 mg is inserted and this can be repeated on one further occasion after 6 hours. This dose should be reduced in multiparous women to 1 mg.

If the cervix is ripe, labour is induced by:

- Artificial rupture of the membranes by forewater rupture
- Oxytocin infusion – if labour does not commence within an hour after rupturing the membranes, then an infusion of oxytocin should be started. Infusions should start at 1–4 mU/min and then incrementally increasing the dose to 32 mU/min. The infusions are increased every half hour depending on the response.

The fetal heart rate should always be monitored, as well as the level of uterine activity. If excessively strong or frequent contractions occur or there is evidence of fetal distress, the infusion should be discontinued.

Complications

- There is an increased incidence of placental abruption in pregnancies complicated by hypertension
- Severe pre-eclampsia is associated with reduced glomerular filtration resulting in oliguria or anuria; liver function may be impaired and intrahepatic haemorrhage may occur leading to liver failure
- Disseminated intravascular coagulation with all its consequences
- Maternal complications such as cerebral infarction, heart failure and adult respiratory distress syndrome.

Eclampsia

The onset of convulsions in a pregnancy complicated by pre-eclampsia denotes the onset of eclampsia. Eclampsia most commonly occurs in primigravidae but may occur in women of higher parity with previously normal histories. Eclampsia is a preventable condition and its occurrence often denotes a failure to recognize the early worsening signs of pre-eclampsia. It carries serious risks of intrauterine death for the fetus and of maternal death from cerebral haemorrhage and renal and hepatic failure.

All cases must be managed in hospital and preferably in hospitals with appropriate intensive care facilities. Any woman admitted to hospital with convulsions during the course of pregnancy, or who is admitted in a coma associated with hypertension, should be considered to be suffering from eclampsia until proved otherwise.

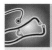

Case study

Not all women admitted with fitting in pregnancy are eclamptic. Marilyn D was a single mother who was brought into an accident and emergency department by two friends with a statement that she had fitted on two occasions. She was booked for confinement at the same hospital and her antenatal records showed that her pregnancy had so far been uncomplicated. She was 34 weeks pregnant and on admission her blood pressure was 140/90. There was a trace of protein in the urine. She was brought into hospital on a Saturday night and her friends stated that they had stopped the car on the way in to hospital and laid Marilyn down on the pavement by the roadside because of the violence of her fits.

After careful assessment and biochemical tests, it was decided to proceed with observation and, within 24 hours, there were no further fits. Further discussion with Marilyn revealed that she had been at a party and subsequent tests revealed that she had taken amphetamines – a diagnosis that was suggested by one of the medical students!

Management of eclampsia

The three basic guidelines for management of eclampsia are:
- Control the fits
- Control the blood pressure
- Deliver the infant.

Control of fits

Various drugs are used to control the fits but the most widely used regimes are as follows.

- Intravenous administration of diazepam 10 mg as a bolus if the women is still fitting after the initial fit. A further 10 mg can be given if this does not control the fit and if the level of consciousness and respiration is not depressed.

- Magnesium sulphate is the drug of choice for the control of fits thereafter. The drug is effective in suppressing convulsions and inhibiting muscular activity. It also reduces platelet aggregation and minimizes the effects of disseminated intravascular coagulation. Treatment is started with a bolus dose of 4 g given over 20 minutes as 20 ml of a 20% solution. Thereafter blood levels of magnesium are maintained by giving a maintenance dose of 1 g/h administered as a solution made up in normal saline with 5 g/500 ml and run at 100 ml/hour. The blood level of magnesium should be measured and monitored. The therapeutic range is 2–4 mmol/l. A level of more than 5 mmol/l causes loss of patellar reflexes and a value of more than 6 mmol/l causes respiratory depression. Magnesium sulphate can be given by intramuscular injection but the injection is often painful and sometimes leads to abscess formation. The preferred route is by intravenous administration.

> ✓ It is not always possible to monitor the blood levels of magnesium. It is, however, important to avoid toxic levels of magnesium, as they may result in complete respiratory arrest. Eclampsia is associated with hyper-reflexia and, on occasions, with clonus, so a guide to the levels of magnesium can be obtained by regular checks on the patellar reflexes. In the event of the suppression of respiration, the effects can be reversed by the administration of 1 g of calcium gluconate given intravenously over 2–3 minutes.

It is important to ensure that a clear airway is maintained and that further fits are prevented. To this end, the patient should be managed as in an intensive care unit and where possible, managed jointly with intensive care staff. Constant nursing attendance is essential by staff accustomed to managing patients with airway problems.

Fluid balance must be strictly observed and urinary output is measured and recorded by the use of an indwelling catheter. As a general principle, total fluid input should be restricted to 100 ml/h. If the urine flow falls to below 30 ml/h, a central venous pressure line should be inserted or, if available under appropriate conditions, a Swan–Ganz catheter to measure pulmonary capillary wedge pressures. If the capillary wedge pressure is low, extra colloid infusion should be given. Fluid overload in these women may induce pulmonary oedema and adult respiratory distress syndrome with lethal consequences.

Control of blood pressure

It is essential to control the blood pressure to minimize the risk of maternal cerebral haemorrhage. The drug of choice is hydralazine given intravenously as 5–10 mg over an interval of 5 minutes and repeated after 15 minutes if the blood pressure is not controlled. It is important not to drop the blood pressure precipitously and one should aim to lower it to 140/90.

An alternative is to use intravenous labetalol, starting with a bolus of 20 mg followed by further doses of 40 mg and 80 mg to a total of 200 mg.

Subsequent blood pressure control can be maintained with a continuous infusion of hydralazine at 5–40 mg/h or labetalol 20–160 mg/h depending on the amount required to control the blood pressure.

Epidural analgesia relieves the pain of labour and also helps to lower the blood pressure by causing vasodilatation in the lower extremities. It also reduces the tendency to fit by relieving pain in labour. However, it is essential to perform clotting studies before inserting an epidural catheter because of the risk of causing bleeding into the epidural space if there is defective clotting.

Delivery of the infant

Once convulsions have occurred or severe and sustained hypertension and proteinuria are established, then the risk to both the mother and the infant of continuing the pregnancy will exceed the risk of delivery. Clearly the risks of prematurity to the infant are high if the gestational age is less than 28 weeks but, if the gestational age is greater than 34 weeks, then there is certainly no point in continuing with the pregnancy and delivery is advisable. It is essential to establish reasonable control of the blood pressure before embarking on any procedures to expedite delivery as the intervention itself may precipitate a hypertensive crisis.

If the cervix is sufficiently dilated to enable artificial rupture of the membranes, labour should be induced by forewater rupture and an oxytocin infusion. If this is not possible, then it is best to proceed to delivery by caesarean section.

Management after delivery

The risks of eclampsia do not stop with delivery and the management of pre-eclampsia and eclampsia continues for up to 7 days after delivery although, after 48 hours, if fitting occurs for the first time, alternative diagnoses such as epilepsy or cortical vein thrombosis must be considered. Up to 45% of eclamptic fits occur after delivery, including 12% after 48 hours.

The following points of management should be observed.

- Maintain the patient in a quiet environment under constant observation.
- Maintain appropriate levels of sedation. If she has been treated with magnesium sulphate, continue the infusion for 24 hours after the last fit.
- Continue antihypertensive therapy until the blood pressure has returned to normal. This will usually involve transferring to oral medication and, although there is usually significant improvement after the first week, hypertension may persist for the next 6 weeks.

Case study

Mrs T was a 28-year-old primigravida and the wife of one of the junior medical staff. Her pregnancy was uneventful until 37 weeks, when she developed hypertension and was admitted to hospital for bed rest. Her blood pressure stayed around 140/90 and there was a trace of protein in the urine. At 38 weeks gestation, labour was induced and she had a normal delivery of a healthy male infant. The following day she was fully mobile but complained to the midwifery staff that she had a frontal headache and indigestion, with epigastric discomfort. She was given aspirin and an antacid but the symptoms persisted. Her hypertension also persisted and later that day she fitted. Unfortunately, she fell against the side of her bed and fractured her zygoma. Although she had not fitted before delivery, it is important to remember that such symptoms in a pre-eclamptic woman are as significant after delivery as they are antenatally.

- Strict fluid balance charts should be kept and blood pressure and urine output observed on an hourly basis. Biochemical and haematological indices should be made on a daily basis until the values have returned to normal.

Although most mothers who have suffered from pre-eclampsia or eclampsia will completely recover and return to normal, it is important to review all such women at 6 weeks after delivery. If the hypertension or proteinuria persist at this stage, then they should be investigated for other factors such as underlying renal disease.

ANAEMIA IN PREGNANCY

Anaemia is a common complication of pregnancy and in some countries may be a major factor in the cause of maternal death. Where parasitic diseases are rife, extremely low levels of haemoglobin concentration, with values as low as 3–4 g/dl, may result in maternal death with relatively small losses of blood from antepartum or postpartum haemorrhage.

The fetus tends to withstand maternal anaemia surprisingly well despite the reduced oxygen-carrying capacity of the mother but becomes more vulnerable if there are further maternal complications such as placental abruption or pre-eclampsia.

Definition

There is no agreed definition of anaemia that is appropriate to all communities but, in the UK, a haemoglobin level of less than 11 g/dl is generally accepted as indicating significant anaemia. Normal levels in pregnancy in the UK have been shown to be 12 g/dl in the first trimester, 11.9 g/dl in the second trimester and 11.4 g/dl in the third trimester. The fall in the second trimester is a reflection of the relatively faster expansion of plasma volume than the total red cell mass, but this does not account for significant degrees of anaemia.

Nutritional requirements

Anaemia in pregnancy may arise from any of the recognized causes of anaemia but the most important causes are those related to an imbalance between the needs of the mother and the growing fetus and the actual supply and absorption of essential nutrients (Fig. 8.8).

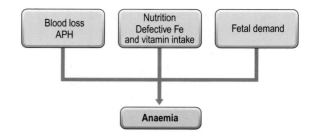

Fig. 8.8 Basic factors in the aetiology of anaemia in pregnancy.

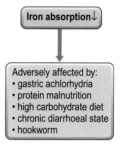

Fig. 8.9 Factors that influence iron absorption.

Essential nutrients for haemoglobin synthesis include protein, iron, vitamin B_6 and vitamin B_{12}, folic acid, ascorbic acid and numerous trace elements such as copper. The dietary requirement of iron is estimated at 15 mg per day so that a good iron content in the diet is essential. Iron absorption tends to increase in pregnancy and iron is absorbed in the ferrous ionized form. Ascorbic acid assists the process of absorption because it acts as a reducing agent. However, iron absorption may be adversely affected by a number of factors (Fig. 8.9) such as gastric achlorhydria, protein malnutrition, and high carbohydrate diets, chronic diarrhoeal states and hookworm infestations. Iron loss from the body is generally minimal during pregnancy as menstrual loss ceases although some natural loss still occurs from hair, nails and sweat. The major reduction in maternal stores is due to the demands of the fetus and of the mother.

Investigations

Routine antenatal care should include the measurement of haemoglobin levels at regular intervals throughout the pregnancy. If the haemoglobin falls to less than 11 g/dl, the following investigations should be performed:

- Complete blood picture: as by far the commonest cause of anaemia in pregnancy is iron deficiency, the most important measurements are mean corpuscular volume (MCV) and mean corpuscular haemoglobin concentration (MCHC) – MCV gives an index of macrocytosis and megaloblastic anaemia and MCHC gives the best index for iron deficiency anaemia
- Serum iron and iron-binding capacity
- Serum folate and serum vitamin B_{12} levels in all cases of persistent anaemia or where there is evidence of macrocytosis
- Other investigations, including urinary culture to exclude urinary tract infection and the examination of the faeces for ova and parasites
- Bone marrow analysis where the diagnosis is in doubt
- Haemoglobin electrophoresis to exclude haemoglobinopathies.

Management

The management of anaemia in pregnancy depends on the diagnosis of the cause. However, the majority of cases are due to nutritional deficiencies and in particular, deficient iron intake to meet the needs of both the mother and the fetus.

The use of prophylactic oral iron and folic acid supplements is generally reserved for those mothers who have poor diets; this may include women from good socioeconomic backgrounds with dietary fads. Iron should be administered in the form of ferrous sulphate, gluconate, succinate or fumarate. For prophylactic purposes, combined preparations containing 150 mg of ferrous sulphate and 0.5 mg of folic acid on a once-daily basis should be sufficient to meet the demands of the mother. However, in the presence of anaemia, up to 200 mg 8-hourly with a folic acid supplement of 5 mg daily should be given orally and this should result in an increase of 1 g/dl over a 7–10-day period. Some women tolerate oral iron therapy poorly and develop gastric irritation and constipation. Constipation is the commonest complaint and can often be resolved by dietary fibre supplementation. However, if toleration is poor and the haemoglobin level does not rise, either because of non-compliance or defective absorption, then parenteral therapy may be necessary.

Parenteral therapy

Parenteral therapy is indicated when iron deficiency anaemia fails to respond to oral therapy. Iron preparations include saccharated iron oxide or, commonly, iron–dextran complexes or an iron– sorbitol–citric acid complex such as Jectofer. All of these compounds may cause severe anaphylactic reactions and a test dose must be given before the full therapeutic dose is administered. The drugs may be administered intravenously in the form of a total dose infusion or, on occasions, by intramuscular injections.

SICKLE CELL SYNDROME

These disorders include the heterozygous state for sickle cell haemoglobin (sickle cell trait; HbAS), homozygous sickle cell disease (HbSS), compound heterozygotes for haemoglobin variants, such as sickle cell HbC disease, and sickle cell thalassaemia.

- **HbSS:** The clinical manifestations of HbSS include chronic anaemia and occasional crises characterized by intravascular sickling leading to vascular occlusions and tissue infarction. Crises are often precipitated by infection and dehydration. Renal complications are common.
- **Sickle cell HbC disease:** This is a milder variant with near-normal haemoglobin levels. However, it may, on occasions, produce massive sickling crises during pregnancy.
- **HbAS.** This trait rarely causes problems unless there are conditions of extreme anorexia, dehydration and acidosis.

In pregnancy, there are special problems and these should be anticipated. All potentially high-risk ethnic groups such as black people of African origin, Indians, Mediterraneans and Saudi Arabs should be offered screening.

The rates of miscarriage, preterm labour and fetal loss are high. These risks can be reduced by regular blood transfusions to maintain a high proportion of HbA in the circulation. During labour, adequate hydration at all times and the prevention of infection by the use of prophylactic antibiotics with the use of blood transfusion to maintain haemoglobin levels throughout pregnancy all play an important role in reducing the occurrence of crises during pregnancy.

THE THALASSAEMIAS

These conditions are genetic disorders associated with a reduced rate of production of one or more of the globulin chains of haemoglobin. They fall into two broad disorders of alpha- and beta-thalassaemia.

The **beta-thalassaemias** are defined by an inability to synthesize adult beta chains. In the heterozygous state they are symptomless but in the homozygous state there is severe and persistent anaemia. These conditions are particularly common in the Mediterranean countries and in India and south-east Asia. The major problems in pregnancy are those related to anaemia and the need for repeated transfusions.

The **alpha-thalassaemias** are characterized by an inability to produce alpha-chains common to haemoglobin A. During pregnancy, these women may become very anaemic. Sometimes the fetus may also become anaemic and hydropic and give rise to severe pre-eclampsia.

If routine screening of the parents indicates a risk of carrying a child with alpha-thalassaemia, the parents should be referred for prenatal diagnosis. Indeed, this is becoming an increasingly important aspect of management of the homozygous forms of either alpha- or beta-thalassaemia.

DIABETES IN PREGNANCY

Diabetes affects 0.2–0.3% of pregnancies and a further 1–2% of pregnant women have evidence of impaired glucose tolerance.

Pregnancy affects maternal diabetes and produces an increase in insulin requirements. At the same time, diabetes has a significant effect on the pregnancy and on plasma levels of insulin and glucose (Fig. 8.10).

With appropriate management and careful regulation of blood glucose levels, perinatal losses can be minimized and will approach levels in the normal population. This management is best undertaken by a combined team of physicians and obstetricians with a special interest in diabetes in pregnancy. Delivery should always be effected in a major obstetric hospital that has first class neonatal services.

Nomenclature

All forms of diabetes are associated with increased perinatal loss unless properly managed. The degree of risk is directly related to the severity of the diabetes.

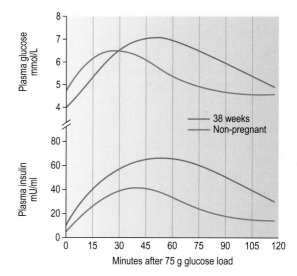

Fig. 8.10 Changes in blood insulin and glucose levels in normal pregnancy.

The presentation has been defined by the British Diabetic Association as follows:

1. **Potential diabetes:** Patients with no evidence of chemical diabetes but who have a family history of diabetes, a previous history of delivering an infant with a birth weight in excess of 4.5 kg or a history of an unexplained fetal death. Glycosuria is not a reliable sign in pregnancy but should be investigated if it is persistent.
2. **Latent or gestational diabetes:** Some women who develop overt diabetes in later life develop chemical or clinical diabetes during pregnancy. This condition is known as gestational diabetes.
3. **Chemical diabetes:** These women have abnormal glucose tolerance but no other manifestations of diabetes. However, the risk of perinatal morbidity and mortality is significantly increased.
4. **Clinical diabetes:** Insulin-dependent diabetes requires careful control throughout pregnancy. Ideally, good control should be established before conception to minimize the risk of miscarriage and congenital abnormalities.

The American classification introduced by White in 1965 also linked management and prognosis to the classification of diabetes and is shown in Table 8.1.

As discussed in Chapter 7, women with potential diabetes should have a glucose tolerance test unless the fasting blood glucose is less than 4.5 mmol/l.

Table 8.1
White classification of diabetes

Class A: Chemical diabetes only; impaired glucose tolerance.
Class B: Diabetes of adult; onset after 20 years of age.
Class C: Diabetes of long duration (between 10 and 19 years) with no evidence of vascular disease.
Class D: Diabetes present since before the age of 10 years and present for 20 years or more with vascular disease, calcification of leg vessels or benign retinopathy.
Class E: Diabetes associated with calcification of limb vessels.
Class F: Diabetic nephropathy.
Class G: The presence of proliferating diabetic retinopathy.

> ❗ Remember that glucose crosses the placenta readily and that maternal hyperglycaemia results in elevated blood glucose levels in the fetus. Insulin, on the other hand does not pass across the placenta and therefore the fetus is entirely dependent on the supply of its own insulin production for the regulation of its blood sugar levels.

An abnormal test using a 75 g loading dose of glucose is defined by the following criteria:

- **Normal test:** a fasting blood glucose level of less than 6 mmol/l and a 2-hour value of less than 7.8 mmol/l
- **Gestational impaired glucose tolerance:** a fasting level between 6 and 7 mmol/l and a 2-hour value of 7.8–11.1 mmol/l
- **Diabetes:** a fasting value of more than 7 mmol/l and a 2-hour value of more than 11.1 mmol/l.

Maternal complications

- **Pregnancy is diabetogenic** and necessitates careful regulation of insulin dosage in order to maintain strict control of blood glucose levels. Poor control leads to the development of hyperglycaemia and on occasions to ketoacidosis and diabetic coma, with the real risk of both maternal and fetal death. Hypoglycaemia is much less common and may result in fetal death only if it is severe and prolonged. It occurs more commonly in early pregnancy, particularly where the pregnancy is complicated by hyperemesis.

- **Hydramnios** is a common complication of the diabetic pregnancy and may result in an unstable lie and premature rupture of the membranes.
- **Pre-eclampsia** is common in the diabetic mother and is worse where control of the diabetes is poor. Where there is diabetic nephropathy, the prognosis for both mother and fetus is poor and these women should think carefully before embarking on a pregnancy.
- **Dystocia** and in particular, **shoulder dystocia** are common features of labour and delivery, as a result of the fact that the fetus may be abnormally large and labour may become obstructed. If there is evidence of potential cephalopelvic disproportion or definite evidence of fetal macrosomia, delivery by caesarean section may be the safest option. On the other hand, good diabetic control throughout pregnancy should optimize the chance of having a normal vaginal delivery.

Fetal complications

Babies born to diabetic mothers tend to be larger than normal; this is due to macrosomia and increased fat deposition (Fig. 8.11). Intrauterine death rates are increased but can be kept to near non-diabetic levels if the diabetic control is good. Diabetic infants are particularly prone to fetal acidosis in labour and therefore should be monitored electronically.

Neonatal complications

- **Hypoglycaemia** is common in the neonate – particularly in the first 48 hours after delivery. There is hyperplasia and hypertrophy of the islets of Langerhans as a consequence of stimulation from maternal blood glucose levels during pregnancy. When this supply of glucose is removed at delivery, the infant is particularly prone to develop

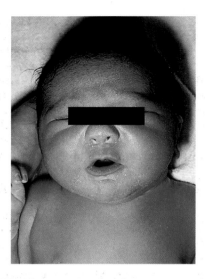

Fig. 8.11 Macrosomic infant born to an insulin-dependent diabetic mother.

hypoglycaemia and it is therefore important to monitor blood glucose levels until feeding is well established.

- **Respiratory distress syndrome** is more common in the 'diabetic' infant when compared with infants of comparable gestational age born to non-diabetic mothers. These infants are also more prone to jaundice, hypocalcaemia and hypomagnesaemia.
- **Congenital abnormalities** occur more frequently in infants born to diabetic mothers, being found in 7% of cases.

Management of diabetes

All grades of diabetes carry a significant risk to the fetus, although the level of risk increases with the severity of the disease. Gestational diabetes is generally managed by dietary control and the diet is designed to limit periods of hyper- or hypoglycaemia. The diet should contain 50% carbohydrate, 20–30% protein and 20–30% fat. The caloric intake should be about 25–30 kcal/kg per day depending on the body weight of the mother. In general, the aim should be keep the blood glucose levels below 7 mmol/l at all times, either by diet alone or by diet and insulin.

Hospital admission is not essential unless there is an additional complication such as pre-eclampsia. Control of blood glucose levels should be implemented by self-measurement of blood glucose with profiles performed every 2 weeks during the first two trimesters and weekly during the third trimester.

All women taking oral hypoglycaemic agents should be changed to short-acting insulin treatment. The usual approach is to give a small dose of a medium- or long-acting insulin in the evenings and to supplement this with small doses of short-acting insulin before each meal. Insulin requirements increase in the later stages of pregnancy and fall rapidly to prepregnancy levels after delivery.

The measurement of glycosylated haemoglobin levels (HbA_1) is a useful method of monitoring compliance and control; HbA_1 should normally constitute less than 7% of the total haemoglobin concentration.

Women with insulin-dependent diabetes should have their control optimized prior to conception and be counselled about the maternal and fetal complications of diabetes in pregnancy. Pregnancy should be deferred if the HbA_1 levels exceed 12% or if there is evidence of ischaemic heart disease, untreated proliferative retinopathy, hypertension or proteinuria.

Antenatal assessment

Antenatal progress should be carefully monitored throughout pregnancy. The patient should be seen regularly at fortnightly or weekly intervals and home visits by a diabetic clinic sister to check for any problems with monitoring blood glucose profiles form an important part of management. Regular ophthalmological examinations are performed to assess retinal vascular changes and serial test of renal function should also be performed.

Fetal growth and development should be monitored by serial ultrasound scans, biophysical profiles and umbilical artery Doppler recordings.

Method of delivery

If good diabetic control is achieved and there are no other complications, it should be possible to allow the pregnancy to proceed to full term, although delivery is usually effected between 38 weeks and term. Induction of labour and vaginal delivery can be achieved with the careful regulation of blood glucose levels during labour and continuous fetal monitoring. If there is any evidence of fetal distress or delay in the progress of labour, delivery should be effected by caesarean section.

THYROID DISEASE IN PREGNANCY

Thyroid disorders of various types complicate approximately 1 in 500 pregnancies. Normal pregnancy carries some of the features of hyperthyroidism, with slight enlargement of the thyroid gland and increased levels of activity. However, this is a normal physiological event and must not be confused with abnormal thyroid states.

Hypothyroidism

Hypothyroidism is the commonest thyroid problem to occur in pregnancy and complicates between 6 and 9/1000 pregnancies.

Most cases have a basis in **autoimmune diseases** such as Hashimoto's disease. As these diseases commonly cause infertility where the disease is untreated, they will usually present with an established diagnosis and the woman will already be on therapy. Hypothyroidism may also be **iatrogenic** as the consequence of thyroidectomy, radio-iodine ablation or excessive doses of antithyroid drugs.

In developing countries where **iodine deficiency** is endemic, it is associated with 30% fetal wastage from miscarriage, stillbirth, neonatal death and congenital abnormalities. Where the mother is receiving adequate replacement therapy, the outcome for the infant is normal.

The diagnosis of hypothyroidism in the mother is made by the presence of low free thyroxine and a raised level of thyroid-stimulating hormone (TSH). Treatment is by thyroid replacement therapy.

Hyperthyroidism

Hyperthyroidism occurs in between 1 in 500 and 1 in 2000 pregnancies and is much less common than hypothyroidism. The commonest cause is Graves' disease; this is associated with an increased risk of fetal malformation, low birthweight and premature labour. If the disease is not well controlled in the mother, it may result in a thyroid crisis, which has a mortality rate of up to 25%. The condition is diagnosed by the presence of high tri-iodothyronine and low TSH or a flat response to thyrotrophin-releasing hormone. Thyroid stimulating or blocking immunoglobulins may cross the placenta and cause fetal thyroid disease.

Treatment is with drug therapy, although it may on occasions be necessary to resort to surgical treatment if the woman is unable to tolerate drug treatment.

The drugs used are carbimazole, methimazole and propylthiouracil (PTU). All of these drugs do cross the placenta, although PTU does so more slowly and is therefore the drug of choice in pregnancy. However, the drugs will also suppress fetal thyroid function and therefore the aim of treatment should be to keep the maternal thyroxine levels at the upper level of normal to minimize fetal thyroid suppression, as maternal thyroxine does not cross the placenta. It is also important to look for signs of hypothyroidism in the neonate.

CARDIAC DISEASE IN PREGNANCY

Normal pregnancy is associated with a 40% increase in cardiac output in the resting state and therefore creates a substantial load on the myocardium if there is underlying cardiac disease that may result in the mother going into cardiac failure. Whatever the lesion, the risk to the mother can be seen summarized on the basis of the New York Heart Association classification (Table 8.2).

Women in classes 1 and 2 can generally be reassured that, with appropriate care, they should progress well. If they are class 3 or 4, their prognosis is generally poor and consideration should be given as to whether they should continue with the pregnancy.

The maternal risk varies also with the nature of the cardiac lesion.

- **Low-risk conditions:** These include septal defects, patent ductus arteriosus, pulmonary and tricuspid lesions
- **Moderate risk:** Mitral stenosis, aortic stenosis; Marfan's syndrome without cardiomyopathy, previous myocardial infarction and coarctation are associated with significant risk
- **High risk:** The conditions with maximum risk include Eisenmenger's syndrome, pulmonary hypertension, Marfan's syndrome involving the aorta and with a cardiomyopathy.

Table 8.2
New York Heart Association classification

Grade 1: Normal exercise tolerance
Grade 2: Breathless on moderate exertion
Grade 3: Breathless on less than moderate exertion
Grade 4: Breathless at rest without significant activity

The risks to the mother are those of cardiac failure and acute pulmonary oedema. Adequate rest and the avoidance of infection are important. Iron supplements should be given to maintain optimal haemoglobin levels. The use of antibiotic cover should be routine in labour and vaginal delivery should be encouraged unless there are other obstetric indications for operative delivery. Care should be undertaken to avoid fluid overload.

Anticoagulant therapy may also be necessary where there has been a valve replacement.

It must be remembered that the risk of cardiac decompensation is maximal during labour and in the first 4 days after delivery.

RESPIRATORY DISORDERS IN PREGNANCY

The majority of chronic respiratory disorders are well tolerated in pregnancy, with the occasional exception in those women who have gross kyphoscoliosis, where the upward displacement of the diaphragm by the expanding uterus may cause respiratory embarrassment to the mother. In these circumstances, it may be necessary to bring forward the date of delivery if significant deterioration of respiratory function occurs.

Asthma

Asthma is an increasingly common disorder and can be expected to affect 5–10% of pregnant women. There is no consistent or predictable effect, as 25% of mothers improve during pregnancy, 25% get worse and the remainder stay the same. Severe asthmatic attacks are rare in late pregnancy. Although the clinical features remain the same in pregnancy, objective assessment with pulmonary function tests is essential to assess the presence of airway deterioration. The presence of a maternal tachycardia in excess of 120 beats/min, a respiratory rate in excess of 30/min and a peak flow of less than 120 l/min indicate that control is inadequate.

Management is no different in pregnancy with the use of beta-agonists and inhaled corticosteroids. Short courses of prednisone should be used where control is poor but control can usually be maintained with inhalation of beclometasone (beclomethasone), budesonide and fluticasone. Uncontrolled asthma has been reported as being associated with an increased incidence of preterm birth, low birthweight and increased perinatal mortality.

EPILEPSY IN PREGNANCY

Epilepsy is the most commonly encountered neurological disease in pregnancy and has a prevalence of 0.6–1.0%. Pregnancy has no consistent effect on maternal epilepsy and 50% remained unchanged, 25% get better and 25% get worse. Because of a reduction of absorption, a reduction of plasma binding, increased liver metabolism and increased plasma volume, serum levels of the anti-epileptic drugs tend to fall and the dosage may need to be increased. Preconceptual counselling may provide an opportunity to try to discontinue drug therapy but up to 50% of women can be expected to relapse.

Status epilepticus is uncommon in pregnancy.

The effect of epilepsy and its treatment on the fetus

All anti-epileptic drugs are potentially teratogenic but the hazards of poorly controlled epilepsy exceed the risk of therapy. Although the risk of teratogenesis is recognized, it should not be overemphasized, as the majority of women, on monotherapy in particular, have a normal outcome to the pregnancy. However, the risk is dose-related and every effort should therefore be made to use the minimum therapeutic dose commensurate with control of fits.

No one anti-epileptic drug is superior for use in pregnancy. Congenital abnormalities include congenital heart defects, orofacial clefts, microcephaly, intrauterine growth restriction and developmental delay. Some 10% of infants born to mothers taking phenytoin have vitamin-K-dependent clotting problems.

Management

The first priority is to maintain control of the fits, using one drug if possible. If there have been no seizures for 2–3 years and the mother presents prenatally, it may be possible to discontinue therapy but the fits may return if drug therapy is discontinued.

The pattern of management is shown in Figure 8.12.

AUTOIMMUNE DISEASE

Antiphospholipid antibodies are expressed by 15–20% of patients with systemic lupus and myeloproliferative disorders and are associated with an increased risk of intrauterine growth retardation, stillbirth, miscarriage and

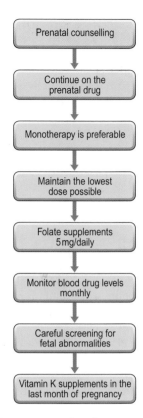

Fig. 8.12 Management of epilepsy in pregnancy.

thrombosis. Lupus anticoagulant prolongs phospholipid-dependent coagulation and is associated with an increased risk of fetal loss in all trimesters. Treatment is with heparin and low-dose aspirin. Conditions such as rheumatoid arthritis tend to improve during pregnancy but there is an increased risk of relapse during the puerperium.

LIVER DISEASE IN PREGNANCY

Intrahepatic cholestasis of pregnancy

This condition has a prevalence of 1–2 cases per 1000 pregnancies and is associated with the development of unexplained pruritus and late-onset jaundice in pregnancy. Initially, the patient notices darkening of the urine and pale stools. There is bilirubinuria and high blood levels of bile salts. The condition is not life-threatening and is pregnancy-related. It carries some risk of obstetric haemorrhage, largely due to hypoprothombinaemia and an increased risk of stillbirth and fetal distress in

labour. Pruritus is often severe and distressing and may be relieved by oral dexamethasone. Postnatally, the condition usually resolves within 4–7 days.

Acute fatty liver of pregnancy

This is a rare and lethal condition involving 1 case in 10 000 pregnancies. It is characterized by microvascular fatty infiltration in the liver and is associated with death from hepatic encephalopathy, genital tract haemorrhage and disseminated intravascular coagulation. Although the condition was once responsible for a 90% maternal death rate, it is now apparent that, if the condition is recognized early and management of the coagulopathy, hypoglycaemia and acidosis is instituted, the death rate can be reduced to less than 25%. Once these problems have been controlled, the pregnancy should be terminated by induction of labour or by caesarean section.

Acute viral hepatitis

Both hepatitis A and hepatitis B are viral diseases, although the method of transmission differs between the two viruses. Hepatitis B may be asymptomatic but the usual symptoms for both infections include nausea, anorexia, vomiting and fever followed by the development of jaundice. Patients with the hepatitis B carrier state may suffer a reactivation of the disease state during pregnancy. Most women will recover within 3–4 months from the time of onset of the disease but a few will progress to the development of chronic hepatitis.

Maternal–fetal transmission in hepatitis A does occasionally occur but is not common, whereas, with hepatitis B, vertical transmission is a significant problem. The infant should be protected with hepatitis B immunoglobulin by intramuscular injection at birth followed by hepatitis B vaccine, preferably within 7 days of delivery and certainly not later than 1 month after birth. The vaccine should be repeated within 6 months.

RENAL DISEASE IN PREGNANCY

Acute pyelonephritis and urinary tract infections

Asymptomatic bacteriuria occurs in about 5% of all pregnant women; hence the need to routinely screen all women antenatally. If the bacteriuria is treated with antibiotics, the risk of later development of acute ascending urinary tract infection can be minimized.

Nevertheless, approximately 1% of all pregnancies are complicated by an episode of acute pyelonephritis. The common organism is *Escherichia coli* and this will usually respond to antibiotics in the form of amoxicillin or cefuroxime with supportive treatment with fluid replacement, pain relief and bed rest.

Chronic renal disease

Pregnancy generally has an adverse effect on maternal renal function in women suffering from chronic renal disease as shown in Table 8.3.

Thus, women with mild impairment generally recover their renal function but those with moderate or severe impairment see a deterioration in renal function that does not improve after completion of the pregnancy.

Maternal renal disease also has a direct effect on the fetus, with an increased incidence of intrauterine growth restriction, preterm delivery and perinatal loss. The prognosis becomes worse with increasing severity of renal impairment.

Lupus nephritis

Woman who suffer from systemic lupus erythematosus and lupus nephritis and who have stable renal disease and controlled hypertension prior to pregnancy can expect a good maternal and fetal outcome. If a flare up of lupus nephritis occurs during pregnancy, it should be treated with corticosteroids and azathioprine. On occasions, if the condition becomes life-threatening to the mother, it may be necessary to use cytotoxic drugs, but this should be avoided if possible.

Polycystic kidney disease

These women usually have uneventful pregnancies but have a higher incidence of pre-eclampsia and severe pyelonephritis. Genetic counselling is obviously important because the disease is an autosomal dominant syndrome.

During pregnancy, renal deterioration may occur as the result of urinary tract infection. Control of hypertension is also important. This condition is not an indication for termination of pregnancy unless there is severe compromise of renal function.

Pregnancy after renal transplantation

Fertility usually returns after renal transplantation. About 5% of these women will conceive although as there is a high miscarriage rate, only 35% of these conceptions will go beyond the first trimester. However, 90% of these pregnancies will be successfully completed. Pregnancy should be delayed for 18–24 months after transplantation and immunosuppression should be maintained at prepregnancy levels. Pregnancy does not appear to affect the rate of rejection. Perinatal outcome is good provided that there is no hypertension or impaired renal function.

Renal calculi

Symptomatic renal stone disease is no more common in pregnancy than in the non-pregnant state. However, women with renal calculi have an increased frequency of urinary tract infections and such infections should be treated for longer than isolated urinary tract infections in women without renal stones. Fluid loading, alkalinization of the urine and pain relief with conservative management should be the first line of management, as this will tend to prevent the precipitation of uric acid and cystine stones. In the absence of comprehensive data concerning safety, lithotripsy should be avoided in pregnancy.

Table 8.3
Maternal renal function and chronic renal disease in pregnancy

	Serum creatinine (mmol/l)	Renal damage
Mild renal impairment	<120	Nil
Moderate renal impairment	124–168	Deterioration 20%
Severe renal impairment	> 177	Deterioration 70%

ESSENTIAL INFORMATION

Hypertension in pregnancy

- Commonest complication of pregnancy in the UK
- Gestational hypertension – hypertension alone after 20 weeks or within 24 hours of delivery in a previously normotensive woman
- Pre-eclampsia – hypertension and proteinuria after 20 weeks
- Eclampsia – pre-eclampsia plus convulsions, to 48 hours after delivery
- Pathogenesis of pre-eclampsia uncertain – increase in angiotensin-II receptors, endothelial dysfunction, decreased antioxidants all contribute
- Management of pre-eclampsia
  - Bed rest
  - Antihypertensive drug therapy
- Management of eclampsia
  - Control of fits
  - Control of blood pressure
  - Deliver infant by induction of labour or caesarean section

Anaemia

- In UK, haemoglobin level < 11 g/dl
- Usually caused by:
  - Inadequate intake of dietary iron
  - Impaired absorption of iron (gastric achlorhydria, malnutrition, chronic diarrhoea, hookworm)
  - Investigations – MCV, HCHC, serum iron and iron-binding, folate and vitamin B; others if cause still obscure
- Management usually with oral iron/folic acid

Diabetes

- Classified into potential, latent/gestational, chemical and clinical
- Management by dietary control (gestational diabetes)or short-acting insulin

Thyroid disease

- Graves' disease may cause fetal malformation, low birthweight, premature labour – treat with drug therapy

Cardiac disease

- NYHA classes 3 and 4 prognosis poor – consider termination
- Antibiotic cover in labour

Respiratory disease

- Assess control of asthma with pulmonary function tests
- Treatment as non-pregnant

Epilepsy

- Anti-epileptic drugs teratogenic but hazards of epilepsy exceed risks of therapy
- First priority to control fits

Liver disease

- In acute viral hepatitis B, infant must be given immunoglobulin at birth and vaccinated within 1st month to prevent vertical transmission of infection

Renal disease

- Treat bacteriuria with antibiotics to prevent acute pyelonephritis
- Moderate–severe chronic renal disease usually worsens during pregnancy and does not improve after delivery
- Renal disease causes increased rates of intrauterine growth restriction, preterm delivery and perinatal loss

9

Antepartum haemorrhage

Haemorrhage from the vagina after the 24th week of gestation is classified as antepartum haemorrhage. The factors that cause antepartum haemorrhage may be present before 24 weeks, but the original distinction between a threatened miscarriage and an antepartum haemorrhage was based on the potential viability of the fetus.

Vaginal bleeding may be due to:

- Haemorrhage from the placental site and uterine cavity
- Lesions of the vagina or cervix
- Fetal bleeding from vasa praevia.

UTEROPLACENTAL HAEMORRHAGE

The major causes of uterine bleeding are:

- Placenta praevia
- Abruptio placentae or accidental haemorrhage
- Uterine rupture
- Unknown aetiology.

Placenta praevia

The placenta is said to be praevia when all or part of the placenta implants in the lower uterine segment and therefore lies in front of the presenting part (Fig. 9.1)

Incidence

Approximately 1% of all pregnancies are complicated by clinical evidence of a placenta praevia. Unlike the incidence of placental abruption, which varies according to social and nutritional factors, the incidence of placenta praevia is remarkably constant.

Placenta praevia occurs more commonly in multiparous women, in the presence of multiple pregnancy and where there has been a previous caesarean section.

Aetiology

Placenta praevia is due to delay in implantation of the blastocyst so that this occurs in the lower part of the

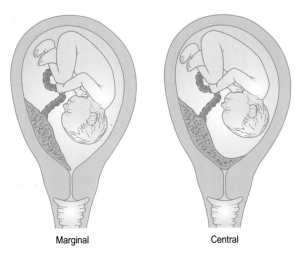

Marginal   Central

Fig. 9.1 Classification of placenta praevia.

uterus. It is commoner in high parity and in conditions where the placental area is large, such as multiple pregnancy or placenta membranacea.

Classification

From the point of view of management, there are three degrees of severity of placenta praevia (Fig. 9.1):

- **Lateral:** The placenta encroaches on the lower uterine segment but does not reach the internal cervical os
- **Marginal:** The placenta encroaches on or covers the internal cervical os before cervical dilatation occurs
- **Central:** The placenta completely covers the os even with cervical dilatation.

Classification is important in relation to management because spontaneous delivery is extremely rare where there is central placenta praevia but normal labour and delivery may occur with lateral or marginal implantation.

An alternative classification is based on grades, with grade 1 being defined by the placenta encroaching on the lower segment but not on the internal cervical os, grade II when the placenta reaches the internal os, grade III with the placenta eccentrically covering the os and grade IV as central placenta praevia. Grades II and III are equivalent to marginal placenta praevia and, as most women who have a marginal placenta are now delivered by caesarean section, there is probably little point in differentiating between grades II and III unless the mother is in labour when the diagnosis is made.

Bleeding results from separation of the placenta as the formation of the lower segment occurs and the cervix effaces. This blood loss occurs from the venous sinuses in the lower segment. Occasionally, fetal blood loss may occur, particularly where one of the placental vessels lies across the cervical os – a condition known as *vasa praevia*.

Symptoms and signs

The main symptom of placenta praevia is painless vaginal bleeding. There may sometimes be lower abdominal discomfort where there are minor degrees of associated placental abruption.

The signs of placenta praevia are:

- Vaginal bleeding
- Malpresentation of the fetus
- Uterine hypotonus.

Development of the lower uterine segment begins at 28 weeks gestation and thus bleeding is likely to occur from 28 weeks onwards. Bleeding is unpredictable and may vary from minor shows to massive and life-endangering haemorrhage.

Case study
Placenta praevia

Janet Y was admitted to hospital at 28 weeks gestation with a substantial painless vaginal haemorrhage in her first pregnancy. The presenting part was high but central and the uterine tone was soft. A diagnosis of placenta praevia was made and she was advised to stay in hospital under observation until delivery. There was no further bleeding and, at 32 weeks gestation, she asked to go home to marry her partner. As this necessitated a 1 hour flight, she was strongly advised against this action so her partner flew to Janet instead and the wedding was arranged in a church close to the hospital. At the wedding, Janet had a further substantial bleed as she walked down the aisle and was rushed back into hospital. The bleeding again subsided but, at 35 weeks gestation, Janet had a massive haemorrhage in the ward to the extent that blood soaked her bed linen and flowed over the side of the bed. The resident staff inserted two intravenous lines and she was rushed to theatre. She was shocked and hypotensive and it was extremely difficult to maintain her blood pressure. A 'crash section' was performed and the diagnosis of central placenta praevia was confirmed. A healthy male infant was delivered. Had Janet been at home, it is very unlikely that she would have survived.

Diagnosis

Clinical findings

Painless bleeding occurs suddenly and tends to be recurrent. When labour starts and the cervix dilates, profuse haemorrhage may occur, although sometimes in a lateral placenta praevia the presenting part compresses the placental site and bleeding is controlled.

Abdominal examination

- **Displacement of the presenting part:** The presence of the placenta in the lower segment tends to displace the presenting part and, when the placenta

is posterior, the head is pushed forward over the pelvic brim and is easily palpable. When the placenta is anterior, the presenting part is difficult to feel. Lateral placement of the placenta results in contralateral displacement of the presenting part. Where there is a central placenta praevia, the fetal head is held away from the pelvic brim and the lie may be transverse or oblique. If the head does not approach the pelvic brim when the placenta is anterior, the presenting part is difficult to palpate.
- **Flaccidity of the uterus:** Uterine muscle tone is usually low and the fetal parts are easy to palpate.

Diagnostic procedures

- **Ultrasound scanning:** This is predominantly used to localize the placenta and has largely replaced other techniques. Errors in diagnosis are most likely to occur in posteriorly situated placentae because of difficulties in identifying the lower segment. Anteriorly, the bladder provides an important landmark for the lower segment and diagnosis is more accurate. Localization of the placental site in early pregnancy may result in inaccurate diagnosis, as fundal development may lead to an apparent upward displacement of the placenta.
- **Magnetic resonance imaging:** This is the most accurate method of placental localization because the internal cervical os can be clearly visualized. However, it is not as yet widely available or used and would only be relevant if the ultrasound image was inconclusive.

Management

When antepartum haemorrhage of any type occurs, the diagnosis of placenta praevia should be suspected and hospital admission advised. The diagnosis should be established by ultrasound imaging. Vaginal examination should be performed only in an operating theatre prepared for caesarean section, with blood cross-matched. There are only two indications for performing a vaginal examination:

- When there is serious doubt about the diagnosis
- When bleeding occurs in established labour.

It is, in fact, often difficult to establish a diagnosis of placentae praevia by vaginal examination where the placenta is lateral, and there is a serious risk of precipitating massive haemorrhage if the placenta is central.

If the placenta is lateral, then it may be possible to rupture the membranes and allow spontaneous vaginal delivery.

Conservative management of placenta praevia involves keeping the mother in hospital with blood cross-matched until fetal maturity is adequate, and then delivering the child by caesarean section. Providing there is no active bleeding, there is no need to keep the mother in bed and she should remain ambulant, as she is as likely to bleed lying supine. Blood loss should be treated by transfusion where necessary so that an adequate haemoglobin concentration is maintained.

Postpartum haemorrhage is also a hazard of the low-lying placenta, as contraction of the lower segment is less effective than contraction of the upper segment.

There is an increased risk of placenta accreta where placental implantation occurs over the site of a previous uterine scar.

> ! Placenta praevia accreta is one of the most lethal conditions in obstetrics. It commonly occurs where the placenta is implanted over a previous section scar. The trophoblast grows into the scar tissue, making it almost impossible to separate the placenta from the uterine wall and, as a consequence, massive bleeding may occur. The only way this bleeding can be controlled is by hysterectomy. The condition carries a high mortality rate. The important management issue is to be prepared. Caesarean section associated with anterior implantation of a placenta praevia and a previous section scar should be performed by an experienced obstetric surgeon with ample supplies of blood on standby.

Abruptio placentae

Abruptio placentae or accidental haemorrhage is defined as haemorrhage resulting from premature separation of the placenta. The term 'accidental' implies separation as the result of trauma, but most cases do not involve trauma and occur spontaneously.

Aetiology

Placental abruption tends to occur more frequently under conditions of social deprivation in association with dietary deficiencies. Folic acid deficiency, in particular, has been implicated.

Out of 7.5 million pregnancies in the USA, the incidence of placental abruption has been recorded as 6.5/1000 births with a perinatal mortality of 119/1000 births.

The incidence of placental abruption is increased in the presence of pre-eclampsia or essential hypertension. It must be remembered that hypertension and proteinuria may develop as a result of abruption.

Whatever factors predispose to placental abruption, they are well-established before the abruption occurs. The fetus is more likely to be male and the birthweight is often low, indicating pre-existing growth retardation. A history of a placental abruption in a previous pregnancy is a predictor for a further abruption. The prognosis for fetal survival is significantly worse in those women who smoke cigarettes during pregnancy. Trauma is a relatively uncommon cause of abruption and in the

Case study
Abruptio placentae

Mandy, a 23-year-old primigravida, was admitted to hospital at 35 weeks gestation with a complaint that she had developed severe abdominal pain followed by substantial vaginal bleeding. On examination, she was restless and in obvious pain. Her blood pressure was 150/90 and the uterus was rigid and tender. Her pulse rate was 100 bpm and she looked pale and tense. The uterine fundus was palpable at the level of the xiphisternum. The fetal lie was longitudinal, with the head presenting. The fetal heart beat could not be detected. An intravenous line was established and blood cross-matched as a matter of urgency. Mandy was given pain relief and her blood picture and clotting profile were examined. Vaginal examination showed that the cervix was effaced and 3 cm dilated and the membranes were bulging through the os. A forewater rupture was performed and blood-stained amniotic fluid was released. Labour ensued and Mandy was delivered 3 hours later of a stillborn male infant. A large amount of clot was delivered with the placenta, and some 50% of the placenta appeared to have been avulsed from the uterine wall.

majority of cases no specific predisposing factor can be identified for a particular episode.

Clinical types and presentation

Three types of abruption have been described (Fig. 9.2):

- Revealed
- Concealed
- Mixed, or concealed and revealed.

Unlike placenta praevia, placental abruption presents with pain, vaginal bleeding and increased uterine activity.

Revealed haemorrhage

The major haemorrhage is apparent externally, as haemorrhage occurs from the lower part of the placenta and blood escapes through the cervical os. Under these circumstances the clinical features are less severe.

Abruption tends to occur after 36 weeks gestation, with the fetal lie longitudinal and the presenting part sitting well into the pelvic brim. In revealed placental abruption, uterine activity may be increased, but this finding is not consistent.

Concealed haemorrhage

In this case the haemorrhage occurs between the placenta and the uterine wall. The uterine content increases in volume and the fundal size appears larger than would be consistent with the estimated date of confinement. Uterine tonus is increased and pain and shock are common features. The uterus may become rigid and tender.

> **!** It is important to realize that initially, even in the presence of substantial intra-uterine haemorrhage where the blood loss is concealed, the blood pressure may be raised and the pulse rate slowed but eventually the patient becomes shocked with the development of tachycardia, hypotension and oliguria. The peripheral circulation becomes vasoconstricted and there may be physical signs of vasoconstriction even before hypotension develops.

In some severe cases, haemorrhage penetrates through the uterine wall and the uterus appears bruised. This is described as a *Couvelaire uterus*. On clinical examination the uterus will be tense and hard and the uterine fundus will be higher than is normal for the gestational age. The patient will often be in labour and in approximately 30% of cases the fetal heart sounds will be absent and the fetus will be stillborn. The prognosis for the fetus is dependent on the extent of placental separation and is inversely proportional to the interval between onset and delivery.

Mixed, or concealed and revealed haemorrhage

In most cases the haemorrhage is both concealed and revealed. Haemorrhage occurs close to the placental

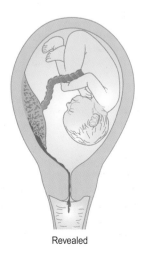
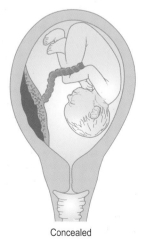
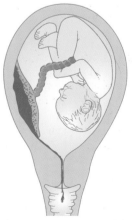

Revealed   Concealed   Concealed and revealed

Fig. 9.2 Types of placental abruption.

edge and, after an interval when the haemorrhage is concealed, blood loss soon appears vaginally.

Differential diagnosis

The diagnosis is made on the history of vaginal bleeding, abdominal pain, increased uterine tonus, proteinuria and the presence of a longitudinal lie. This must be distinguished from placenta praevia, where the haemorrhage is painless, the lie unstable and the uterus hypotonic. Occasionally, some manifestations of placental abruption may arise where there is a low-lying placenta. In other words, placental abruption can arise where there is low placental implantation and, on these occasions, the diagnosis can only really be clarified by ultrasound location of the placenta.

The diagnosis should also be differentiated from other acute emergencies such as acute hydramnios, where the uterus is enlarged, tender and tense but there is no haemorrhage. Other acute abdominal emergencies such as perforated ulcer, volvulus of the bowel and strangulated inguinal hernia may simulate concealed placental abruption, but these problems are rare during pregnancy.

Management

The patient must be admitted to hospital and the diagnosis established on the basis of the history and examination findings (Fig. 9.3). Mild cases may be treated conservatively and the placental site localized to confirm the diagnosis. If the haemorrhage is severe, resuscitation is the first prerequisite.

It is often difficult to assess the amount of blood loss accurately and intravenous infusion should be started with normal saline, Hartmann's solution or blood substitutes until blood is cross-matched and transfusion can be commenced. Fluid replacement should be monitored by the use of a central venous pressure line. Unlike placenta praevia, any significant abruption should be treated by delivering the fetus as soon as possible.

If the fetus is alive and there are no clinical signs of fetal distress, or if the fetus is dead, surgical induction of labour is performed as soon as possible and, where necessary, uterine activity is stimulated with a dilute Syntocinon infusion. If the fetus is alive, it should be monitored and caesarean section should be performed if signs of fetal distress develop. If induction is not possible because the cervix is closed, then delivery

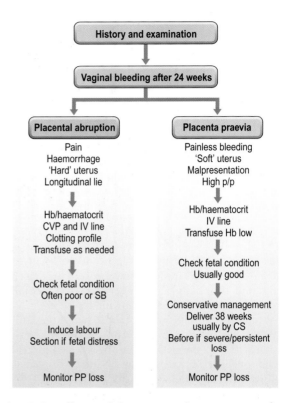

Fig. 9.3 Differential diagnosis and management of antepartum haemorrhage.

should be effected by caesarean section. Pain relief is achieved by the use of opiates. Epidural anaesthesia should not be used until a clotting screen is available.

Complications

The complications of placental abruption are summarized in Figure 9.4.

Afibrinogenaemia

In afibrinogenaemia, severe placental abruption results in significant placental damage and the release of thromboplastin into the maternal circulation. This in turn may lead to intravascular coagulation and to defibrination, with the development of hypo- and afibrinogenaemia. The condition may be treated by the infusion of fresh frozen plasma, platelet transfusion and fibrinogen transfusion but can only be reversed by delivering the fetus. It may lead to abnormal bleeding if operative delivery is attempted or may result in

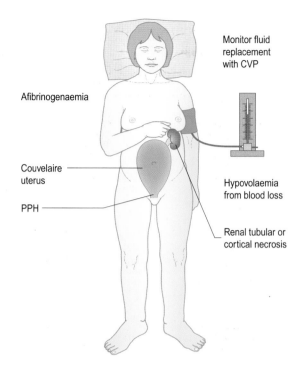

Fig. 9.4 Complications of placental abruption. CVP, central venous pressure; PPH, postpartum haemorrhage.

uncontrollable postpartum haemorrhage unless the clotting defect has been corrected.

Renal tubular or cortical necrosis

This is a complication that must always be considered as a possibility and it is essential to keep careful fluid balance charts and to take particular note of urinary output. This complication may, on occasion, necessitate haemodialysis or peritoneal dialysis, but it is becoming increasingly rare.

OTHER CAUSES OF ANTEPARTUM HAEMORRHAGE

These are summarized in Figure 9.5.

Unexplained antepartum haemorrhage

In many cases, it is not possible to make a definite diagnosis of abruption or placenta praevia.

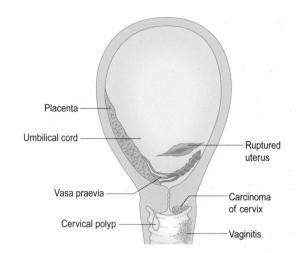

Fig. 9.5 Non-placental causes of antepartum haemorrhage.

These cases involve a significant increase in perinatal mortality and it is therefore important to monitor placental function and fetal growth. The pregnancy should not be allowed to proceed beyond term.

Rarely, the bleeding may be fetal in origin and arises from the rupture of an aberrant placental vessel known as a vasa praevia. The only way that this can be diagnosed is by detecting the presence of fetal haemoglobin in the vaginal blood loss.

Vaginal infections

Vaginal moniliasis or trichomoniasis may cause blood-stained discharge and, once the diagnosis is established, should be treated with the appropriate therapy.

Cervical lesions

Benign lesions of the cervix such as cervical polyps are treated by removal of the polyp. Cervical erosions are best left untreated.

Carcinoma of the cervix is occasionally found in pregnancy. If the pregnancy is early, termination is indicated. If the diagnosis is made late in pregnancy, the diagnosis should be established by biopsy and the lesion treated according to the staging.

ESSENTIAL INFORMATION

- Vaginal bleeding after 24 weeks.

Placenta praevia

- Lower segment implantation
- Incidence 1%
- Classification – marginal, central and lateral.
- Diagnosis – painless loss, unstable lie, soft uterus.
- Diagnosis confirmed by ultrasound or MRI
- Management – conservative until 37 weeks
- Hospital admission for all major degrees
- Blood held – cross-matched
- Caesarean section unless marginal
- Prognosis for the fetus – good.

Placental abruption

- Incidence 0.5–1.0%
- Diagnosis – uterus hypertonic
- Normal fetal lie
- Commonly associated with maternal hypertension
- Management – replace blood loss
- Check for DIC
- Deliver the infant if abruption severe
- Prognosis for fetus poor
- Maternal complications
- Afibrinogenaemia
- Renal tubular necrosis
- Scar dehiscence and uterine rupture

Unexplained causes

- Cervical and vaginal lesions
- Vasa praevia

10 Congenital abnormalities and infections in pregnancy

There are a very large number of congenital abnormalities and genetic syndromes documented in the literature but most clinicians encounter very few of them. Genetic counselling has become an important specialty in its own right. Only those conditions that are encountered relatively commonly will be considered in this section.

CONGENITAL ABNORMALITIES

Incidence

The incidence of serious congenital abnormalities has been estimated at 25–30/1000 births and this figure has remained relatively constant in England and Wales since 1920. Congenital abnormalities account for 25% of all stillbirths and 20% of all deaths in the first week. The commonest five groups of defect include neural tube defects (3–7/1000), congenital heart disease (6/1000), severe mental retardation (4/1000), Down's syndrome (1.5/1000) and hare lip/cleft palate (1.5/1000; Table 10.1).

While the total number of infants born with congenital defects is small, the overall incidence of chromosomal abnormalities is high, as about 30% of early miscarriages show significant chromosomal abnormalities.

Neural tube defects

The neural tube defects are the commonest of the major congenital abnormalities and include anencephaly, microcephaly, spina bifida with or without myelomeningocele, encephalocele, holoprosencephaly and hydranencephaly (Fig. 10.1). The incidence is approximately 1/200 and the chance of having an affected child after one previous abnormal child is 1/20. Infants with anencephaly or microcephaly do not usually survive. Many die during labour and the remainder within the first week of life. Infants with open neural tube defects often survive – particularly where it is possible to cover the lesion surgically with skin. However, the defect may result in paraplegia and bowel and bladder incontinence. The child often has normal

Table 10.1
Major congenital abnormalities

Abnormality	Approximate incidence (/1000 births)
Neural tube defects	3–7
Congenital heart disease	6
Severe mental retardation	4
Cerebral palsy	2
Down's syndrome	1.5
Cleft lip/palate	1.5
Talipes	1–2
Abnormalities of limbs	1–2
Deafness	0.8
Blindness	0.2
Others, including urinary tract anomalies	2
Total	**15–30**

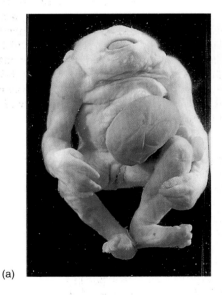

(a)

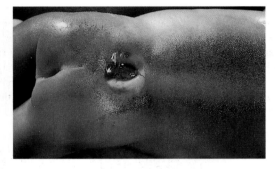

(b)

Fig. 10.1 Two common abnormalities of the central nervous system. (a) Anencephaly. (b) Spina bifida with open neural tube defect.

intelligence and becomes aware of the problems posed for the parents. Closed lesions generally do not cause problems and may escape detection until after birth.

Although there is some evidence that multivitamin supplementation may reduce the incidence of this condition, the major effort at the present time is directed toward screening techniques that enable recognition of the abnormality and termination of the pregnancy where there is a lethal abnormality.

Folic acid dietary supplementation is indicated both before and during pregnancy in those women who have experienced a pregnancy complicated by a neural tube defect.

Screening by α-fetoprotein

This glycoprotein is made in the fetal yolk sac and in the fetal liver and enters the amniotic fluid via fetal urine. Maternal serum alpha-fetoprotein (AFP) enters the maternal circulation by diffusion across the placenta. Maternal serum levels rise until 30 weeks gestation and, between 15 and 20 weeks, the levels increase by about 15% per week. Assessment is therefore critically gestational-age-dependent.

Serum AFP levels are usually expressed as multiples of the median: values over 2.3–2.5 times the median are considered to be abnormal.

All women should be offered screening by measurement of serum α-fetoprotein between 15 and 19 weeks gestation. Women who would not accept termination of an abnormal pregnancy should not have the test performed unless it is specifically requested.

An abnormally high value should be investigated by:

- Checking the gestational age by ultrasound scan
- Checking for multiple pregnancy by scan
- Screening by scan for neurological abnormality.

Improvements in the precision of ultrasound diagnosis of neural tube defects have meant that scanning procedures have largely replaced the measurement of liquor alpha-fetoprotein and hence the need for amniocentesis. However, there are occasions where visualization of the spine may be difficult and amniocentesis is therefore advisable. Under these circumstances, the measurement of amniotic fluid acetylcholinesterase will improve diagnostic precision. This enzyme is not normally found in amniotic fluid and is released into amniotic fluid when fetal cerebrospinal fluid has access to the amniotic sac, as with open neural tube defects and anencephaly.

The mother should be advised that there is a risk of miscarriage from the procedure of amniocentesis; it is estimated to be about 1% above the risk of spontaneous miscarriage in the second trimester.

> **!** There are many other causes of raised maternal AFP levels: these include bleeding in early pregnancy, fetal death, fetal abdominal wall defects, congenital nephrosis, bowel obstruction, renal tract abnormalities, sacrococcygeal tumours and placental and umbilical cord tumours. Most of these abnormalities can be diagnosed by high-resolution ultrasound imaging.

Congenital cardiac defects

The next group to be considered is that of congenital cardiac defects. Some of these infants present with intrauterine growth retardation and oligohydramnios but in many cases the diagnosis is established after delivery. With improvements in real-time ultrasound imaging, recognition of many cardiac defects has become possible, but early recognition is essential if any action is to be taken. A four-chamber view of the fetal heart is shown in Figure 10.2.

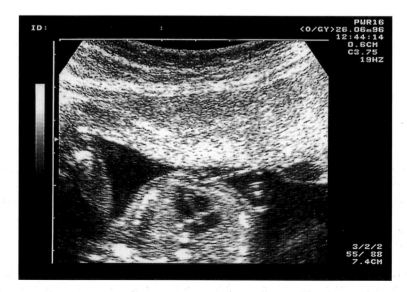

Fig. 10.2 Four-chamber ultrasound view of the fetal heart.

The most common defects are ventricular and atrial septal defects, pulmonary and aortic stenosis, coarctation and transpositions, including the tetralogy of Fallot. These lesions can generally now be recognized on the four-chamber views recorded during detailed 18-week gestation scans.

Defects of the abdominal wall

Defects of the abdominal wall can be diagnosed by ultrasound imaging. They include **exomphalos**, where the bowel extrudes outside the abdominal cavity (Fig. 10.3) and **ectopia vesicae**, where the bladder is everted and opens on to the surface of the abdominal wall. The latter condition has a poor prognosis but exomphalos has a good prognosis if the condition is recognized antenatally. Under these circumstances, delivery is best effected by elective caesarean section followed by immediate repair of the child's abdominal wall defect. This minimizes the risk of damage to the gut and liver and also of infection.

Cerebral palsy

This is a disorder of movement and posture caused by a non-progressive insult to the immature brain. There is persistence in infantile behaviour and reflexes and, as the central nervous system matures, the manifestations change and the degree of handicap tends to increase. It affects 2/1000 term infants and up to 50/1000 infants with birth weights of below 1500 g, particularly in twin pregnancies. The aetiology is complex but includes disorders of development, intrauterine infections, disturbance of normal fetal nutrition and oxygenation before or during labour as well as postnatal events such as kernicterus, meningitis and trauma. Fewer than 15% of cases are thought to arise from intrapartum asphyxia.

Other conditions amenable to diagnosis by amniocentesis

X-linked diseases

This group (Fig. 10.4) includes Duchenne's muscular dystrophy and haemophilia. If the mother is a carrier and the karyotype demonstrates a male fetus, then the child will have a 50/50 chance of having Duchenne's muscular dystrophy and therefore abortion should be offered.

However, this diagnostic precision can now be improved by cordocentesis under ultrasound control, as direct blood samples can be obtained from the umbilical and placental blood vessels. Serum creatinine kinase is grossly elevated in the affected infant.

Metabolic disorders and others

Conditions such a phenylketonuria, which may result in severe mental retardation, are now amenable to prenatal diagnosis by identifying enzyme deficiencies in cultured fetal cells. The conditions that can be reliably diagnosed in this way are listed in Table 10.2

Conditions associated with visible abnormalities such as absent eyes, limb deformities, hare lip and encephalocele may also be diagnosed antenatally by ultrasound scanning.

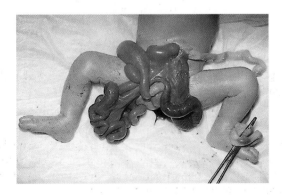

Fig. 10.3 Bowel extrusion associated with exomphalos.

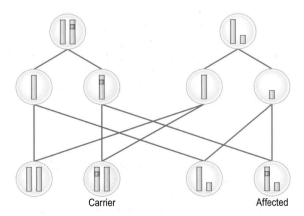

Carrier   Affected

Fig. 10.4 Transmission of recessively inherited X-linked disorder. The abnormal gene is carried on the female X chromosome.

Table 10.2
Inherited metabolic disorders most commonly diagnosed antenatally

Disorder	Deficient enzyme
Sphingolipidoses	
Tay–Sachs disease	Hexoseaminadase A
Gaucher's disease	Glucocerebrosidase
Metachromatic leukodystrophy	Arylsulphatase
Krabbe's leukodystrophy	Galactosyloceramide β-galactosidase
Pompe's disease (glycogen storage)	α-1-4-glucosidase
Mucopolysaccharidoses	
Hurler's disease	α-L-iduronidase
Hunter's disease	Sulphoiduronide sulphatase
Sanfilippo disease	Heparan sulphate sulphatase
Galactosaemia	Galactose-1-phosphate uridyl transferase
Homocystinuria	Cystathionine synthetase
Maple syrup urine disease	Ketoacid decarboxylase
Methylmalonic acidaemia	Methylmalonic CoA mutase

> **!** It has to be emphasized that most of these conditions are extremely rare. In conversation, a now retired senior professor of paediatrics with an extensive clinical practice pointed out that, in a professional lifetime, he had seen only six metabolic and genetic disorders out of the 2000 or more syndromes described in the literature.

Chromosomal abnormalities

A considerable number of chromosomal abnormalities has been identified from the culture and karyotype of fetal cells in the amniotic fluid and include structural and numerical abnormalities of the karyotype. The commonest abnormality is that associated with trisomy 21 or Down's syndrome.

Down's syndrome

This syndrome is characterized by the typical abnormal facial features, mental retardation of varying degrees of severity, and congenital heart disease (Fig. 10.5). The karyotype includes an additional chromosome on group 21 and this presents as a trisomy 21, although it sometimes occurs at number 22. The incidence overall is 1.5/1000 births. However, the risk increases with

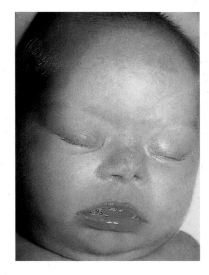

Fig. 10.5 Facial appearance of infant with Down's syndrome.

advancing maternal age and over the age of 30 years is 1/300, while over the age of 45 years it is about 1/40. The underlying reason may be related to an increased frequency of non-disjunction at meiosis.

About 6–8% of affected infants have the disease as a result of a translocation and the extra 21 chromosome is carried on to another chromosome, usually in group 13–15. The mother or the father will usually show evidence of being a translocation carrier. If the mother is a carrier the risk of recurrence is 1/10. Thus, all women over the age of 35 years or with a family history of mongolism should be offered amniocentesis with a view to termination of the pregnancy, if the karyotype is abnormal. Not all societies accept that termination of pregnancy is indicated for Down's syndrome.

As discussed in Chapters 7 and 11, the diagnosis can also be suspected from screening of nuchal thickness by ultrasound and established by chorion villus sampling, either transcervically or transabdominally, at 10–14 weeks gestation.

Amniocentesis is usually also offered to women who have a previous history of Turner's syndrome (45XO) or Klinefelter's syndrome (47XXY), although the risk of recurrence is low.

globulin may help to prevent infections where contact with rubella has occurred, but the evidence is equivocal.

The diagnosis of rubella during pregnancy can be made on the clinical manifestations of the infection, which include a fine macular rash, lymphadenopathy in the cervical lymph nodes and mild pyrexia (Fig. 10.7). The diagnosis can be confirmed in the acute phase by virus isolation from a throat swab or from blood culture but usually the diagnosis is established by determination of the level of antibodies in the mother. A fourfold increase in antibody titre in consecutive blood samples taken 2 weeks apart constitutes evidence of recent rubella infection in the mother. In the infant, cord blood measurements will show similar antibody titres to the mother and the presence of raised levels of immunoglobulin IgM will strongly suggest infection acquired in utero.

MATERNAL INFECTIONS THAT MAY AFFECT FETAL DEVELOPMENT

Rubella

The effect of maternal rubella infection has been discussed in a previous chapter. Congenital malformations include microcephaly, cataracts, deafness, congenital heart disease and osteitis. From 0–4 weeks the risk is 33%, between 5 and 8 weeks 25%, between 9 and 12 weeks 9%, between 13 and 16 weeks 4% and between 17 and 30 weeks 1% (Fig 10.6). Injections of gamma-

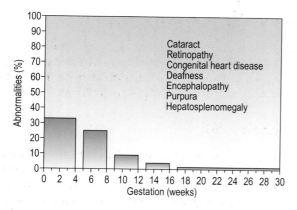

Fig. 10.6 Incidence of congenital defects and rubella in relation to gestational age.

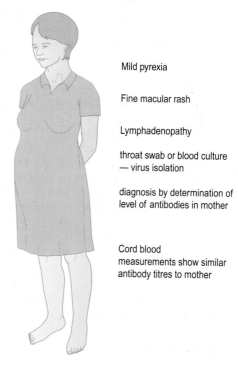

Fig. 10.7 Clinical manifestations of maternal rubella infection.

> ! The diagnosis of rubella acquired in early pregnancy is particularly important as these infections have potentially dire consequences. Rubella acquired in the first 14 weeks of pregnancy will inevitably result in infection in the fetus. At least 40% of infected fetuses will be damaged, often having major defects. Infection in weeks 4–12 of pregnancy affects the lens of the eye, causing cataracts and infection; from weeks 5–12 it also damages the heart as well as causing fetal growth restriction, thrombocytopenia, hepatosplenomegaly and vasculitis. Because of the consequences of rubella infection, termination of pregnancy should be offered where there is evidence of infection during the first 14 weeks of pregnancy.

Hepatitis B

There are two types of viral hepatitis – infective hepatitis (virus A) and serum hepatitis (virus B). Virus A is associated with a short incubation period and virus B with a long incubation time. Hepatitis B surface antigen is known as Australia antigen.

The risk to the fetus of maternal infection appears to be minimal in cases of hepatitis A. In cases of hepatitis B, the infant may become infected by swallowing maternal blood or amniotic fluid during labour and about 25% of these infants subsequently develop hepatitis. Up to 90% of the infants will become carriers of the virus unless the mother also carries antibodies to the virus (HbeAB positive) in which case only 5% of the infants will be affected. Transplacental transmission occurs in about 5% of cases.

Australia-antigen-positive women are managed with particular precautions as cross-infection may occur from maternal faeces, urine, maternal blood or amniotic fluid. These patients should be managed with barrier nursing, taking special precautions with the disposal of excreta.

The risk of vertical transmission is substantially reduced by the concurrent administration of immunoglobulin and vaccination after delivery.

Chronic infection with the hepatitis C virus is also found in pregnant women but the transmission rate to neonates is relatively low at about 5%.

Herpes simplex

Herpes infections are due to two antigenic types of herpes virus, HSV1 and HSV2. Type 1 is now responsible for 50% of genital tract infections, but also occurs in non-genital sites such as the mouth, eyes and central nervous system. Type 2 infections are sexually transmitted.

Genital herpes is associated with a fivefold increase in the incidence of miscarriage during the first 20 weeks. Genital infection at term results in a 40% incidence of infection in the fetus and this may be manifest in skin vesicles and in infections involving the brain, liver and adrenals.

At the present time it is generally considered advisable to deliver the infant by caesarean section to minimize the risk of infection acquired during vaginal delivery if there are active genital tract lesions and this is the primary attack.

Other infections with predominantly fetal effects

Cytomegalovirus

It has been estimated that 4% of women acquire this infection during pregnancy. Both the placenta and fetus may be affected by the viraemia, which may result in the development of microcephaly and be the cause of mental retardation of infants in the first 6 years of life. The diagnosis can be established by the presence of a rising antibody titre. Newborn screening is based on raised cord blood IgM levels (> 20 mg/dl). In primary infections, some 30–40% of infants will be affected but only 5–7% of these infants will be affected at birth with growth restriction, jaundice, hepatosplenomegaly, rash, chorioretinitis, intracranial calcification, encephalitis or microcephaly.

Pregnancy bacteriuria

Bacteria in the mother is associated with an increase in low-birthweight infants. Urine specimens yielding more than 10^5 colonies/ml are considered bacteriuric and should be treated with appropriate antibiotic therapy.

Toxoplasmosis

Toxoplasma gondii is a protozoon which is found throughout the world. The mode of infection involves the domestic cat. Congenital toxoplasmosis may occur if the mother acquires the infection during pregnancy. Reports in the literature on the incidence are highly variable but, at the present time, the UK prevalence is about 2/1000. In France the prevalence is generally higher. Maternal infection may be a cause of recurrent miscarriage. The risk to the fetus of infection increases with advancing gestation and the abnormalities that may arise in the fetus include hydrocephalus, mental retardation and retinochoroiditis. Treatment to the mother should be initiated as soon as the presence of the infection is confirmed, as this will minimize the risk of abnormalities. The drugs used include spiramycin, pyrimethamine, sulfadiazine and folinic acid.

Chlamydiosis

The intracellular bacterium *Chlamydia trachomata* is a cause of neonatal conjunctivitis and trachoma. The infection can be diagnosed by immunoassay and treated with 7–14 days of erythromycin.

Varicella zoster

Most women of child-bearing age are immune to *Varicella zoster* (> 85%) but, following the primary infection known as chicken pox, the virus may remain latent in the sensory nerve ganglia and become reactivated as herpes zoster or shingles.

First-trimester infection is associated with an increased risk of miscarriage and, rarely, embryopathy with intrauterine growth retardation, limb scarring, eye defects, microcephaly and neurological abnormalities. The major risk to the fetus comes from intrapartum infection, which is most likely to occur when delivery is within 4 days of the onset of symptoms in the mother. Infection in the newborn develops 2–3 weeks after delivery and has a 20% mortality. Infants born within this time from mothers who are known not to be immune should be given immunoglobulin.

The incidence of abnormalities arising in the fetus is 2% if the infection arises between 13 and 20 weeks.

If the mother comes into contact with chicken pox during her pregnancy, blood should be taken for IgG and, if this confirms past immunity, she can be reassured that there is no risk to the fetus.

Listeriosis

Listeria monocytogenes is found in soil, unwashed vegetables, birds, insects and crustaceans. The organisms can be transmitted transplacentally or by inhalation of amniotic fluid by the infant at delivery. The incidence varies greatly from one country to another. There is an increased risk of intrauterine death and miscarriage and untreated neonatal infection has a 90% mortality rate in the infant. The diagnosis can be established by blood and urine cultures and should be suspected in any women presenting with a flu-like illness with conjunctivitis, pharyngitis, loin pain and diarrhoea.

Listeriosis tends to be most common in the third trimester. While the organism is sensitive to ampicillin, rifampicin and vancomycin, the best approach to management is prevention.

> ! Pregnant women should be advised to thoroughly cook raw food from animal sources, thoroughly wash raw vegetables before eating them and keep uncooked meats separate from other foods. They should avoid the consumption of raw milk and soft cheeses.

Parvovirus B19

Parvovirus infections are common in children and, as a consequence, at least half the female population are immune by the time they achieve child-bearing age. Infection arising in pregnancy can result in infection in the fetus and may cause severe anaemia and myocarditis, leading to gross hydrops and fetal death. As 30–40% of maternal infections are subclinical, the diagnosis is often only made with the development of fetal hydrops and death. Where maternal infection is diagnosed, regular fetal surveillance by ultrasound is recommended as the early recognition of the development of hydrops can enable treatment of fetal anaemia by transfusion with fetal salvage.

Human immunodeficiency virus infection

Human immunodeficiency virus (HIV) is a retrovirus that affects human lymphocytes and other cells in the central nervous system. There are three levels of manifestation of HIV infection:

- **Asymptomatic:** A positive test for HIV but no clinical symptoms
- **Acquired immunodeficiency syndrome (AIDS)-related complex (ARC):** This includes persistent generalized lymphadenopathy, weight loss, lethargy, fever and joint pains

- **AIDS:** This includes the clinical symptoms plus opportunistic infections, such as *Pneumocystis carinii*, and the presence of Kaposi's sarcoma.

Infection is usually asymptomatic and incubation takes 15–58 months. Transmission is sexual or blood-borne and transplacental. There is no evidence to suggest that airborne infection occurs.

Incidence

The incidence of AIDS varies widely in different countries but continues to rise globally. In the USA AIDS was originally largely confined to homosexual or bisexual individuals, but this group now accounts for only about half of cases. The remaining 50% of cases occur in intravenous drug abusers and in people receiving blood products or blood transfusions or who become infected by heterosexual contacts. Obviously, these clinical incidence figures will continue changing and already vary considerably according to geographic location.

In pregnancy, there is no evidence that HIV infection is clinically accelerated. AIDS and ARC depress the T-helper cell population. It does not affect fertility.

There is a higher incidence of preterm labour and low-birthweight infants in affected mothers, but there are complicating social factors. There are three routes of infection of the child:

- Transplacental
- At birth
- Breast milk.

Incidental perinatal transmission occurs in 30–50% of cases.

Vertical transfer of HIV occurs in 30% of untreated pregnancies.

Risk of infection cannot be judged on maternal history alone, as some 50–70% of HIV-positive women give no self-identified risk factors. This has led to recommendations that all pregnant women should be screened. In the UK this is now routinely carried out along with screening for syphilis and hepatitis with the informed consent of each mother and with an appropriate counselling service available for those who are found to be positive.

Fetal AIDS

This syndrome is manifested by intrauterine growth retardation, microcephaly, prominent forehead and blue sclerae.

Prognosis

The outlook for survival in infected children is very poor, with a high mortality rate. There is some evidence that the extent of maternal illness may determine the risk of infection in the baby.

Care of HIV-seropositive women in pregnancy and labour

All HIV-positive pregnant women should be managed jointly with a physician who specializes in HIV. It is not considered essential to nurse these mothers in isolation unless there is abnormal haemorrhage or infective complications. Early signs and symptoms include malaise, fevers, night sweats and weight loss. There are numerous gastrointestinal and dermatological symptoms, including Kaposi's sarcoma. Delivery by elective caesarean section reduces the incidence of vertical transmission and is now the recommended mode of delivery.

During the second stage of delivery, staff should wear full protective clothing with face protection and overshoes, with double gloves for suturing.

Fetal blood sampling should be avoided whenever possible.

The placenta should be double-bagged and incinerated. The newborn infant should undergo the investigations shown in Table 10.3.

Breastfeeding appears to double the risk of transmission of HIV and therefore these women should generally be advised against breastfeeding.

Drug therapy

The use of zidovudine administered to the mother during pregnancy has been shown to significantly reduce fetal transmission and is now considered standard care. Zidovudine is given to the mother antenatally in a

Table 10.3
Neonatal investigations in babies at risk of HIV

- Full blood count
- Urine culture for cytomegalovirus
- Hepatitis B and C serology
- HIV serology
- Virology
- Immunology including T lymphocyte subsets
- Immunoglobulin levels

dose orally of 100 mg 5 times daily and intravenously during labour at an infusion rate of 1 mg/kg body weight per hour until delivery occurs. The neonate is given 2 mg/kg orally 6-hourly for the first 6 weeks of life.

Malaria

Malaria occurs in over 200 million people per year and results in more than 1 million deaths per year. It is a common complication of pregnancy in those countries where the disease is endemic.

Women who live in endemic areas show an increased prevalence of the severe forms of the disease.

The severity of disease is related to the species of parasite, the level of parasitaemia and the immune status of the individual. *Plasmodium falciparum* is the most virulent of the organisms, as it attacks all forms of the erythrocyte. The parasite grows in the placenta and placental malaria occurs in anywhere between 15–60% of cases. Congenital malaria is rare in the infants born to mothers who have immunity as protective immunoglobulin G crosses the placenta.

However, acute malaria in the previously unexposed woman is a medical emergency and may result in miscarriage, fetal death and premature labour.

Mothers travelling to endemic areas should take prophylaxis or, preferably, not go to the area until the pregnancy is completed. They should also be advised to keep their skin covered and to use insecticides to minimize the risk of being bitten by mosquitoes.

Drug treatment of the acute attack will depend on the nature of the infection. Prophylaxis is given in the form of chloroquine phosphate at a dose of 300 mg each week, starting 1 week before travel and continuing for 4 weeks after leaving the area. Where chloroquine-resistant strains exist, a combination of chloroquine and pyrimethamine with sulfadoxine can be used, or proguanil and mefloquine. These drugs need to be taken with a folic acid supplement. Although chloroquine can cause retinal and cochleovestibular damage in high doses in both the mother and the fetus, it has never been shown to be associated with an increased incidence of birth defects where it has been taken for prophylaxis.

ESSENTIAL INFORMATION

Congenital abnormalities

- 25–30/1000 births in England and Wales
- Account for 25% of stillbirths, 20% of neonatal deaths
- Commonest are neural tube and cardiac defects (6–7/1000)
- Chromosomal defects (1.5/1000)
- Incidence of trisomy 21 increases with maternal age
- Most structural defects can be demonstrated by ultrasound
- Metabolic disorders may need fetal blood sampling
- Chromosomal defects need confirmation by amniocentesis
- Defects can also be diagnosed by chorion villus sampling

Maternal infections affecting the fetus

- Incidence of congenital defects in rubella varies in relation to gestational age at time of infection
- Hepatitis B transmission occurs by contamination by faeces, amniotic fluid inhalation
- Delivery by caesarean section is recommended for patients with active herpes (type 2) infections; 40% incidence of neonatal infection
- Cytomegalovirus can cause microcephaly and mental retardation
- Toxoplasmosis affects 2/1000 births – infection acquired from domestic cats
- Listeriosis causes miscarriage and stillbirth – avoid eating raw meat and soft cheeses
- Vertical transmission of HIV can be reduced from 30% to less than 5% by drug treatment, delivery by caesarean section and avoiding breastfeeding
- Malaria is worse in pregnancy – prophylaxis is essential

Normal labour

Labour or *parturition* is the process whereby the products of conception are expelled from the uterine cavity after the 24th week of gestation. *Premature labour* is defined as labour occurring before the commencement of the 37th week of gestation. *Prolonged labour* is defined as labour lasting in excess of 24 hours in a primigravida and 16 hours in a multigravida. This definition is based on the fact that labours exceeding these times are more likely to be associated with increased fetal and maternal morbidity and mortality.

STAGES OF LABOUR

Labour is described in three stages that are defined as follows:

- **The first stage** commences with the onset of labour and terminates when the cervix has reached full dilatation and is no longer palpable
- **The second stage** or stage of expulsion begins at full cervical dilatation and ends with expulsion of the fetus
- **The third stage** or placental stage begins with the delivery of the child and ends with the expulsion of the placenta.

ONSET OF LABOUR

The onset of labour is defined as the time of onset of regular, painful uterine contractions, which produce progressive effacement and dilatation of the cervix. It is often difficult to be certain of the exact time of onset of labour because of the occurrence of 'false labour' where the onset of painful contractions is not associated with progressive dilatation of the cervix. Also, in rare cases of cervical stenosis, the normal contractions of labour produce thinning and effacement of the cervix but do not result in cervical dilatation. However these exceptions do not interfere with the general definition.

Thus, the clinical signs of the onset of labour include:

- The onset of regular, usually painful contractions that produce progressive cervical dilatation

- The exhibition of a vaginal show – the passage of blood stained mucus.
- Rupture of the fetal membranes – this is variable and may occur at the time of onset of contractions or it may be delayed until the delivery of the fetus.

> ! Making a decision about the time of onset of labour has important implications for the subsequent management of labour. An assumption that labour is abnormally prolonged may result from an erroneous decision as to the time of onset of labour.

The initiation of labour

The mechanism of the onset of labour remains uncertain despite extensive research. There are many factors that change at the time of the onset of labour. Furthermore, the inhibition and promotion of certain factors can both delay or accelerate the process of parturition. It is unlikely that any one factor is sufficient to provide an explanation for the onset of labour as intervention at any one of several biochemical points can either stimulate or delay it.

It is likely that there is a cascade of events regulated and controlled by the fetoplacental unit. During pregnancy, uterine activity is present but is minimal. At the end of gestation, there is a gradual downregulation of those factors that keep the uterus and cervix quiescent and an upregulation of procontractile influences.

At term, the fetus increases its production of cortisol and this cortisol reduces the production of placental progesterone and increases the production of oestrone and oestradiol. Progesterone suppresses uterine activity and oestradiol increases it.

These changes also result in increased production of prostaglandins by the placenta and thus a further increase in myometrial activity.

These changes also stimulate oxytocin release, which also enhances myometrial activity.

At the cellular level, the myocytes both contract and shorten, unlike the process in striated muscle, where cells contract but then return to their precontraction length. The formation of gap junctions between myocytes allows communication between the cells and thus the production of co-ordinated contractions.

Gap junctions are composed of connexins (Cx), which are expressed throughout pregnancy but maximally during labour. Furthermore, ion channels within the myometrium play an important role in influencing activity by influencing the influx of calcium ions into the myocytes and promoting contraction of the myometrial cells.

The situation is further complicated by other hormones produced in the placenta that also act directly or indirectly on the myometrium, such as relaxin, activin A, follistatin, hCG and corticotrophin-releasing hormone (CRH).

The cervix contains myocytes and fibroblasts and serves to contain the products of conception. Towards term, the cervix becomes softened as there is a decrease in the amount of collagen and an increase in proteolytic enzyme activity. Increased production of hyaluronic acid reduces the affinity of fibronectin for collagen and, in conjunction with the affinity of hyaluronic acid for water, there is a consequent softening and ripening of the cervix.

Increasing cervical compliance allows progression of labour with reduced intrauterine pressure. The cervix also contracts during labour up to 3–4 cm dilatation but, in the active phase of labour, cervical dilatation occurs secondary to uterine contractions alone. In other words, the cervix is passively stretched by the increasing strength of the uterine contractions.

UTERINE ACTIVITY IN LABOUR – THE POWERS

The uterus exhibits infrequent, low-intensity contractions throughout pregnancy. As full term approaches, uterine activity increases in both the frequency and strength of contractions. With the onset of labour, intrauterine pressures rise to 20–30 mmHg during contractions that occur every 10–15 minutes and last approximately 30–40 seconds. Normal resting tonus in labour starts at around 10 mmHg and increases slightly during the course of labour. Contractions increase in intensity to reach pressures of 50 mmHg – around 5 kPa – in terms of active pressure in the first stage of labour (Fig. 12.1).

In the second stage, with the additional effect of voluntary expulsive efforts, intrauterine pressure may rise to 100 mmHg.

> ! In late pregnancy, strong contractions can sometimes be palpated that do not produce cervical dilatation, even when the cervix is normal and these do not constitute true labour.

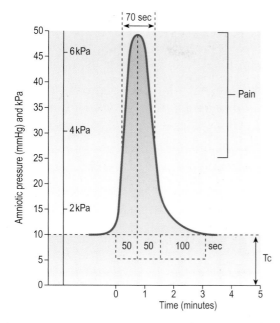

Fig. 12.1 Uterine contractions reach pressures of 50 mmHg (6.5 kPa) with first stage of labour. Contractions become painful when amniotic pressure exceeds 25 mmHg (3.2 kPa).

Throughout labour, contractions produce effacement and dilatation of the cervix as the result of shortening of myometrial fibres in the upper uterine segment and stretching and thinning of the lower uterine segment (Fig. 12.2). This process is known as *retraction*. The lower segment becomes elongated and thinned as labour progresses and the junction between the upper and lower segment rises in the abdomen. Where labour becomes obstructed, the junction of the upper and lower segments may become visible at the level of the umbilicus; this is known as a *retraction ring*.

Contractions are initiated by a pacemaker in the left uterine cornus and spread downwards through the myometrium. Contractions occur first in the fundus of the uterus, where they are stronger and last longer than in the lower segment. This phenomenon is known as *fundal dominance* and is essential to progressive effacement and dilatation of the cervix. As the uterus and the round ligaments contract, the axis of the uterus appears to straighten, pulling the longitudinal axis of the fetus towards the anterior abdominal wall in line with the inlet of the true pelvis.

The realignment of the uterine axis promotes descent of the presenting part as the fetus is pushed directly downwards into the pelvic cavity (Fig. 12.3).

THE PASSAGES

The shape and structure of the bony pelvis has already been described. Because of softening of the sacroiliac ligaments and the pubic symphysis, some expansion of the pelvic cavity can occur.

The soft tissues also become more distensible than in the non-pregnant state and substantial distension of the pelvic floor and vaginal orifice occurs during the descent and birth of the head. This commonly results in tearing of the perineum and of the vaginal walls and sometimes in tearing and disruption of the external anal sphincter.

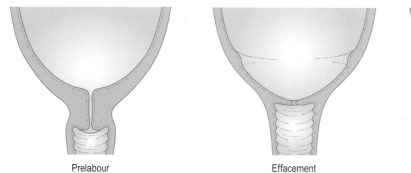
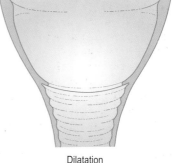

Prelabour   Effacement   Dilatation

Fig. 12.2 Effacement and dilatation of the cervix in labour with formation of the lower uterine segment.

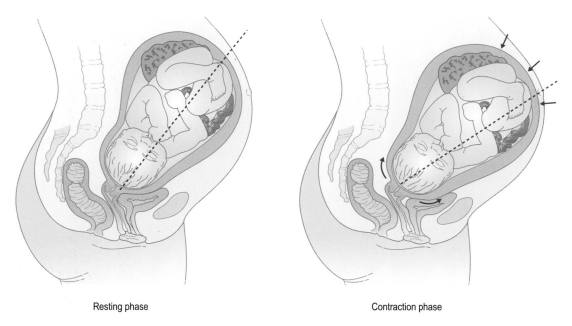

Resting phase   Contraction phase

Fig. 12.3 Change in direction of the fetal and uterine axis during contractions in labour.

THE MECHANISM OF LABOUR

The head normally engages in the pelvis in the transverse position and the passage of the head and trunk through the pelvis follows a well-defined pattern. The passage of the fetal head in normal labour requires that the head presents by the vertex and is well flexed, as not all diameters can enter the pelvic brim. A deflexed or extended head, such as occurs in the occipitoposterior position, or a brow presentation may either delay (with an occipitoposterior position) or prevent (with the brow presentation) entry of the head into the pelvic brim.

The process of normal labour therefore involves the adaptation of the fetal head to the various segments and diameters of the maternal pelvis and the following processes occur (Fig. 12.4):

1. **Descent** occurs throughout labour and is both a feature and a prerequisite for the birth of the baby. Engagement of the head normally occurs before the onset of labour in the primigravid woman but may not occur until labour is well established in a multipara. Descent of the head provides a measure of the progress of labour.

2. **Flexion** of the head occurs as it descends and meets the pelvic floor, bringing the chin into contact with the fetal thorax. Flexion produces a smaller diameter of presentation, changing from the occipitoposterior diameter, when the head is deflexed, to the suboccipitobregmatic diameter when the head is fully flexed.

3. **Internal rotation:** The head rotates as it reaches the pelvic floor and the occiput normally rotates anteriorly from the lateral position towards the pubic symphysis. Occasionally, it rotates posteriorly towards the hollow of the sacrum and the head may then deliver as a face-to-pubes delivery.

4. **Extension:** The acutely flexed head descends to distend the pelvic floor and the vulva, and the base of the occiput comes into contact with the inferior rami of the pubis. The head now extends until it is delivered. Maximal distension of the perineum and introitus accompanies the final expulsion of the head, a process that is known as *crowning*.

5. **Restitution:** Following delivery of the head, it rotates back to be in line with its normal relationship to the fetal shoulders.

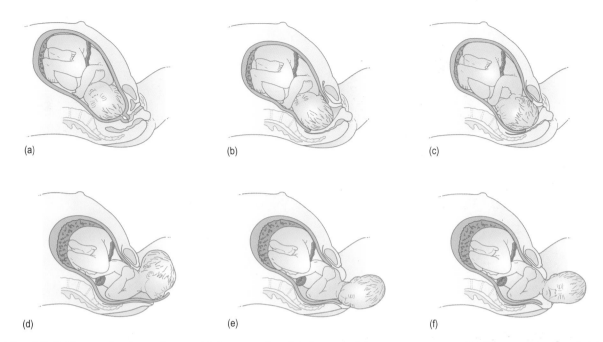

Fig. 12.4 The mechanisms of normal labour involve: (a) descent of the presenting part; (b) flexion of the head; (c) internal rotation; (d) distension of the perineum and extension of the fetal head; (e) delivery of the head; (f) delivery of the shoulders.

6. **External rotation:** When the shoulders reach the pelvic floor, they rotate into the anteroposterior diameter of the pelvis. This is accompanied by rotation of the fetal head so that the face looks laterally at the maternal thigh.

7. **Delivery of the shoulders:** Final expulsion of the trunk occurs following delivery of the shoulders. The anterior shoulder is delivered first by traction posteriorly on the fetal head so that the shoulder emerges under the pubic arch. The posterior shoulder is delivered by lifting the head anteriorly over the perineum and this is followed by rapid delivery of the remainder of the trunk and the lower limbs.

> **!** The occiput normally rotates anteriorly but, if it rotates posteriorly, it deflexes and presents a larger diameter to the pelvic cavity. As a result, the second stage may be prolonged and the damage to the perineum and vagina is increased.

THE THIRD STAGE OF LABOUR

The third stage of labour starts with the completed expulsion of the baby and ends with the delivery of the placenta and membranes (Fig. 12.5).

A fourth stage of labour is sometimes described as the time interval following expulsion of the placenta up to 6 hours after delivery. The implication of describing a fourth stage is to draw attention to the increased risk of abnormal haemorrhage that exists in the first few hours after delivery.

Once the baby is delivered, the uterine muscle contracts, shearing off the placenta and pushing it into the lower segment or the vault of the vagina.

The classic signs of placental separation include a show of bright blood, apparent lengthening of the umbilical cord and elevation of the uterine fundus within the abdominal cavity. The uterine fundus becomes tent shaped instead of globular and sits on top of the placenta as it descends into the lower segment.

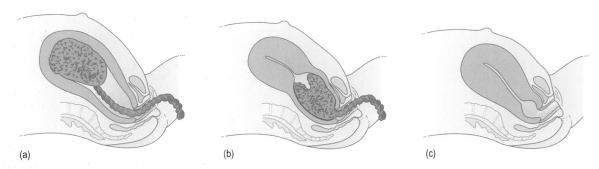

Fig. 12.5 The normal third stage: (a) separation of the placenta from the uterine wall; (b) expulsion into the lower uterine segment and upper vagina; (c) complete expulsion of the placenta from the genital tract.

The signs of placental separation may be compressed and obscured by the use of oxytocic drugs administered at the delivery of the anterior shoulder.

As the placenta is expelled, it is accompanied by the fetal membranes, although the membranes often become torn and may require additional traction or uterine exploration to complete their removal.

The whole process lasts between 5 and 10 minutes. If the placenta is not expelled within 30 minutes, the third stage should be considered to be abnormal.

PAIN IN LABOUR

Contractions in labour are commonly although not invariably associated with pain, particularly as they increase in strength and frequency (Fig. 12.1). The cause of pain is uncertain but it may be due to compression of nerve fibres in the cervical zone or to hypoxia of compressed muscle cells. Pain is felt in the lower abdomen and as lumbar backache and becomes apparent when the intrauterine pressure exceeds 25 mmHg.

THE MANAGEMENT OF NORMAL LABOUR

The primary aim of intrapartum care is to deliver a healthy baby to a healthy mother. The preparation of the mother for the process of parturition begins well before the onset of labour. It is important for the mother and her partner to understand what actually happens during the various stages of labour. Strategies to deal with pain in labour, including psychoprophy-laxis with controlled respiration, should be introduced during antenatal classes, as well as educating the mother about the regulation of expulsive efforts during the second stage of labour.

Antenatal classes should also include instructions about neonatal care and breastfeeding, although this is a process that requires reinforcement in the postdelivery period.

The mother should be advised to come into hospital, or to call the midwife in the event of a home birth, when contractions are at regular 10–15 minute intervals, when there is a show or if and when the membranes rupture. If the mother is in early labour, she should be encouraged to take a shower and to empty her bowels and bladder. Shaving of the pubic hair is no longer considered necessary unless there is a likelihood of delivery by caesarean section, in which case the abdomen should be shaved down to the pubic hairline.

It is common practice in the United Kingdom to organize 'domino' (*dom*iciliary *in* and *o*ut) deliveries, whereby the mother is discharged home 6 hours after delivery, provided that the delivery is uncomplicated.

Examination at the commencement of labour

On admission, the following examination should be performed:

- **Full general examination**, including temperature, pulse, respiration, blood pressure and state of hydration; the urine should be tested for glucose, ketone bodies and protein

- **Obstetrical examination of the abdomen:** inspection, palpation and auscultation to determine the fetal lie, presentation and position, and the station of the presenting part, as well as to determine the presence of a fetal heartbeat
- **Vaginal examination** in labour should be performed only after cleansing of the vulva and introitus and using an aseptic technique with sterile gloves and an antiseptic cream. Once the examination is started, the fingers should not be withdrawn from the vagina until the examination is completed.

The following factors should be noted:

- The consistency, effacement and dilatation of the cervix
- Whether the membranes are intact or ruptured and, if ruptured, the colour of the amniotic fluid
- The nature and presentation of the presenting part and its relationship to the level of the ischial spines
- Assessment of the bony pelvis and in particular of the pelvic outlet.

General principles of the management of the first stage of labour

The guiding principles of management are:

- Observation and intervention if the labour becomes abnormal
- Pain relief during labour and emotional support for the mother
- Adequate hydration throughout labour.

Observation – the use of the partogram

The introduction of graphic records has proved to be a major advance in the management of labour because it enables the early recognition of a labour that is becoming dysfunctional. The partogram (Fig. 12.6) is a single sheet of paper on which there is a graphic representation of progress in labour. The partogram should be started as soon as the mother is admitted to the delivery suite and this is recorded as zero time regardless of the time at which contractions started. However, the point of entry on to the partogram depends on a vaginal assessment at the time of admission to the delivery suite. The value of this type of record system is that it draws attention visually to any aberration from normal progress in labour.

The use of partograms at an applied level was first introduced in remote obstetric units in Africa, where recognition that progress in labour is becoming abnormal enables early transfer to specialist units before serious obstruction occurs.

This has led to a major reduction in maternal mortality. One colleague recounted a story to the authors of seeing an ambulance in the Sudan returning to a base hospital after a 2-day journey with two women, both of whom had died in obstructed labour. Earlier recognition of these obstructed labours could have prevented this tragedy.

Fetal condition

The fetal heart rate is charted as beats/minute and decelerations of heart rate that occur during contractions are recorded by an arrow down to the lowest heart rate recorded on the partogram. These records are an adjunct to the actual recording of fetal heart rate.

The time of rupture of the membranes and the nature of the amniotic fluid (i.e. whether it is clear or meconium-stained) are also recorded. Moulding of the fetal head and the presence of caput are also noted as they provide an indicator of obstructed labour.

Progress in labour

Progress in labour is measured by assessing the rate of cervical dilatation and descent of the presenting part. To assess the rate of progress, vaginal examination should be performed on admission to hospital and every 4 hours during the first stage of labour. Cervical dilatation is recorded in centimetres along the scale of 0–10 of the cervicograph and a plot of the cervical dilatation is recorded. The graph for progress in a normal labour is recorded on the chart.

Dilatation of the cervix occurs in two well-defined phases. The *latent phase* starts at the onset of labour and ends at 3 cm dilatation. This takes up some two thirds of the whole time of labour.

This is followed by the *active phase* that extends from the end of the latent phase until the onset of the second stage when full cervical dilatation has been reached.

If the dilatation of the cervix lags more than two hours behind the expected rate of dilatation, the labour is considered to be abnormal. The rate of dilatation increases rapidly during the active phase of labour

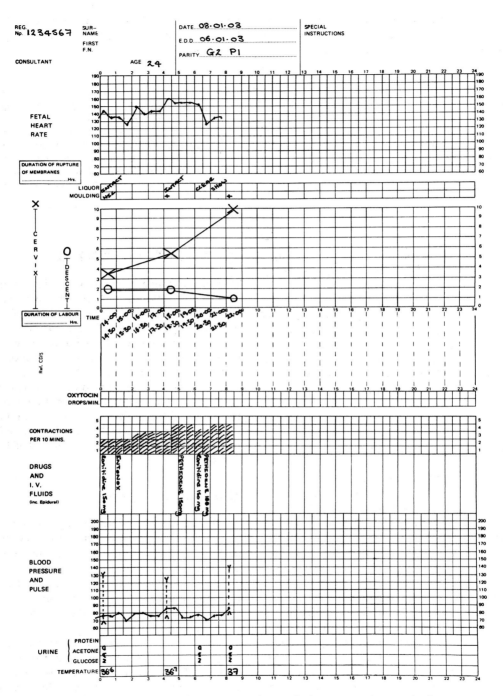

Fig. 12.6 The partogram is a complete visual record of measurements made during delivery (courtesy of Catherine Tamizian).

although it slows again near the phase of full cervical dilatation. The station of the head is also charted on the partogram using the following definitions (Fig. 12.6):

- If the head is high, the level is five-fifths above the pelvic brim
- If the head is just descending into the pelvic brim, it is four-fifths above the brim
- If less than half the head is through the brim, it is three fifths above the brim
- If more than half the head is through the brim it is two-fifths above the brim
- If just the base of the skull is palpable abdominally, it is one-fifth above the brim.

The station of the head is plotted on the 0–5 gradation of the partogram.

Descent is also recorded by assessing the level of the presenting part above or below the level of the ischial spines.

The nature and frequency of the uterine contractions are recorded on the chart by shading in the number of contractions per 10 minutes. Dotted squares indicate contractions of less than 20 seconds duration, cross-hatched squares are contractions between 20 and 40 seconds duration, while contractions lasting longer than 40 seconds are shown by complete shading of the squares.

Fluid and nutrition during labour

In most maternity units in the UK, caesarean section rates now exceed 20%. The issue of what can be taken by mouth becomes particularly important. If there is a likelihood that the mother will need operative delivery under general anaesthesia, then it is clearly important to avoid oral intake at any significant level during the first stage of labour. Delayed gastric emptying may result in vomiting and inhalation of vomitus if general anaesthesia for operative delivery is needed. On the other hand, most operative deliveries are now achieved under epidural anaesthesia and therefore there is a case for giving some fluids and light nutrition orally if labour is progressing normally and a vaginal delivery can be anticipated. Intravenous fluid replacement should be considered after 6 hours in labour if delivery is not imminent. Remember that the major cause of acidosis and ketosis is dehydration. If delivery is not imminent at the end of 6 hours, an intravenous infusion should be commenced with the alternative administration of normal saline 500 ml alternating with 500 ml of Hartmann's solution, the total not exceeding 1500 ml in 12 hours.

> The classic signs of dehydration in labour include tachycardia, mild pyrexia and loss of tissue turgor. Remember that labour can be hard physical work and that the environmental temperature of delivery rooms is often raised to meet the needs of the baby rather than the mother, leading to considerable insensible fluid loss.

PAIN RELIEF IN LABOUR

There are a number of strategies used in labour for the relief of pain. Essentially, these techniques are aimed at reducing the level of pain experienced in labour whilst invoking minimal risk for the mother and baby.

The level of pain experienced in labour varies widely with each mother. Some women experience very little pain whilst others suffer from abdominal and back pain of increasing intensity throughout their labours. Thus, any programme for pain relief must be tailored to the needs of the individual. Often a combination of methods will provide the best results. The only technique that can provide complete pain relief is epidural analgesia.

Narcotic analgesia

In the past, a variety of narcotic agents have been used for pain relief in labour and such agents are still widely used, particularly where epidural analgesia is not available.

Pethidine is the most widely used narcotic agent and is given in doses of 50–150 mg intramuscularly; the effects last about 2–3 hours, after which time the dose can be repeated.

Current evidence suggests that pethidine has a weak analgesic action but tends to reduce anxiety and discomfort. The unwanted side effects include nausea, vomiting and respiratory depression in both the mother and the baby. The effect on the neonate is particularly important when the drug is given within 2 hours of delivery. Pethidine is often administered with phenothiazines to reduce nausea.

Other opioids occasionally used in labour include papaveretum 10–20 mg, diamorphine 5–10 mg, pentazocine 30–60 mg, phenazocine 1–2 mg or oxymorphone 1–1.5 mg by intramuscular injection. However, the use of all these compounds, with the possible exception of pethidine, is becoming increasingly uncommon as the use of epidural analgesia increases.

The search for more effective agents continues and a new agent, remifentanil, has recently been evaluated. This is an ultra-short-acting opioid that produces superior analgesia to pethidine and has less effect on neonatal respiration.

Because some mothers are unsuitable for regional analgesia, opiates are likely to continue to play a significant role in pain relief in labour .

Inhalational analgesia

These agents are commonly reserved for use in the late first stage and in the second stage. The most widely used agent is Entonox, which is a 50/50 mixture of nitrous oxide and oxygen. The gas can be self-administered and is inhaled as soon as the contraction starts. Entonox is used in the UK by about 75% of mothers in labour and is effective in about 40%.

Other inhalation agents include trichloroethylene 0.3–0.5%, and methoxyflurane 0.35%, in air. These compounds take longer to achieve adequate analgesic concentrations because they have a high degree of solubility in body fat. They are effective in only 10% of women and their use has now been largely abandoned.

Nitrous oxide has been shown to have adverse effects on birth attendants if exposure is prolonged; these effects include decreased fertility, bone marrow changes and neurological changes. Forced air change every 6–10 hours is effective in reducing the nitrous oxide levels and should be mandatory in all delivery rooms.

Non-pharmacological methods

Transcutaneous electrical nerve stimulation (TENS) involves the placement of two pairs of TENS electrodes on the back on each side of the vertebral column at the levels of T10–L1 and S2–S4. Currents of 0–40 mA are applied at a frequency of 40–150 Hz. This can be effective in early labour but is often inadequate by itself in late labour. For the technique to be effective, antenatal training of the mother is essential.

Other non-invasive methods include massage and relaxation techniques.

Regional analgesia

Epidural analgesia is the most widely used form of regional analgesia. It is also the most effective way of relieving the pain of contractions, with complete relief of pain in 95% of labouring women.

The procedure may be instituted at any time and does not interfere with uterine contractility. It may reduce the desire to bear down in the second stage of labour.

A fine catheter is introduced into the lumbar epidural space and a local anaesthetic agent such as bupivacaine is injected (Fig. 12.7). The addition of an opioid to the local anaesthetic greatly reduces the dose requirement of bupivacaine, thus sparing the motor fibres to the lower limbs and reducing the classic complications of hypotension and abnormal fetal heart rate.

The procedure involves:

- Insertion of an intravenous cannula and preloading with no more than 500 ml of saline or Hartmann's solution
- Insertion of the epidural cannula at the L3–L4 interspace and injection of the local anaesthetic agent at the minimum dose required for effective pain relief

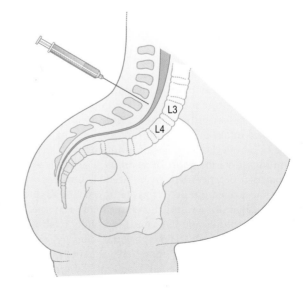

Fig. 12.7 Epidural anaesthesia is induced by injection of local anaesthetic agents into the lumbar epidural space.

- Monitor blood pressure, pulse rate and fetal heart rate and adjust maternal posture to achieve the desired analgesic effect.

The complications of epidural analgesia include:

- Hypotension – this can be avoided by preloading and the use of low-dose anaesthetic agents and opioid solutions
- Accidental dural puncture – occurs in fewer than 1% of epidurals
- Postdural headache – about 70% of mothers will develop a headache if a 16 or 18 gauge needle is used. A postdural headache that persists for more than 24 hours should be treated with an epidural blood patch.

Contraindications to regional anaesthesia include:

- Maternal refusal
- Coagulopathy
- Local or systemic infection
- Uncorrected hypovolaemia
- Inadequate or inexperienced staff or facilities.

> **!** Many women set out in labour without requesting any form of pain relief. However, as labour progresses, the realization that labour can be painful will change the requirements of the mother. It is therefore essential to have an epidural service that can be readily available so that the labour is not too far advanced before the epidural can become established.

Other forms of regional anaesthesia

Spinal anaesthesia is commonly used for operative delivery, particularly as a single-shot procedure. It is not used for the general control of pain in labour because of the superior safety of epidural analgesia.

Paracervical blockade involves the infiltration of local anaesthetic agents into the paracervical tissues. This is rarely used for obstetric procedures.

Pudendal nerve blockade involves infiltration around the pudendal nerve as it leaves the pudendal canal and the inferior haemorrhoidal nerve (Fig. 12.8). It was a

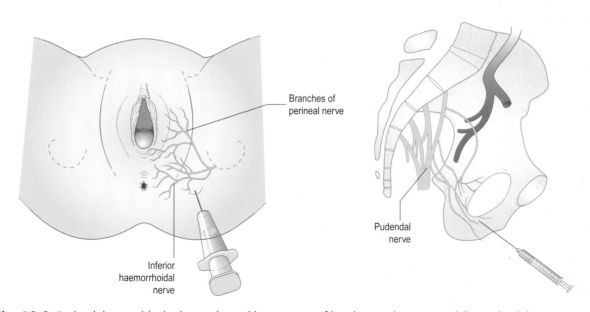

Branches of perineal nerve

Inferior haemorrhoidal nerve

Pudendal nerve

Fig. 12.8 Pudendal nerve blockade is achieved by injection of local anaesthetic around the pudendal nerve at the level of the ischial spine. Additional infiltration is used to block branches of the inferior haemorrhoidal and perineal nerves.

widely used form of local anaesthesia in the past but is now less frequently used as it has been replaced by epidural anaesthesia.

Infiltration directly into the perineal tissues over, for example, an episiotomy site is still widely used, particularly for the repair of perineal wounds. Great care must be taken to avoid a direct intravenous drug at the time of infusion and to limit the total amount of agent injected. Toxic symptoms such as cardiac arrhythmias and convulsions may result from anaesthetic over-dosage.

POSTURE IN LABOUR

Some women prefer to remain ambulant or to sit in a chair during the first stage of labour. However, most women prefer to lie down as labour advances into the second stage, although some will prefer to squat to use the forces of gravity to help expel the baby. This posture carries an increased risk of causing severe perineal damage if the delivery is uncontrolled. In the past, women who wish to have epidural anaesthesia were advised to remain supine because of temporary motor impairment. This problem can now be reduced by the use of low-dose anaesthesia combined with opiates.

Water births

Immersion of the mother in a water bath is a common option for pain relief, on the basis that flotation improves support of the pregnant uterus. However, delivery should not occur in the bath, as it may result in the baby inhaling the bath water with the first breath, with changes in the lungs that are characteristic of drowning.

FETAL MONITORING

The term 'fetal distress' is used to describe certain changes in the fetal heart rate, the passage of meconium-stained liquor (fetal bowel motion) and excessive fetal movements that have traditionally been used to describe the signs of fetal asphyxia. However, these signs all occur in normal circumstances, so at best they represent changes that occur in response to a transitory situation. Diminution of fetal movements may also indicate fetal jeopardy and cessation of movements may indicate death.

Intermittent auscultation

During labour, the fetal heart rate can be monitored every 15 minutes using a Pinard fetal stethoscope and contractions are monitored by manual palpation. There are, however, no trials that address the issue of how frequently intermittent auscultation should be performed. The general recommendation is that the heart rate should be recorded every 15 minutes in the first stage and after each contraction in the second stage.

The clinical guidelines for the use of electronic fetal monitoring produced by the Royal College of Obstetricians and Gynaecologists in May 2001 concluded that there is no place for either admission cardiotocogram or routine cardiotocography using electronic monitoring where the labour is classified as low risk. However, there are specific indications for electronic fetal monitoring; these are shown in Table 12.1.

Table 12.1	
Indications for the use of continuous electronic fetal monitoring	
Maternal	**Fetal**
Previous caesarian section	Fetal growth restriction
Pre-eclampsia	Prematurity
Post-term pregnancy	Oligohydramnios
Prolonged rupture of the membranes	Abnormal Doppler artery velocimetry
Induced labour	Multiple pregnancy
Diabetes	Meconium-stained liquor
Antepartum haemorrhage	Breech presentation
Other maternal medical diseases	

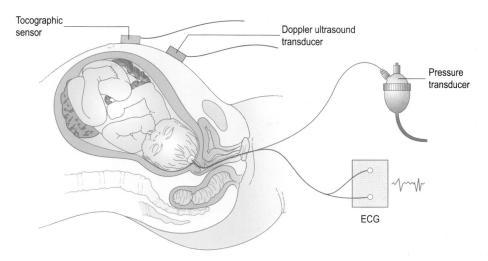

Fig. 12.9 Monitoring during labour – contractions are recorded by intra- and extrauterine tocography; the fetal heart rate is recorded externally by Doppler ultrasonography or by direct application of an ECG electrode to the presenting part.

Fetal cardiotocography

Electronic fetal monitoring enables continuous monitoring of the fetal heart rate and the frequency and strength of uterine contractions (cardiotocography; CTG). The heart rate of the fetus is usually calculated using a Doppler ultrasound transducer, which is applied externally to the maternal abdomen. The signals that are detected are those of cardiac movement and what is actually measured is the time interval between cardiac cycles. Traditionally, this is converted to heart rate. The heart rate can also be measured from the R wave obtained from the fetal electrocardiogram by direct application of an electrode to the presenting part.

Uterine pressure is recorded either with a pressure transducer applied over the anterior abdominal wall or by inserting a fluid-filled catheter or a pressure sensor into the uterine cavity through the cervical canal (Fig. 12.9).

Basal heart rate

The definition of normality in the pattern of the fetal heart rate is easier than defining what is abnormal. The normal heart rate varies between 110 and 160 beats per minute. There is some variation in this, some

definitions defining normality as 110–180 beats/min (Fig. 12.10).

A rate faster than 160 is defined as *fetal tachycardia* and a rate less than 110 is *fetal bradycardia*. The heart rate exhibits variations from the baseline, which is known as *baseline variability*. Although there is variability on a

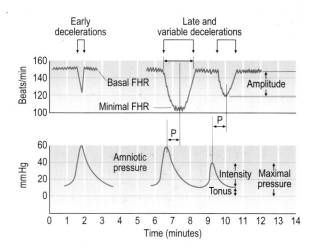

Fig. 12.10 Patterns of fetal heart rate change and amniotic pressure change in labour.

beat-to-beat basis, this is not what is recorded by the standard cardiotocograph and cannot be recorded at the standard paper speed of 1 cm/min. Baseline variability is a record of the oscillations in heart rate around the baseline heart rate and normally varies between 10 and 25 beats/min.

A 'silent' fetal heart rate with a variability of less than 5 beats/min is abnormal and may indicate fetal jeopardy (Table 12.2).

Transient changes in fetal heart rate

Accelerations

Accelerations are defined as increases in heart rate of more than 15 beats/min for more than 15 seconds and are associated with fetal movements. Accelerations are a reassuring sign of good fetal health.

Decelerations

Decelerations are defined as decreases in heart rate of more than 15 beats/min for more than 15 seconds. These are defined both by their relationship to uterine contractions and by their intensity; some patterns of change are generally considered to have clinical significance in relation to hypoxia (Fig. 12.10).

Early decelerations

Based on the early classifications, these are sometimes known as type 1 decelerations and are synchronous with uterine contractions. The nadir of the deceleration occurs at the peak of the contraction and the decrease in heart rate is generally less than 40 beats/min. These decelerations are generally due to head compression and cord compression and are commonly considered to be physiological. They are a common form of deceleration seen in labour.

Late decelerations

Sometimes defined as type II decelerations, the onset of the slowing of heart rate occurs well after the contraction is established and does not return to the normal baseline until at least 20 seconds after the contraction is completed.

Late decelerations are a less common form of deceleration and have more sinister connotations, as they are indicative of fetal hypoxia.

Variable decelerations

Variable decelerations vary in timing and amplitude, hence their name. An early deceleration where the heart rate falls by more than 40 beats/min is also classified as a variable deceleration. The commonest cause is cord compression and the changes may be considered to be pathological if the cord compression is persistent.

> ! The interpretation of the CTG now forms a major focus for litigation in cases of cerebral palsy and mental handicap. It is essential that, where electronic monitoring is employed, any birth attendant responsible for intrapartum care should understand how to interpret the CTG and should be able to take the appropriate action. The action needed where there is a significant abnormality of heart rate will be either to take a fetal blood sample for acid–base status or to expedite delivery.

The fetal electrocardiogram

The fetal electrocardiogram (ECG) can be recorded from scalp electrodes or by the placement of maternal abdominal electrodes. Although the QRS complex is usually clearly visible, other details of the ECG are often obscured by electrical noise.

Modern filtering and computer averaging techniques have now largely overcome these problems so that continuous real-time monitoring of all the variables of the fetal ECG morphology and time intervals is possible.

Table 12.2 Fetal heart rate definitions		
Definition		**Heart rate (beats/min)**
Baseline rate		
Normal		110–160
Tachycardia	– Moderate	160–180
	– Severe	> 180
Bradycardia	– Moderate	100–110
	– Severe	< 100
Baseline variability		
Normal	> 5	
Reduced	3–5	
Absent	< 3	

Two features have emerged using these techniques. First, the relationship between the height of the T wave and the QRS height has been shown to be related to acidosis and second, the relationship between the lengths of the PR interval and the RR interval has been shown to change in the presence of asphyxia.

The fetal ECG can also be used to identify the nature of fetal arrhythmias, although this does not involve the use of averaging techniques.

Fetal acid–base balance

Where abnormalities of fetal heart rate occur in labour, they may provide an indication of fetal acidosis but, to confirm these findings, the fetal acid base status should be examined.

Fetal blood sampling was introduced in the late 1960s by Eric Saling in Berlin and the technique is now a standard part of labour ward management.

Fetal blood is obtained directly from the scalp or buttocks through an amnioscope. The instrument is inserted through the cervix, which must be at least 2 cm dilated. The mother is put into the lithotomy position or may lie in the lateral supine position. The latter is preferable as it will avoid the risk of inducing supine hypotension. A small stab incision is made in the fetal scalp and blood is collected into a heparinized capillary tube. The sample is then analysed in a blood gas analyser.

A pH between 7 and 7.25 in the first stage of labour indicates mild acidosis; normal pH lies between 7.25 and 7.35. If the pH is less than 7.25, sampling should be repeated within the next hour. If there is sufficient sample, a full blood gas analysis should be performed, as a raised P_{CO_2} may indicate a respiratory acidosis that may correct itself if the posture of the mother is changed.

A value of less than 7.20 in the first stage of labour generally indicates a significant degree of acidosis and should be considered as an indication for delivery, unless delivery is imminent with the cervix near full dilatation.

MANAGEMENT OF THE SECOND STAGE OF LABOUR

The onset of the second stage of labour is heralded by a desire to bear down and, on occasions, to vomit. The recognition that the second stage of labour has been reached can be confirmed by vaginal examination; the cervix is no longer palpable as it has reached full dilatation.

The second stage of labour normally lasts up to 2 hours in the primigravida and up to 1 hour in the multiparous woman. If progress is delayed beyond these times, it is important to look for a reason for the delay, such as cephalopelvic disproportion, fetal malposition or poor expulsive forces.

Progress in the second stage is assessed by descent of the presenting part and by the degree of distension of the perineum.

The desire to bear down may not be present or may be weakened by epidural analgesia; in this situation the onset of the second stage of labour can only be identified by vaginal examination and the recognition of full cervical dilatation.

Practical procedures – preparation for delivery

The attendant scrubs and puts on a sterile gown and gloves. The mother is commonly placed in the left lateral supine position or semi-sitting position. Some women are delivered in the lithotomy position, particularly where instrumental delivery is likely to be necessary, and other women elect to deliver in the squatting position, either in a birthing chair or on their own. As the head is pushed down with each contraction, it distends the perineum and anus.

The anus is covered with a pad and the descent of the occiput is controlled with the left hand, the head being kept well flexed until crowning occurs, when it is allowed to extend as the perineum sweeps over the face. This process helps to minimize perineal damage. As the head delivers, the eyes and nasopharynx are cleared, using either a swab or, in the case of the nasopharynx, a suction pipette. Aspiration is particularly important when the amniotic fluid is meconium-stained in order to prevent meconium aspiration when the first breath occurs (Fig. 12.11).

If the perineum appears to be tearing, an episiotomy is performed, the incision being made in the mediolateral direction from the midpoint of the posterior margin of the introitus (Fig. 12.12). With the next contraction, the head is gently pulled towards the perineum until the anterior shoulder is delivered under the subpubic arch and then pulled anteriorly to deliver the posterior shoulder and the remainder of the trunk.

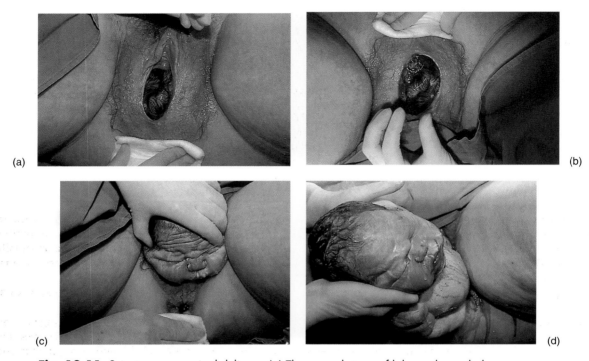

(a)

(b)

(c)

(d)

Fig. 12.11 Spontaneous vaginal delivery. (a) The second stage of labour, the scalp becomes visible with contractions and expulsive efforts by the mother. (b) Crowning of the head. (c) At delivery, the head is in the anteroposterior position. (d) Delivery of the head and shoulders.

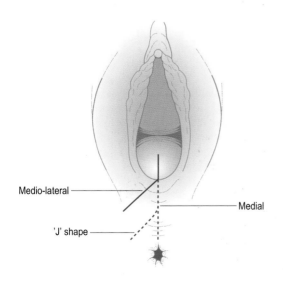

Medio-lateral

Medial

'J' shape

Fig. 12.12 Sites for episiotomy incisions: the object is to avoid extension of the incision or tear into the anal sphincter or rectum.

The umbilical cord is clamped twice and cut between the two clamps. There is no need to rush at this stage as a small delay will enable further blood in the placenta to be expressed into the baby's circulation. The infant will normally cry immediately after birth but if respiration is delayed for more than 1 minute, the nasopharynx should be aspirated again and the baby's lungs inflated with oxygen using a face mask in the first instance. If the onset of respiration is further delayed, endotracheal intubation and ventilation becomes necessary.

The condition of the baby is assessed at 1, 5 and 10 minutes (if the baby is depressed) using the Apgar scoring system (Table 12.3).

MANAGEMENT OF THE THIRD STAGE

The mother is turned on to her back if she is not already in the supine position. A dish is placed under the cord and below the introitus and the buttocks to collect any blood loss. The left hand is rested on the abdomen, on

Table 12.3
Evaluation of the Apgar score

	0	1	2
Colour	White	Blue	Pink
Tone	Flaccid	Rigid	Normal
Pulse	Impalpable	<100 beats/min	>100 beats/min
Respiration	Absent	Irregular	Regular
Response	Absent	Poor	Normal

the uterine fundus. An oxytocic drug such as Synto-metrine, a combination of 0.5 mg ergometrine and 5 IU oxytocin, is given intramuscularly or intravenously with the crowning of the head or birth of the anterior shoulder. On occasion either 5 or 10 IU of Syntocinon is given. This will cause the uterus to contract firmly shortly after delivery of the fetus and thus minimize the risk of postpartum haemorrhage.

As soon as the uterus is contracted, cord traction is applied with the right hand while monitoring fundal descent and applying counterpressure against the uterus (Fig. 12.13). This is known as the Brandt–Andrews technique. Assisted delivery of the placenta is usually completed within 5 minutes of delivery.

The placenta and membranes are checked to see if any cotyledons are missing and whether the membranes are complete. The blood loss is recorded.

Repair of perineal damage

If there is an episiotomy or tear, this is now repaired. Vaginal tears generally occur directly posteriorly towards the anus, whereas the episiotomy wound is usually directed mediolaterally to avoid damage to the anal sphincter.

The episiotomy or tear may be first-degree, second-degree, third-degree or fourth-degree.

A first-degree tear describes damage to vaginal and perineal skin. The second-degree tear involves the posterior vaginal wall and the underlying levator and perineal muscles but not involving the anal sphincter. Third-degree tears involve the anal sphincter, with either total or partial damage to the sphincter. The fourth degree involves the anal sphincter and a tear into the rectal mucosa.

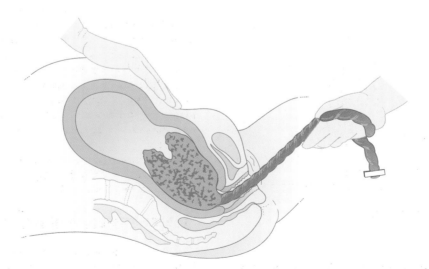

Fig. 12.13 Brandt–Andrews technique for assisted delivery of the placenta: the uterine fundus must be contracted before this technique is attempted.

It is always essential to check that the anal sphincter is intact, as primary repair is the treatment of choice. The sphincter ends often retract and are difficult to see but can be palpated as a small pit in the perianal zone.

The woman is placed in the lithotomy position so that a good view of the extent of the wound can be obtained.

The wound is infiltrated with local anaesthesia and a tagged pack is inserted into the vagina to keep the operative field clear of blood (Fig. 12.14).

Closure of the vaginal wound requires a clear view of the apex of the incision, as it is important to close the wound from the apex down to the introitus. The vaginal wound can be closed by interrupted absorbable sutures or by continuous locking sutures. Apposition of the perineal muscles is completed by the insertion of interrupted absorbable suture, and haemostasis is secured.

The perineal skin may be closed by non-absorbable sutures, which are removed 5 days later, or by absorbable sutures, either interrupted or continuous subcuticular sutures, which do not need to be removed.

If the tear is third- or fourth-degree, repair should be performed by an experienced obstetrician in an operating theatre under good surgical lights. The ends of the sphincter are identified and an overlap repair is performed.

On completion of the procedure:

• Remove the pack
• Ensure that the vagina is not constricted and that it admits two fingers easily
• Perform a rectal examination and make sure that none of the sutures have penetrated the rectal mucosa. If this occurs, the suture must be removed. If it is left in situ, it may result in the formation of a rectovaginal fistula.

> **!** Accurate repair of an episiotomy is important. Over-vigorous suturing of the wound or shortening of the vagina may result in dyspareunia and sexual dysharmony with the partner. Failure to recognize and repair damage to the anal sphincter may result in varying degrees of incontinence of flatus and faeces.

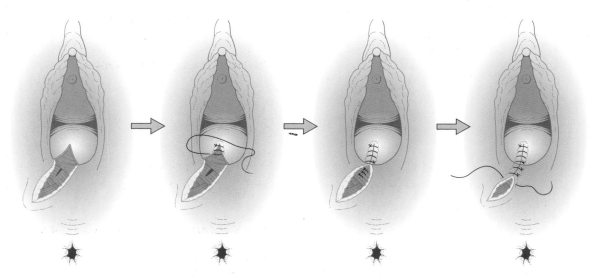

Fig. 12.14 Repair of the episiotomy: the posterior vaginal wall may be closed with continuous or interrupted sutures; apposition of the cut levator muscle ensures haemostasis before skin closure. (a) Episiotomy wound. (b) Continuous suture of posterior vaginal wall. (c) Interrupted sutures into the cut edge of the levator. (d) Interrupted suture into the perineal skin.

ESSENTIAL INFORMATION

- Normal labour:
  - Labour resulting in vaginal delivery
  - < 24 h in a primigravida
  - < 12 h in multigravida
- Three stages
  - First stage – onset to full dilatation
  - Second stage – full dilatation to delivery
  - Third stage – delivery to expulsion of the placenta
- Onset of labour
  - Regular painful contractions

Initiation of labour

- Complex interaction of fetal and maternal factors
- Principal components:
  - Interaction of progesterone/oestradiol
  - Increased fetal cortisol
  - Local activity of prostaglandins
- Effects on myometrium of relaxin, activin A, follistatin, hCG and CRH
- A 'show'
- Rupture of fetal membranes

Uterine activity

- Increasing strength/frequency contractions
- Normal resting tonus increases slightly during labour
- Contractions cause shortening of myometrial cells
- Effacement and dilatation of the cervix
- Fundal dominance necessary for progression

The passages

- Softening of pelvic ligaments
- Increased distensibility of pelvic floor

The mechanism of normal labour

The fetal head adapts by:
- Descent throughout labour
- Flexion – to minimize diameter of presentation
- Internal rotation – as head reaches pelvic floor
- Extension – with delivery of head
- Restitution – head in line with shoulders
- External rotation – shoulders descend into pelvis
- Delivery of shoulders

The third stage

Following delivery:
- Placenta shears off uterine wall
- Uterus expels placenta into lower segment
- Oxytocic drugs given with delivery of the anterior shoulder
- Assisted delivery of placenta
- Check placenta

Separation associated with:

- Lengthening of cord
- Elevation of uterine fundus
- Show of blood

Management of labour

- Observation and use of partogram
- Fluid balance and nutrition in labour
- Pain relief:
  - Narcotic agents
  - Inhalation analgesia
  - Non-pharmacological methods
  - Regional analgesia

Fetal monitoring in labour

- Fetal cardiotocography
- Basal heart rate
- Transitory changes
- Accelerations
- Decelerations
- The fetal electrocardiogram
- Fetal acid–base changes
- Scalp blood sampling

Management of the second stage

- Delivery of the head
- Controlled descent
- Minimizing perineal damage
- Clamping the cord
- Evaluation of Apgar score

Management of the third stage

- Recognition of placental separation
- Assisted delivery of the placenta with cord traction
- Routine use of oxytocic agents with crowning of the head

Repair of perineal damage

- Four degrees of perineal damage
- Third and fourth degree tears should be repaired by experienced staff
- Following repair, check:
  - No retained swabs
  - No rectal suture
  - Vagina not abnormally constricted

These drugs have various rather sinister maternal side effects and hence must be used with caution. The side effects include palpitations and tremor, ischaemic arrhythmias, pulmonary oedema and sometimes sudden death.

The most commonly used drugs are ritodrine, salbutamol and terbutaline. The drugs should not be used where there is a known history of cardiovascular disease.

The drugs are administered diluted in 5% dextrose or dextrose/saline and the infusion rate should be incrementally increased every 10–20 minutes until contractions are reduced to one every 15 minutes, or until the maternal heart rate has reached 140 beats/min. Careful monitoring of maternal pulse rate, blood pressure and plasma electrolytes is essential.

Beta-adrenergic drugs can cause hypokalaemia and hyperglycaemia.

The dosage can be reduced slowly after the administration of corticosteroids to the mother to minimize the risk of neonatal respiratory distress syndrome. It is unlikely that any benefit will accrue to the fetus if the gestational age exceeds 34 weeks. It may also be necessary to continue the treatment until the mother can be transferred to a tertiary care centre. The value of oral therapy remains unproven.

Prostaglandin synthetase inhibitors

Drugs such as indocid (indomethacin) inhibit prostaglandin production and thus uterine activity. These drugs are very effective in preventing the progression of labour. However, they also result in in-utero closure of the ductus arteriosus and may therefore adversely affect the fetal circulation. Nevertheless, there may be occasions when they are the drug of choice and where the premature delivery of the infant constitutes a greater risk than the not invariable early closure of the ductus.

Indomethacin also reduces liquor volume by its effect on fetal renal function, so may be of additional benefit in cases of polyhydramnios.

Magnesium sulphate

In vitro, magnesium sulphate can completely inhibit uterine activity. It achieves this effect by changing the uptake of calcium in smooth muscle cells.

The hazards of magnesium sulphate administration are respiratory depression, cardiac arrest, pulmonary oedema, paralysis, tetany, hypotension and paralytic ileus.

These side effects can be avoided by carefully programmed administration of the compound and the avoidance of administration to women with muscle disorders and renal impairment.

Magnesium is always administered as magnesium sulphate, with an initial loading dose of 4–6 g over 30 minutes followed by 2–3 g/h with an increase of 0.5 g/h until uterine quiescence or side effects are achieved. A maximum plasma concentration of 7 mg/dl should be achieved and, if this is not effective, the regime should be discontinued. The effectiveness of magnesium sulphate in delaying the onset of labour when used prophylactically is uncertain.

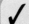
Loss of deep tendon reflexes indicates magnesium toxicity.

Calcium antagonists

The effect of slow calcium channel blockers in inhibiting uterine activity is not in doubt. There has been some evidence in animal studies using very large doses of these compounds, in particular nifedipine, that they may cause rib fusions in the fetus if given during the period of organogenesis. However, if the drugs are administered in the late second and third trimesters, this is well past this period and there is no evidence that they pose a threat.

Nifedipine is administered with a starting dose of 20 mg followed by 10–20 mg 4–6-hourly thereafter. Severe side effects are rare.

Calcium antagonists are not licensed for use in pregnancy in the UK.

Corticosteroids

The use of corticosteroids in the prevention of respiratory distress is based on the action of these compounds in enhancing the production of surfactant, thus enabling rapid expansion of the alveoli at the time of delivery and the establishment of normal respiratory function. Controlled trials on the antenatal effects of corticosteroids in preterm infants have shown that there are significant reductions in respiratory distress syndrome, periventricular haemorrhage and necrotizing enterocolitis.

The dosage of betametasone (betamethasone) or dexamethasone is given on the basis of 12 mg 12-hourly by intramuscular injection on three occasions. Optimal benefit can be achieved if delivery is postponed for at least 24 hours and up to 7 days. Over 34 weeks gestation, the administration of corticosteroids is not justified. The production of phosphatidylcholine can also be enhanced by the administration of thyrotrophin-releasing hormone (TRH) to the mother.

> **!** Failure to prescribe corticosteroids before delivery between 28 and 34 weeks may now be considered to be negligent.

Method of delivery

On many occasions, it may not be either possible or desirable to inhibit labour. There are only a few occasions, when the gestation is over 34 weeks, when the benefits of intervention outweigh those of allowing the labour to proceed. If the contractions are strong and frequent and the cervix is more than 5 cm dilated on admission, there is little likelihood in any case that labour can be stopped. Furthermore, if the membranes have ruptured and there has been any antepartum bleeding, it may be safer for the fetus to be delivered and the only decision to be made is whether short-term inhibition of contractions to enable the administration of corticosteroids is worthwhile.

There is no proven evidence that the use of forceps or a wide episiotomy improves fetal outcome in the presence of a vertex presentation, although it is important that delivery should be as gentle and controlled as possible. If the perineum is tight, it is not sensible to allow the soft, premature skull to be battered on the perineum for a long period and a sudden expulsive delivery may produce intracranial bleeding. In other words, while routine forceps delivery is not now advocated, a gentle controlled delivery should be the norm.

However, in the presence of a breech presentation, delivery by caesarean section is the preferred option unless the gestational length is greater than 34 weeks. Although there are no randomized studies of any size available, several large studies on the outcome comparing vaginal breech delivery and delivery by caesarean section overwhelming favour delivery by caesarean section in terms of perinatal mortality and in terms of long term neurological deficits. The reason for this is that up to 34 weeks, the head is relatively larger than the trunk so that the fetal trunk may be pushed through an incompletely dilated cervix resulting in delays in delivery and sudden compression and decompression of the head.

PREMATURE RUPTURE OF THE MEMBRANES (PROM)

Preterm labour is associated with PROM, but spontaneous rupture of the membranes may not result in the premature onset of labour. Factors that determine when the membranes rupture are:

- The tensile strength of the fetal membranes, which may be weakened by infection
- The support of the surrounding tissues, which is reflected in the dilatation of the cervix – the greater the dilatation of the cervix, the greater the likelihood that the membranes will rupture
- The intra-amniotic fluid pressure.

Pathogenesis

Premature rupture of the membranes has been shown to be associated with first and second trimester haemorrhage and, less predictably, with smoking. However, the most common factor is infection. Various organisms have been described in this context; these include group B haemolytic streptococci, *C. trachomatis* and those organisms causing bacterial vaginosis.

Management

The risks to the mother and baby are those of infection. However, long-term drainage of amniotic fluid may result in fetal pulmonary dysplasia. The difficulty is to decide both when to deliver the fetus and how to effect delivery, as the uterus is sometimes resistant to the action of oxytocic agents.

The mother will usually observe the sudden loss of amniotic fluid from her vagina. On admission to hospital, a speculum examination should be performed to confirm the presence of amniotic fluid, although sometimes it can be difficult to confirm the diagnosis. The use of Nitrazine sticks is of limited value and tests using more specific markers based on the presence of alpha-fetoprotein and insulin-like growth factor (IGF) are not widely used because of their cost.

 Avoid digital examination if the woman is not in labour, to reduce the risk of introducing infection.

Where there is doubt, it is better to assume that the membranes have ruptured and to continue observation until there is no evidence of continuing drainage of fluid and ultrasound confirms the presence of normal quantities of amniotic fluid in the amniotic sac.

If there is clear evidence of amniotic fluid in the vagina, swabs should be taken for culture. Maternal infection may result in uterine tenderness and pyrexia as well as the presence of a purulent vaginal discharge. Monitoring for the presence of maternal sepsis is best performed by the measurement of C-reactive protein. Persistent levels above 20 mg/l suggest the presence of infection.

 Corticosteroids may cause an increase in maternal white blood count.

If there is a positive culture or evidence of maternal infection, the appropriate antibiotic should be administered. If there is persistent infection, labour should be induced using an oxytocic infusion. If there is no evidence of infection, conservative management with erythromycin cover should be adopted. Tocolysis is generally ineffective in the presence of ruptured membranes if contractions are already well established. In any case, it is rarely indicated after 28 weeks gestation as the infant probably has a better chance of survival if delivered. Most women with PROM will deliver spontaneously within 48 hours.

PROLONGED PREGNANCY

The terms 'prolonged pregnancy', 'post-dates pregnancy' and 'post-term pregnancy' are all used to describe any

Case study
Premature rupture of the membranes

Janet S was 26 weeks into her second pregnancy when she noted that her underwear was wet. She had had one previous pregnancy, which had been terminated at 14 weeks gestation. She was living with her partner, who was unemployed. She smoked 10 cigarettes a day and lived on social security.

On admission to hospital, abdominal examination revealed a pregnancy consistent with her ultrasound dates at 26 weeks. The fetus was presenting by the breech. Speculum examination revealed the presence of clear amniotic fluid in the vagina. The cervix was closed. Swabs taken from the fluid were negative on culture.

A conservative approach to management was adopted. One week later, Janet began to have contractions. A decision was made to inhibit the contractions using a beta-sympathomimetic agonist in the form of ritodrine by the intravenous route.

A further swab was taken and on this occasion a growth of *Streptococcus faecalis* was obtained. Janet was started on ampicillin pending the return of the sensitivity report. The contractions moderated in frequency and she was given two injections of dexamethasone over the next 24 hours. Thirty six hours later, contractions started again and, on this occasion, the decision was made to deliver the child by caesarean section, in view of the breech presentation. Delivery was made through a classic vertical incision as there was no formation of the lower uterine segment. The baby weighed 860 g at birth and, apart from some mild respiratory difficulties over the first week of life, made an uneventful recovery and appeared to be progressing normally at the end of the first year of life.

pregnancy that exceeds 294 days from the first day of the last menstrual period in a woman with a regular 28-day cycle.

The term 'postmaturity' refers to the condition of the infant and has characteristic features (Table 13.1). These

Table 13.1
Postmaturity syndrome

Clinical features

- Dry, peeling and cracked skin, particularly on the hands and feet
- Absence of vernix caseosa and lanugo (fine hair)
- Loss of subcutaneous fat
- Meconium staining of the skin

Complications

- Increased perinatal mortality
- Intrapartum fetal distress
- Increased operative delivery rate
- Meconium aspiration

are all indicators of intrauterine malnutrition and may therefore occur at any stage of the pregnancy if there is placental dysfunction.

The accurate diagnosis of prolonged pregnancy varies with the method of dating. On the basis of the date of the last menstrual period, the incidence is about 10% but by using accurate ultrasound dating this figure can be reduced to 1%. This provides a strong case for routine ultrasound dating in early pregnancy, before 18 weeks gestation.

Aetiology

Prolonged pregnancy can be considered as one end of the spectrum of normal pregnancy. However, the condition may be familial and is sometimes associated with abnormalities of the adrenal–pituitary axis, as in anencephaly.

Evidence in many large studies does suggest an increase in perinatal mortality after 42 weeks; this is partly associated with difficult labours associated with macrosomia, which is at least three times commoner than in infants born at term.

Management

Prolonged pregnancy still constitutes the commonest indication for induction of labour. A routine policy of induction of labour is not advisable because of the risk of failed induction and the need for caesarean section should labour become prolonged or fetal or maternal distress develop.

Postmaturity is often associated with oligohydramnios, an increased incidence of meconium in the amniotic fluid and an increased risk of intrauterine aspiration of meconium-stained fluid into the fetal lungs. Unexpected stillbirth in such prolonged pregnancies is a particular tragedy for the mother, as she and her obstetrician will always live with the knowledge that the child would almost certainly have survived had action been taken earlier.

On the other side of the balance is the knowledge that unnecessary intervention is associated with higher morbidity and mortality in both mother and the fetus. It is therefore particularly important to take the mother's views into consideration. Often, social arrangements have been made that are disrupted by an abnormally prolonged pregnancy. The obstetrician is ill-advised to fail to take action if the mother requests delivery and the pregnancy is ultrasound-dated. On the other hand, if the mother does not want any intervention, careful observation of the fetus should be undertaken, with cardiotocograms and biophysical profiles on a twice-weekly basis.

Should the decision be made to induce labour, this may in itself prove difficult, as the cervix is often unripe and closed, with a Bishop's score of less than 3. In these circumstances, cervical ripening with prostaglandins should be attempted. If this fails and the infant is large, it may on occasions be preferable to deliver the child by elective caesarean section.

Careful observation during labour is mandatory, as these are high-risk pregnancies. Prompt aspiration of the nasopharynx at birth should be routine, although it will not prevent meconium aspiration where this has already occurred in utero.

INDUCTION OF LABOUR

Labour is induced when the risk to the mother or child of continuing the pregnancy exceeds the risks of inducing labour. The incidence of induction varies widely according to the practice of the obstetrician.

Indications

The major indications for induction of labour are:

- Pre-eclampsia
- Prolonged pregnancy (in excess of 42 weeks gestation)

- Placental insufficiency and intrauterine growth restriction
- Antepartum haemorrhage – placental abruption and antepartum haemorrhage of uncertain origin
- Rhesus isoimmunization
- Diabetes mellitus
- Chronic renal disease.

Prolonged pregnancy is defined as pregnancy exceeding 294 days from the first day of the last menstrual period in a woman with a 28-day cycle. The perinatal mortality rate doubles after 42 weeks and trebles after 43 weeks compared with 40 weeks gestation. However, routine induction of labour has a minimal effect on the perinatal mortality rate. Conservative management of prolonged pregnancy involves frequent monitoring of the fetus with ultrasound assessment of liquor volume and induction if there is evidence of fetoplacental compromise. However, many women request induction of labour on the basis of the physical discomfort of the continuing pregnancy.

Cervical assessment

Clinical assessment of the cervix enables prediction of the likely outcome of induction of labour. The most commonly used method of assessment is the Bishop score (Table 13.2). This score involves clinical examination of the cervix.

A score of more than 6 is strongly predictive of labour following induction. A score of less than 5 indicates the need for cervical ripening.

Methods of induction

The method of induction will be determined by whether membranes are still intact and cervical assessment.

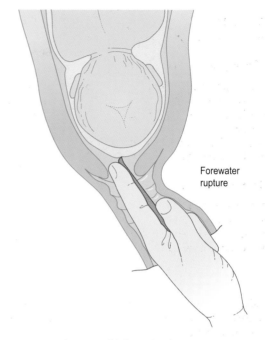

Forewater rupture

Fig. 13.4 Induction of labour by forewater rupture.

Forewater rupture

Rupture of the membranes should be performed under conditions of full asepsis in the delivery suite. Under ideal circumstances, the cervix should be soft, effaced and at least 2 cm dilated. The head should be presenting by the vertex and should be engaged in the pelvis. In practice, these conditions are often not fulfilled, and the degree to which they are adhered to depends on the urgency of the need to start labour. The mother is placed in the supine or lithotomy position and, after swabbing and draping the vulva, a finger is introduced through the cervix, and the fetal membranes are separated from the lower segment – a process known as 'stripping the membranes'. The bulging membranes are then ruptured with Kocher's forceps, Gelder's forewater amniotomy forceps or an amniotomy hook (Fig. 13.4). The amniotic fluid is released slowly and care is taken to exclude presentation or prolapse of the cord. The fetal heart rate should be monitored following rupture of the membranes.

Table 13.2 Bishop's score			
Score	**0**	**1**	**2**
Consistency	Fim	Medum	Soft
Position	Posterior	Mid	Anterior
Dilatation	0	1–2 cm	3–4 cm
Length	3 cm	2 cm	1 cm
Station	< –3	< –2	–1

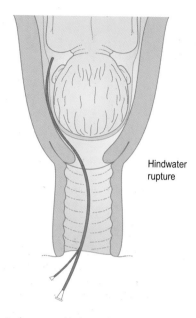

Hindwater
rupture

Fig. 13.5 Induction of labour by hindwater rupture.

Hindwater rupture

An alternative method of surgical induction involves rupture of the membranes behind the presenting part. This is known as hindwater rupture. A sigmoid-shaped metal cannula known as the Drewe–Smythe catheter is introduced through the cervix and penetrates the membranes behind the presenting part (Fig. 13.5). The theoretical advantage of this technique is that it reduces the risk of prolapsed cord. In reality, the risk is even lower with forewater rupture than with spontaneous rupture of the membranes, and the technique of hindwater rupture is now rarely used.

Medical induction of labour following amniotomy

Various pharmacological agents can be used to stimulate uterine activity. It is common practice to combine surgical induction with a Syntocinon infusion. A suitable regimen would begin at 1 mU/min and increase by 3 mU/min every 15 minutes until adequate contractions become established.

The principal hazards of combined surgical and medical induction of labour are:

- **Hyperstimulation:** Excessive and prolonged uterine contractions reduce uterine blood flow and result in fetal asphyxia. Therefore, contractions should not occur more frequently than every 2 minutes and should not last in excess of 1 minute. The Syntocinon infusion should be discontinued if excessive uterine activity occurs or if there are signs of fetal distress.
- **Prolapse of the cord:** This should be excluded by examination at the time of forewater rupture, or subsequently if signs of fetal distress occur.
- **Infection:** A prolonged induction–delivery interval increases the risk of infection in the amniotic sac with consequent risks to both infant and mother. If the liquor becomes offensive and maternal pyrexia occurs, the labour should be terminated and the infant delivered.

Medical induction of labour and cervical ripening

This is the method of choice where the membranes are intact or where the cervix is unsuitable for surgical induction. The two most commonly used forms of medical induction are:

- Syntocinon infusion
- Administration of prostaglandins by various routes.

Syntocinon infusion

This induces uterine contractions but is a relatively ineffective method of inducing labour unless combined with surgical induction.

Prostaglandins

The most widely used form is prostaglandin E_2. This is used to ripen the cervix and may be administered:

- **Orally:** Doses of 0.5 mg are increased to 2 mg/h until contractions are produced
- **By the vaginal route:** The most commonly used method is to insert prostaglandin pessaries or xylose gel into the posterior fornix. Nulliparous women with an unfavourable cervix (Bishop's score of less than 2) are given an initial dose of 2 mg and multiparous women and nulliparae with a Bishop's score of more than 4 an initial dose of 1 mg. This is

repeated if necessary after 6 hours and again the following day up to a maximum dose of 4 mg until labour is established or the membranes can be ruptured and the induction continued with oxytocin.

BREECH PRESENTATION

The incidence of breech presentation depends on the gestational age at the time of onset of labour. At 32 weeks, the incidence is 16%, falling to 7% at 38 weeks and 3–5% at term. Thus it is clear that the fetus normally corrects its own presentation and attempts to correct the presentation before 38 weeks are generally unnecessary.

Types of breech presentation

The breech may present in one of three ways:

- **Frank breech:** The legs lie extended along the fetal trunk and are flexed at the hips and extended at the knees. The buttocks will present at the pelvic inlet. This presentation is also known as an extended breech.
- **Flexed breech:** The legs are flexed at the hips and the knees with the fetus sitting on its legs so that both feet present to the pelvic inlet.
- **Knee or footling presentation-** one thigh is flexed and one is extended so that the foot descends through the cervix into the vagina.

The position of the breech is defined using the fetal sacrum as the denominator. At the onset of labour the breech enters the brim of the true pelvis with the bitrochanteric diameter (9.25 cm) being the diameter of engagement. This is slightly smaller than the biparietal diameter in the full-term fetus. The type of breech presentation has a significant impact on the risk of vaginal breech delivery. The more irregular the presenting part, the greater is the risk of a prolapsed cord or limb. A foot pressing into the vagina below the cervix may stimulate the mother to bear down before the cervix is fully dilated and thus lead to entrapment of the head (Fig. 13.6).

Causation and hazards of breech presentation

Breech presentation is common before 37 weeks gestation but most infants will turn before term (as previously discussed). Breech presentation may, how-

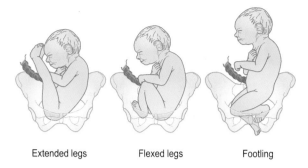

Extended legs   Flexed legs   Footling

Fig. 13.6 Types of breech presentation.

ever, be associated with factors such as multiple pregnancy, congenital abnormalities of the maternal uterus, fetal malformation and placental location, either placenta praevia or cornual implantation.

There is also evidence to suggest that persistent breech presentation may be associated with the inability of the fetus to kick itself around from breech to vertex and that there may therefore be some neurological impairment of the lower limbs (Box 13.3).

 There is a high incidence of neurological impairment in breech babies even when delivered by caesarean section.

Delivery by the breech carries some specific hazards to the infant as compared with normal vertex presentation, particularly in preterm infants and in infants with a birthweight in excess of 4 kg; these are as follows.

- There is an increased risk of cord compression and cord prolapse because of the irregular nature of the presenting part. This is particularly the case where the legs are flexed or there is a footling presentation.

 Box 13.3
Causation of breech presentation

- Gestational age
- Placental location
- Uterine anomalies
- Multiple pregnancy
- Neurological impairment of the fetal limbs

- Entrapment of the head behind the cervix is a particular risk with the preterm infant, in whom the bitrochanteric diameter of the breech is significantly smaller than the biparietal diameter of the head. This means that the trunk may slip through an incompletely dilated cervix, resulting in entrapment of the larger head. If the delivery is significantly delayed, the child may be asphyxiated and either die or suffer brain damage.
- The fetal skull does not have time to mould during delivery and therefore, in both premature and mature infants, there is a significant risk of intracranial haemorrhage.
- Trauma to viscera may occur during the delivery process, with rupture of the spleen or gut.

Management

Antenatal management

Because of the risks to the fetus of breech birth, the best option would appear to be to avoid vaginal breech delivery. However, this is not always possible and the important decision to be made relates to the assessment of the size of the fetus and the size and shape of the maternal pelvis.

Maternal size and shape can be assessed by pelvic examination and by the use of X-ray pelvimetry with erect lateral views of the pelvis. Pelvimetry can also be performed using magnetic resonance imaging (MRI) although it must be remembered that images with MRI are acquired with the mother lying supine, as distinct from X-ray pelvimetry where the images are obtained with the mother standing. The diameters obtained in the anteroposterior plane of the pelvis are therefore smaller with MRI.

Fetal size is difficult to assess but, if fetal gestational age is less than 32 weeks and more than 28 weeks, the birthweight will be less than 1.5 kg and delivery by caesarean section is the preferred option. If the fetal weight as assessed clinically and by ultrasound is calculated to be in excess of 4 kg, then delivery by section is the preferred option but it must be remembered that such estimates are notoriously unreliable.

External cephalic version

Indication

Breech presentation persisting after 37 weeks gestation.

Contraindications

External cephalic version should not be attempted where there is a history of antepartum haemorrhage, where there is placenta praevia or a previous uterine scar or where the pregnancy is multiple. It is also pointless to turn the infant if the intention is to deliver the child by elective caesarean section.

Technique

The mother rests supine with the body slightly tilted down to disimpact the breech. The presentation is confirmed by clinical examination and, if necessary, by ultrasound. The fetal heart rate is checked. In some centres, a tocolytic agent is given to relax the uterus but in many cases this is not necessary and it is not recommended as a routine part of the procedure (Fig. 13.7).

The presenting part is disimpacted from the pelvic brim and the fetus is gently rotated, keeping the head flexed. The fetal heart rate should be checked during the procedure.

It is essential not to use excessive force and, if there is evidence of fetal bradycardia, the fetus should be returned to the original presentation if the version is not past the halfway point.

Complications

The risks of the procedure are cord entanglement, placental abruption and rupture of the membranes.

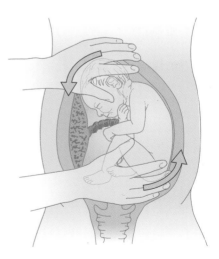

Fig. 13.7 External cephalic version: pressure is applied in the opposite direction to the two fetal poles.

Persistent fetal bradycardia may necessitate urgent delivery by caesarean section. There is some recent evidence to suggest that, even where external version is successful, labour is often incoordinate and there is an increased incidence of fetal distress, leading to a high section rate.

Method of delivery

Vaginal breech delivery

The first stage of labour should be no different from labour in a vertex presentation. Epidural analgesia is the preferred method of pain relief but is not essential. The woman should be advised to come into hospital as soon as contractions commence or the membranes rupture and vaginal examination should be performed on admission to exclude cord presentation or prolapse (Fig. 13.8). The presence of meconium-stained liquor has exactly the same significance as with a vertex presentation.

Technique

When the cervix is fully dilated, the mother is encouraged to bear down with her contractions until the fetal buttocks and anus come on view. To minimize soft tissue resistance, a wide episiotomy should be performed under either local or epidural anaesthesia, unless the pelvic floor is already lax and offers little

resistance. The legs are then lifted out of the vagina and traction is applied downwards and backwards. The anterior arm can usually be delivered easily by sliding the fingers over the shoulder and sweeping the arm downwards. The trunk is then moved laterally until the posterior arm can be delivered. The trunk is then allowed to hang for about 30 seconds to allow the head to enter the pelvis and then the legs are grasped and swung upwards through an arc of 180° until the child's mouth comes into view. The mouth is sucked clear of fluid to allow respiration to commence and Wrigley's forceps are applied to the aftercoming head to enable a gentle and controlled delivery of the head and to protect against sudden expansion and expulsion (Fig. 13.9).

Syntometrine is given at this stage by intramuscular injection (unless contraindicated) and the delivery of the head is completed.

The cord is then clamped and divided and the third stage is completed in the usual way.

The essence of good breech delivery is that progress should be continuous and handling of the fetus must be as gentle as possible.

Caesarean section

Delivery by caesarean section is indicated if the estimated birthweight is less than 1500 g or is greater than 4 kg or there is an additional complication such as severe pre-eclampsia, placental abruption, placenta praevia or a previous caesarean section. If the birthweight is calculated to be less than 700 g, the perinatal outcome both in terms of mortality and morbidity is poor irrespective of the method of delivery.

Although there has been no large randomized trial of caesarean section for very-low-birthweight infants, descriptive studies in some very large series show much improved outcome where the infant is delivered in this way. Caesarean section is currently the method of choice for delivery of very-low-birthweight infants presenting as a breech.

Normally, the technique used is lower segment caesarean section. However, with a preterm infant, the lower segment may not have formed and under these circumstances the preferred method is a midline incision through that part of the lower segment that is formed; a classic incision may on occasions be the incision of choice. In very-low-birthweight infants, the buttocks and trunk are substantially narrower than the head and entrapment of the head may occur at the time

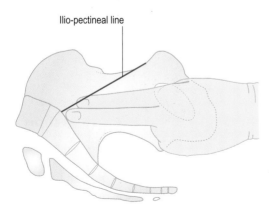

Ilio-pectineal line

Fig. 13.8 Clinical assessment of the pelvis and breech presentation.

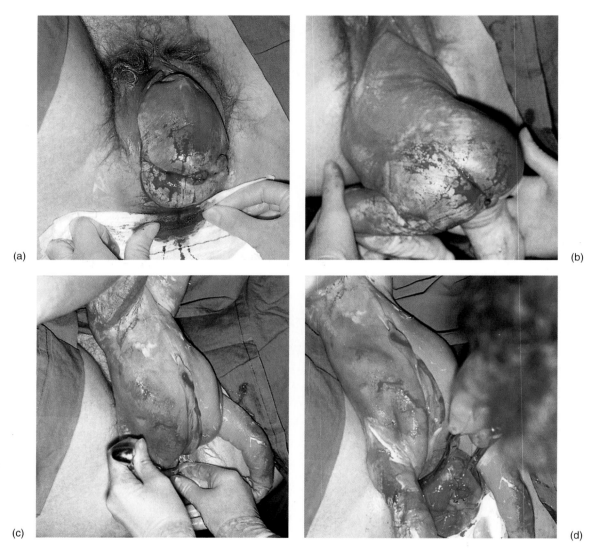

Fig. 13.9 Breech presentation. (a) Buttock on view. (b) Trunk expelled. (c) Rotation of trunk. (d) Forceps applied to aftercoming head.

of delivery through the uterine incision unless an adequate incision is made.

CAESAREAN SECTION

This operation is the process whereby the child is removed from the uterus by direct incision through the abdominal wall and the uterus.

Lower segment caesarean section

The most commonly performed procedure is the *lower segment caesarean section*, where the bladder is reflected from the lower segment (Fig. 13.10a) and a transverse incision is made (Fig. 13.10b). The presenting part is then delivered through the lower segment (Fig. 13.10c). The wound is closed in two layers, taking care to exclude the decidua (Fig. 13.10d).

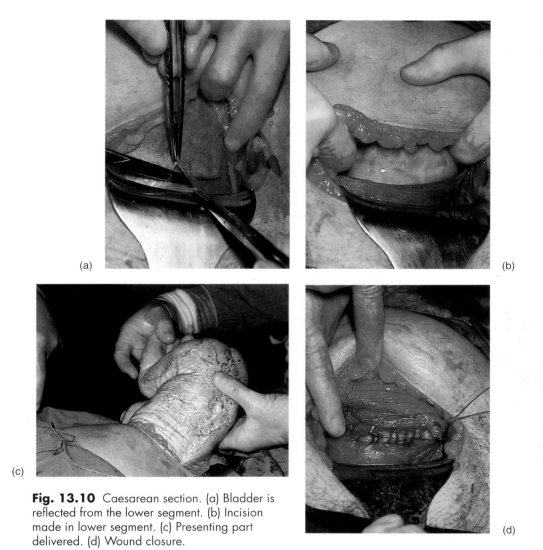

Fig. 13.10 Caesarean section. (a) Bladder is reflected from the lower segment. (b) Incision made in lower segment. (c) Presenting part delivered. (d) Wound closure.

Upper segment or classic caesarean section

In this procedure, a vertical incision is made in the upper segment of the uterus and the child is delivered through this incision. This technique is not widely used because it has a much higher morbidity postoperatively, and a much higher incidence of subsequent rupture of the scar.

Caesarean hysterectomy

Caesarean section and hysterectomy are sometimes performed at the same time – where there is uterine rupture, uncontrollable postpartum haemorrhage or, occasionally, cervical malignant disease.

Indications for caesarean section

It is not particularly helpful to state an incidence figure for caesarean section because it varies widely from country to country. In the UK, it is about 20%, and the vast majority of the procedures are performed by the lower segment technique. The common indications for caesarean section are:

- Obstructed labour
- Placenta praevia and antepartum haemorrhage
- Fetal distress
- Severe pre-eclampsia
- Intrauterine growth restriction and placental failure
- Breech presentation and other malpresentations
- Failed induction – prolonged labour
- Diabetes mellitus
- Prolapsed cord
- Other rare indications such as cervical dystocia.

The rise in the caesarean section rate over the last 20 years has led to a reassessment of the old dictum 'once a section always a section'. In those women with a non-recurrent indication for repeat caesarean section, a vaginal delivery rate of 50–70% can be anticipated. The major concern is the risk of dehiscence of the uterine scar, although this is only 1%. The risk is higher where delivery has been effected by a classic upper uterine segment incision, and the rupture tends to occur before the onset of labour.

The decision to allow labour to proceed after a previous caesarean section must take into account the indication for the original operation, the presentation and size of the present baby and the wishes of the mother. It is important that any woman who has a uterine scar should be delivered where there is ready access to an operating theatre. Blood should be taken for cross-matching, and all labours should be monitored. Signs of impending or actual scar dehiscence or rupture include pain over the scar, maternal tachycardia, fetal distress, incoordinate uterine activity, vaginal bleeding and collapse.

Complications

The immediate complications are those of haemorrhage, shock and the complications of anaesthesia. There may also be damage to the bladder or ureters. Rarely, the fetus may sustain lacerations during the incision of the uterus. Late complications include:

- Secondary postpartum haemorrhage
- Infection – uterine, vesical and wound
- Pulmonary embolus
- Deep vein thrombosis.

FACE PRESENTATION

Face presentation occurs in 1/500 deliveries. The head is hyperextended so that the occiput rests on the cervical spine. It sometimes occurs as a continuing extension of a deflexed head in the occipitoposterior position or from a brow presentation. It is occasionally associated with fetal abnormalities such as anencephaly, or cervical tumours such as cystic hygromas. In modern obstetric practice, where the majority of mothers have an ultrasound scan for congenital abnormalities by 18 weeks gestation and where such abnormalities are now commonly terminated, it is rare to see such conditions as causative at full-term delivery.

The positions in a face presentation are the same as with the vertex presentation but in this presentation the chin is the denominator.

Diagnosis

The diagnosis can occasionally be made antenatally but is usually made in labour. Antenatally, the head is high and feels larger than normal, with a deep groove between the head and the back. The diagnosis can be confirmed by ultrasound or X-ray. However, most cases are diagnosed in labour when the cervix is sufficiently dilated to enable palpation of facial features such as orbital hollows and the orbital ridges, as well as the nose and the mouth (Fig. 13.11).

Management

Labour may proceed normally, as the diameters of presentation are the biparietal diameter and the submentobregmatic diameter. The risk to the fetus may result from the stretching of the intracranial membranes during the process of moulding, resulting in intracranial haemorrhage. However, this is rare and does not justify routine delivery by caesarean section. Facial bruising and oedema are common but usually resolve quickly and the mother should be reassured that there are no long-term sequelae.

The labour should proceed at the same rate as a vertex presentation. If there is undue delay, it is preferable to proceed to caesarean section. However, only about 15% require delivery by section.

The mechanism of labour involves the anterior rotation of the chin under the pubic arch and, as the head rotates during delivery, it flexes as it emerges through the introitus.

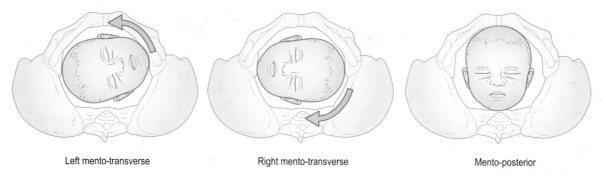

| Left mento-transverse | Right mento-transverse | Mento-posterior |

Fig. 13.11 Position of the face presentation; the denominator is the chin.

> **!** If the chin rotates posteriorly, pointing into the sacral curve, it will become impacted as the head cannot extend any further and spontaneous delivery is impossible. It is sometimes possible to rotate the head manually or with forceps but at this stage, most obstetricians will opt for caesarean section.

BROW PRESENTATION

Brow presentation (Fig. 13.12) occurs when the head is partially extended and lies between a normal vertex presentation and a face presentation. In some cases, a brow presentation will extend further into a face presentation but if it becomes impacted as a brow at the pelvic brim, the presenting diameter, the verticomental diameter, is too large to allow spontaneous delivery unless the head is small or the pelvis large. The condition is rare and occurs in 1/1500 deliveries.

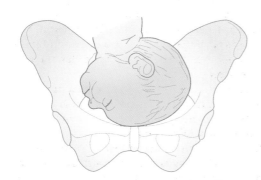

Fig. 13.12 Brow presentation at delivery.

Diagnosis and management

The diagnosis is nearly always made in labour. The head remains high and is easily palpable abdominally.

On vaginal examination, the brow is palpable between the bridge of the nose, the supraorbital ridges and the anterior fontanelle. While it is sometimes possible to flex the head digitally, this is uncommon and the preferred method of delivery is by caesarean section.

UNSTABLE LIE, TRANSVERSE LIE AND SHOULDER PRESENTATION

An unstable lie is one that is constantly changing. It is commonly associated with multiparity, where the maternal abdominal wall is lax, low placental implantation or uterine anomalies such as a bicornuate uterus, uterine fibroids and polyhydramnios.

Complications

If an unstable lie resulting in a transverse lie persists until the onset of labour, it may result in prolapse of the cord or a shoulder presentation and a prolapsed arm, or a compound presentation when both an arm and a leg may present (Fig. 13.13).

Management

No action is necessary in an unstable lie until 37 weeks gestation unless the labour starts spontaneously. It is important to look for an explanation by ultrasound scan for placental localization, the presence of any

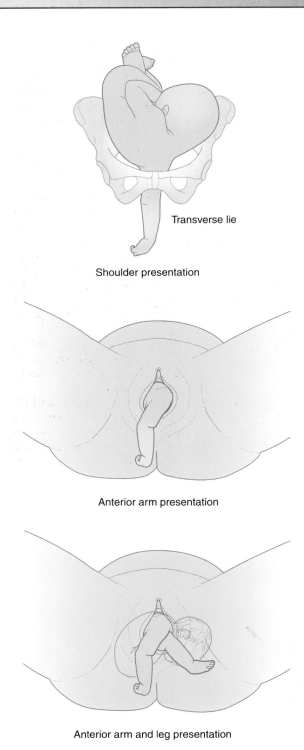

Transverse lie

Shoulder presentation

Anterior arm presentation

Anterior arm and leg presentation

Fig. 13.13 Prolapse of the arm into the vagina, sometimes resulting in a shoulder presentation.

pelvic tumours and the presence of fetal abnormalities. However, it must be remembered that, in most cases, no obvious cause is found.

After 37 weeks, an attempt should be made to correct the lie by external cephalic version. It may be advisable to admit the mother to hospital after 39 weeks gestation if the unstable lie persists.

Assuming that no specific factor such as a low-lying placenta can be identified, the approach may take one of three courses:

- Keep the mother in hospital and correct the lie until labour starts spontaneously
- Stabilizing induction is performed by first correcting the lie to a cephalic presentation, starting an oxytocic infusion and rupturing the membranes as soon as the head enters the pelvic brim
- If labour becomes established spontaneously, the mother should be advised to come in to hospital immediately. If the membranes rupture spontaneously and the cord prolapses or a transverse lie cannot be corrected, the mother should be delivered immediately by caesarean section. If there are any other complicating factors, it may on occasions be advisable to deliver the mother at term by planned elective section (Box 13.4).

In general terms, it is technically easier to perform an external cephalic version when the fetus faces the maternal pelvis rather than when it faces the thorax, as version in these circumstances tends to extend the head.

If the mother arrives in established labour with a shoulder presentation or prolapsed arm, no attempt should be made to correct the presentation or to deliver the child vaginally – delivery should be effected by caesarean section. Sometimes, if the arm is wedged into the pelvis, it may be safer to deliver the child through a classic or midline upper segment incision rather than through a lower segment incision as, in these cases, there may be little lower segment formed.

> **i** **Box 13.4**
> Management of unstable lie
>
> - Exclude causes that are fixed
> - Hospitalization at 37 weeks
> - Stabilizing induction at term
> - Be prepared for cord prolapse

CORD PRESENTATION AND CORD PROLAPSE

Cord presentation (Fig. 13.14) occurs when any part of the cord lies alongside or in front of the presenting part. The diagnosis is usually established by digital palpation of the pulsating cord, which may be felt through the intact membranes. When the membranes rupture, the cord prolapses and may appear at the vulva or be palpable in front of the presenting part.

Predisposing factors

Any condition that displaces the head or presenting part away from the cervix or where the presenting part is irregular and forms poor contact with the cervix will predispose to cord presentation or prolapse. Under these circumstances, if the membranes are ruptured artificially to induce labour, the cord may prolapse. In fact it is no more likely and is probably less hazardous for cord prolapse to occur after artificial rupture of the membranes than after spontaneous rupture because the patient will be near an operating theatre and can be delivered rapidly.

Management

The diagnosis of cord presentation is sometimes made prior to rupture of the membranes and prolapse of the cord but this is the exception rather than the rule. It may be reasonable on occasions to manage cord presentation conservatively, particularly where the cord lies high alongside the presenting part and is difficult to reach, but there are no circumstances where conservative management can be employed when the cord prolapses unless spontaneous delivery is imminent.

If the cord prolapses through a partially dilated cervix, delivery should be effected as soon as possible, as the presenting part will compress the cord. Furthermore, exposure to cold air will induce vasospasm in the cord arteries, as will handling of the cord, and this will lead to fetal asphyxia.

Prolapse of the cord is an obstetric emergency and, unless spontaneous delivery is imminent, the woman should be placed in the knee chest position to reduce pressure on the cord or the presenting part should be digitally displaced to achieve the same effect. There is no point in trying to replace the cord, as this is usually physically impossible.

Delivery should then be effected by caesarean section unless the cervix is fully dilated and delivery can be achieved rapidly by forceps or breech extraction and by encouraging maternal expulsive efforts.

Despite the acute asphyxial insult to the fetus, which is likely to be depressed at birth, the long-term prognosis in these infants is good. Provided there is no pre-existing impairment to gaseous transfer, the fetus can effectively withstand an acute asphyxial episode without suffering long-term damage.

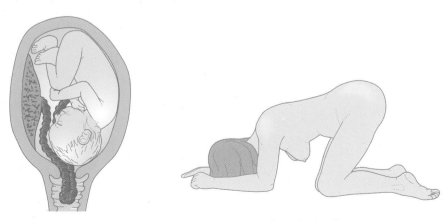

Knee–chest position

Fig. 13.14 Cord prolapse (left); pressure on the cord can be minimized by placing the mother in the knee–chest position.

MALPOSITION OF THE FETAL HEAD

The occipitoposterior position

This is the commonest malposition and, at the time of onset of labour, some 10–20% of all cephalic presentations have the occiput pointing posteriorly in the pelvis, either as a direct occipitoposterior position or, more commonly, with the occiput pointing towards the sacroiliac joints on either side as an oblique right or left occipitoposterior position.

During labour, the head may rotate to the transverse and then anterior position or rotate posteriorly to become a direct occipitoposterior position, or it may remain arrested in the oblique occipitoposterior position. In fact only about 5% remain arrested in this way: the rest rotate either anteriorly or posteriorly and deliver spontaneously.

Where the occiput remains in the posterior position, the head may obstruct, as it is deflexed and the presenting diameter, the occipitoposterior diameter, is 11 cm, larger than the presenting diameter in an occipito-anterior position. The persistence of an occipitoposterior position is often associated with the shape of the pelvis: an android or anthropoid pelvis may be the cause of the non-rotation of the fetal head. The charac-

teristic features of a 'posterior' labour are that it is often prolonged and almost invariably painful and associated with severe backache (Fig 13.15).

Diagnosis

This malposition may be diagnosed on abdominal palpation but the diagnosis can only be confirmed on vaginal examination after the onset of labour and when some cervical dilatation has occurred.

> ✓ In occipitoposterior-position babies the anterior abdominal wall looks flattened below the level of the umbilicus and the fetal limbs may be readily visible. The head tends to engage late and occipitoposterior position is the commonest cause of non-engagement of the fetal head at term in the primigravid woman.

On vaginal examination, once the cervix has dilated beyond 3–4 cm, the sagittal suture can be felt and the posterior fontanelle lies posteriorly in the pelvis.

The head may sometimes rotate to the transverse position and, if it arrests in that position, will need to be rotated prior to delivery.

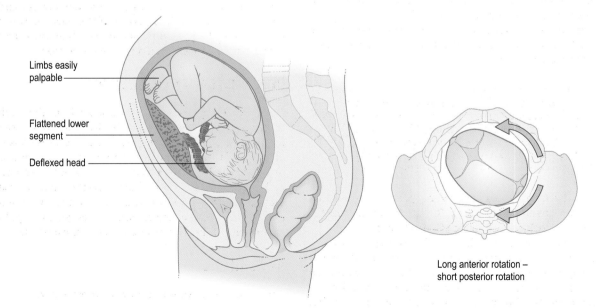

Limbs easily palpable

Flattened lower segment

Deflexed head

Long anterior rotation – short posterior rotation

Fig. 13.15 Clinical findings in the occipitoposterior position (left); the head may rotate anteriorly or posteriorly or may arrest in the occipitoposterior position (right).

The cervix may dilate asymmetrically, leaving a thickened lip of cervix anteriorly because of poor application of the fetal head to the cervix.

Management

The diagnosis is usually first made in labour and, even if it is made antenatally, there is no point in attempting to correct the position at this stage as, in many cases, it will correct itself. Labour will sometimes progress rapidly, the head rotating anteriorly and delivering normally, or it may rotate posteriorly and deliver in a persistent occipitoposterior position.

> **!** Because of the deflexed head and the relatively large presenting diameter, delivery in the posterior position may result in over-distension of the perineum, resulting in third-degree tears.

Labour may be prolonged and painful and it is important to recognize this early, to ensure that adequate pain relief and fluid replacement are given. If uterine activity is incoordinate and progress is slow, as manifest by cervical dilatation of less than 1 cm/h, then it may be justifiable to use a low-dose oxytocin infusion but uterine activity must be monitored at all times if this procedure is to be implemented.

If labour becomes abnormally prolonged and the head remains unengaged, delivery by caesarean section is the preferred method.

> **!** When performing caesarean section for OP position the head sometimes becomes impacted in the pelvis and it may be difficult to disimpact. It is then advisable to disimpact the head vaginally before extracting it abdominally.

If the head is engaged in the pelvis, it should be rotated manually or using Kjelland's forceps to the anterior position and extracted with forceps.

The head is rotated through the shortest distance to achieve this objective, although, if the head rotates easily, it is preferable to rotate it to the anterior position rather than posteriorly. Sometimes it is possible to rotate the head with a suction cup (ventouse); this has the advantage of occupying little space in the pelvis and causing minimal soft tissue damage.

Forceps rotation and delivery requires a high degree of operator skill if damage to the mother and the fetus is to be avoided. Maternal injuries in particular include damage to the vaginal walls, with spiral tears and damage to the bladder and rectum.

Deep transverse arrest

The head normally engages in the pelvis in the transverse diameter and then the occiput rotates anteriorly and emerges under the pubic arch.

If the pelvis is android in shape and narrows or 'funnels' towards the pelvic outlet, the head will arrest at the level of the ischial spines and will mould and elongate as it is driven into the pelvis. The presenting part may appear to be deeper in the pelvis than it really is and vaginal delivery may be impossible. This scenario must be distinguished from arrest in progress in the second stage of labour where the pelvis is normal in size and shape and the delay is due to poor uterine activity and poor expulsive efforts and not to the position of the head. Provided the head is engaged in the pelvis, it can be easily rotated to the anterior position, either manually or with forceps or ventouse, and then extracted with forceps or ventouse.

There is no longer any place for 'heroic' procedures using excessive force to extract and rotate the head. Such procedures may result in tears in the falx cerebri and tearing of major cerebral vessels. If the head does not rotate easily, the procedure should be abandoned and delivery should be effected by caesarean section.

INSTRUMENTAL DELIVERY

Obstetric forceps were first introduced in the 17th century by the Chamberlain family, and have been modified and adapted in various forms. Forceps consist of a pair of fenestrated blades with a handle connected to the blades by a shank (Fig. 13.16). The blades normally exhibit both a pelvic and cephalic curve so that they can adapt both to the fetal skull and to the maternal sacral curve. The instruments are designed for application only to the fetal head and not to the buttocks.

Indications

The common indications for forceps delivery are:

- Delay in the second stage of labour: This occurs most frequently as a result of pelvic floor resistance

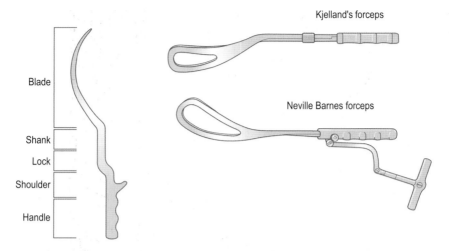

Kjelland's forceps

Neville Barnes forceps

Blade

Shank

Lock

Shoulder

Handle

Fig. 13.16 Forceps parts (left) and commonly used forceps (right); the absence of the pelvic curve in Kjelland's forceps enables rotation of the fetal head.

and a tight perineum but may, however, also be caused by:

– Poor maternal expulsive efforts
– Cephalopelvic disproportion
– Malposition or malpresentation of the head
– Removal of the urge to bear down during epidural anaesthesia

• Fetal distress
• Maternal distress and maternal conditions necessitating minimal expulsive effort from the mother
• Forceps are applied to the aftercoming head in a breech presentation and may also be used to extract the fetal head at caesarean section.

Prerequisites to forceps delivery

When there is an indication for forceps delivery, the mother should be placed in the lithotomy position, and the thighs and perineum should be cleaned and draped. It is then important to check:

• That the cervix is fully dilated
• That the bladder is not overdistended and requiring catheterization
• The position, presentation and status of the fetal head; it must be engaged and not palpable in the abdominal cavity.

Anaesthesia

This is commonly achieved with regional anaesthesia – epidural, spinal, sacral block or pudendal nerve block. On some occasions, general anaesthesia may be indicated.

Method of delivery

Low forceps (outlet forceps)

If the head is in the direct occipitoanterior position, below the level of the ischial spines and resting on the pelvic floor, low forceps delivery is performed.

The forceps used where no rotation of the head is required are:

• **Neville Barnes forceps:** These have an axis traction handle, which allows considerable force to be applied, but this attachment is now rarely used
• **Simpson's forceps:** These are similar to the Neville Barnes forceps but with no axis traction handle.

Both these forceps have cephalic and pelvic curves.

The two blades of the forceps are designated according to the side of the pelvis to which they are applied. Thus, the left blade is applied to the left side of the pelvis (Fig. 13.17a). There is a fixed lock between the blades (Fig. 13.17b). Intermittent traction is applied in the direction of the pelvic canal (Fig. 13.17c) until

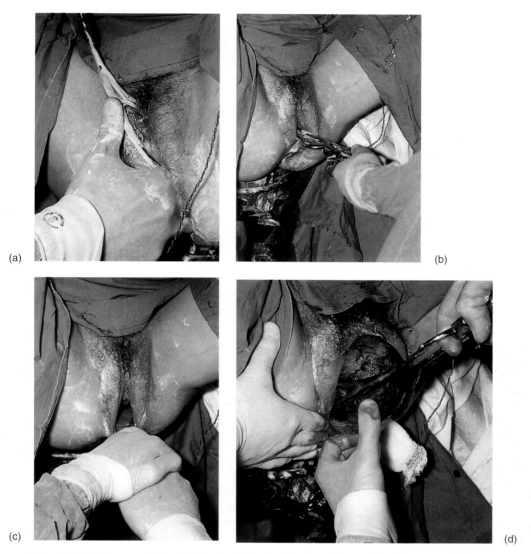

Fig. 13.17 Forceps. (a) Left blade for left side of pelvis. (b) Fixed lock between blades. (c) Application of intermittent traction in direction of pelvic canal. (d) Delivery of head by anterior extension.

the occiput is in view and then the head is delivered by anterior extension (Fig. 13.17d). An episiotomy is usually, although not invariably, performed.

Mid-cavity forceps

Arrest of the head sometimes occurs in the mid-cavity when the presenting part reaches the level of the ischial spine. At this level, the position of the head is usually transverse or posterior.

The position of the head must first be corrected, by either manual or forceps rotation, to a direct antero-posterior position before application of traction.

Kjelland's forceps have a sliding lock and minimal pelvic curve so that rotation of the forceps will not lead to damage by the blades during the process of rotation.

High forceps

This type of delivery, where the head lies well above the level of the ischial spines, is very rarely performed. In fact, if the head can be palpated above the pelvic brim, this is a contraindication to vaginal delivery.

Trial of forceps

Occasionally, a situation arises where there is borderline disproportion, and this is an indication for a trial of forceps. This should be attempted only where there is a high expectation that vaginal delivery will be achieved without significant trauma to the mother or fetus.

A trial of forceps delivery should always be undertaken in an operating theatre with preparation made to proceed to caesarean section.

Careful assessment of the pelvis and presenting part should be made before proceeding to apply the forceps blades. If firm traction does not produce steady descent of the head, then the blades should be removed and the child should be delivered by caesarean section. It may be necessary to disimpact the head vaginally before section.

Ventouse delivery

An alternative to forceps delivery is the application of a suction cup to the fetal scalp and extraction by traction. The indications for vacuum extraction are the same as those for forceps delivery. The metal suction cups of the vacuum extractor are of three different sizes – 30, 40 and 50 mm. The vacuum inside the cup is slowly increased to 0.8 kg/cm^2, and the scalp forms a 'chignon' inside the cup. Traction is applied with the contractions and rotation of the head will generally occur as it is pulled on to the pelvic floor.

Laceration of the scalp and caput or haematoma formation may occur with this procedure but the instrument rarely causes any damage to the mother. Forceps, if incorrectly applied, may result in considerable laceration of the mother, including uterine and bladder or bowel damage. Fetal damage may involve facial bruising, facial nerve damage, skin abrasions and intracranial haemorrhage. Use of the ventouse is contraindicated in face presentation.

ABNORMALITIES OF UTERINE ACTIVITY

The view of what constitutes an abnormal labour has changed substantially over the last two decades. The

definition of prolonged labour now relies more on the rate of progress than on absolute times. Nevertheless, it must be remembered that 90% of primigravid women deliver within 16 hours and 90% of multigravid women within 12 hours. It is now rare to see a labour that lasts in excess of 24 hours. When labour becomes prolonged and progress is abnormally slow, the possibility of cephalopelvic disproportion must be considered but, in many cases, poor progress is associated with abnormal uterine activity.

Uterine activity can be quantified either by the use of Montevideo units or by the computer calculation of the area under the contraction wave as measured by tocography.

Montevideo units are calculated by multiplying the peak pressure of the contractions expressed in millimetres of mercury by the number of contractions in a 10-minute period. When the area under the contraction is measured by computer over a 15-minute period, the activity is expressed in kilopascals per 15 minutes. In fact, the two measurements have a good correlation. Steer has calculated that a level of uterine activity of less than 700 kPa/15 min represents hypotonic uterine activity and levels in excess of 1800 kPa/15 min represent hypertonic uterine activity.

Progress in normal labour depends on uterine polarity associated with fundal dominance and progressive cervical dilatation.

Lack of progress in labour may result from weak contractions but normal polarity – *hypotonic uterine inertia* – or strong and abnormal contractions with abnormal polarity – *hypertonic uterine inertia*.

On occasions, there may be hypertonic uterine activity with normal polarity that will result in a precipitate labour lasting less than 2 hours (Fig. 13.18).

Hypotonic uterine activity

In this condition, the resting uterine tone is low, contractions are infrequent and often irregular, and progress is slow. This type of inertia results in delays in the latent phase and does not usually cause distress to the mother or the fetus.

Hypertonic uterine activity

This is a rare abnormality commonly resulting from reversed polarity of the uterine contractions. The contraction is commonly initiated in the lower segment or it may on occasions be asymmetrical, resulting in a

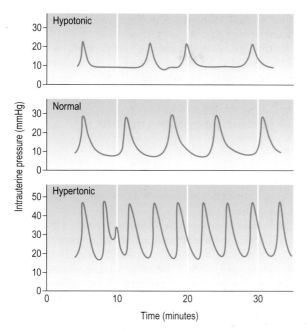

Fig. 13.18 Abnormalities of uterine action which normally result in prolonged labour.

Case study
Primary dysfunctional labour – hypertonic uterine inertia

A 23-year-old primigravida was admitted to hospital in labour with regular and painful contractions. There was no evidence of any antepartum haemorrhage. The cervix was found to be 2.5 cm dilated. However, 4 hours later the cervix was 4 cm dilated and the rate of progress was significantly delayed. The cervicogram is shown in Figure 13.19. An epidural catheter was inserted and epidural analgesia commenced. The membranes were ruptured artificially and clear amniotic fluid was released. Progress in labour continued to be slow and 3 hours later a dilute oxytocin infusion was started. This resulted in rapid progress to full dilatation and vaginal delivery some 2 hours later.

double peak in the contraction wave. Resting uterine tone is also raised so that the level at which the pain of the contraction is felt is earlier in the contraction cycle and the pain persists for longer. Cervical dilatation is slow and the woman suffers from severe backache and pain that radiates into the lower abdomen. This type of inertia is uncommon and, when it does occur, is commonly associated with placental abruption. This diagnosis must always be considered when this type of labour occurs as the abruption may initially be concealed.

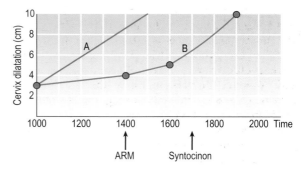

Fig. 13.19 Slow progress in the first stage of labour. The action time is line A, and line B is the actual cervical dilatation.

Constriction ring dystocia

This is a variant of hypertonic uterine activity where the constriction becomes localized and forms a constriction band around part of the fetus. It usually occurs after the membranes have ruptured and where there has been an attempt at some form of intrauterine manipulation such as internal podalic version. As these manoeuvres are now rarely performed, the complication is rarely seen.

Management

Abnormalities of uterine activity are usually recognised by the failure of progress in labour. As incoordinate uterine activity may also be associated with cephalo-pelvic disproportion, it is essential to exclude this possibility by careful assessment of the size and shape of the maternal pelvis and the size of the fetus.

The general principles of management of abnormal uterine activity involve:

- Adequate pain relief, particularly in the presence of hypertonic uterine inertia and principally with epidural analgesia
- Adequate fluid replacement by intravenous infusion of dextrose saline or Hartmann's solution
- Stimulation of coordinated uterine activity using a dilute infusion of oxytocin.

In the presence of hypotonic uterine inertia, uterine activity may be stimulated by encouraging mobilization of the mother and, if the membranes are intact, by artificial rupture of the membranes; an oxytocic infusion will also usually stimulate labour and delivery.

If the uterine activity is hypertonic, rupture of the membranes as well as cautious use of a low-dose oxytocin infusion may produce normal uterine activity. If progress continues to be slow and there is evidence of fetal distress, delivery should be effected by caesarean section.

Constriction ring dystocia can only be reversed by the use of beta-sympathomimetic agents, or ether or halothane anaesthesia.

CERVICAL DYSTOCIA

This is a very rare cause of prolonged and obstructed labour. The cervix may be scarred by previous surgery such as a previous cone biopsy or repeated cautery and, occasionally, the condition may be congenital. Although uterine activity is normal, the cervix fails to dilate and feels rigid and tense on pelvic examination. If labour is allowed to continue, it may lead to annular detachment of the cervix or to uterine rupture. When the condition is recognized, the fetus should be delivered by caesarean section.

PRECIPITATE LABOUR

Occasionally, at one end of the spectrum of normal labour, vigorous but normal uterine activity may produce rapid cervical dilatation and precipitate delivery. The hazards of such labours are that the child may be delivered in a rapid and uncontrolled manner and in an inconvenient environment such as into a toilet! Any labour lasting less than 2 hours is classified as precipitate.

Fetal morbidity and mortality may be related to the lack of resuscitation facilities. Maternal morbidity may arise from severe perineal damage and from postpartum haemorrhage.

Precipitate labour tends to repeat itself with subsequent labours and, where there is such a history, the mother should be admitted to hospital near term to await the onset of labour.

Uterine hyperstimulation

The commonest contemporary cause of uterine hyperstimulation is the uncontrolled use of excessive amounts of oxytocic drugs. In extreme cases, this may result in uterine tetany with a continuous contraction. Leading up to this state, there will be frequent strong contractions and insufficient time between contractions to allow a return to normal baseline pressures. The condition can be rapidly corrected by turning off the oxytocin infusion. In fact, the condition should not arise if uterine activity is properly monitored by external or internal tocography. Contractions should not occur more frequently than five in 10 minutes or more than 1700 kPa/15 min.

Hyperstimulation may also lead to uterine rupture, particularly where there is a uterine scar from a previous section or myomectomy. Such a rupture may sometimes occur even in the presence of normal uterine activity.

TRIAL OF LABOUR AND CEPHALOPELVIC DISPROPORTION

The term 'trial of labour' is reserved for labour where borderline cephalopelvic disproportion is suspected. This may arise because the fetus is abnormally large or where the pelvis, and in particular the pelvic inlet, is small, or a combination of both factors.

The head will not generally be engaged at the onset of labour but may engage with moulding into the pelvis. The pelvis can only be truly tested in the presence of strong uterine contractions.

Management

When the possibility of cephalopelvic disproportion is suspected, labour should be carefully monitored. Regular observations must be recorded of uterine activity, the descent of the presenting part, the rate of cervical dilatation and the condition of both the mother and the fetus.

In primigravid women, the uterus may become exhausted late in the first stage and contractions may cease or become attenuated and cervical dilatation remains arrested at 8–9 cm. If there is no change in cervical dilatation over a period of 4–6 hours, the trial of labour should be abandoned. Similarly, if clinical signs of fetal distress or maternal exhaustion develop, the labour should be terminated by caesarean section.

> Multiparous women are at increased risk of uterine rupture if the labour becomes obstructed. Delay in progress in a multigravid patient should always be treated with caution as it is likely to be associated with malposition or cephalopelvic disproportion and there is a greater risk of uterine rupture with the injudicious use of oxytocic agents.

Case study
Secondary arrest

A 38-year-old multigravid woman was admitted in labour at term. After good initial progress in labour, significant arrest occurred at 8 cm dilatation (Fig. 13.20). Vaginal examination confirmed the presence of an occipitoposterior position associated with marginal cephalopelvic disproportion. The cervix eventually became fully dilated and the head was rotated and delivered with forceps.

Shoulder dystocia

Shoulder impaction occurs where there is a large infant or a small pelvis and particularly where the trunk is large, as with diabetic macrosomia. The head is usually delivered without difficulty and, therefore, the condition is one of some urgency as it can only be recognized at this stage. The neck and shoulders do not appear. Unless delivery is achieved within 5–7 minutes, the child will die from asphyxia.

Delivery can usually be achieved with firm traction posteriorly to disimpact the anterior shoulder (Fig. 13.21) and then with traction anteriorly to deliver the posterior shoulder (Fig. 13.22). Firm downward pressure should be applied suprapubically to disempact the anterior shoulder. The danger of this procedure is that excessive traction on the brachial plexus results in Erb's palsy.

Occasionally, the shoulders are disimpacted by rotation through 45° so that either the anterior or posterior shoulder may be disengaged.

Shoulder dystocia should be anticipated where the estimated fetal weight is over 5 kg, where there is evidence of macrosomia or where there is a history of previous dystocia. Such patients should be delivered where experienced obstetric and paediatric support is readily available (Box 13.5).

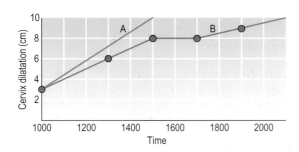

Fig. 13.20 Secondary arrest of cervical dilatation at 8 cm associated with the occipitoposterior position.

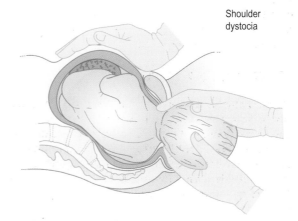

Shoulder dystocia

Fig. 13.21 Disimpaction of the anterior shoulder.

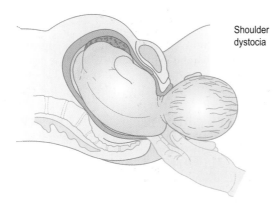

Shoulder dystocia

Fig. 13.22 Impacted shoulders: it is sometimes necessary to rotate the fetus to disimpact the posterior shoulder.

<blockquote>
ℹ️ **Box 13.5**
Difficulty delivering shoulders – action to be taken

- Summon help including paediatrician, senior obstetrician and anaesthetist
- Place mother in the lithotomy position with the hips flexed and abducted as far as possible (McRobert's manoeuvre)
- Apply suprapubic (not fundal) pressure from the posterior aspect of the anterior shoulder to displace it laterally and downwards by suprapubic pressure
- Make or extend episiotomy
- Rotate shoulders into the oblique by applying pressure to the anterior aspect of the most accessible shoulder (Woods manoeuvre)
- Deliver the posterior arm by flexing it at the elbow and sweeping across the chest by grasping the wrist
</blockquote>

ABNORMALITIES OF THE THIRD STAGE OF LABOUR

The third stage of labour starts immediately after the delivery of the infant and ends with expulsion of the placenta. This is normally accomplished within 10–15 minutes and should be complete within 30 minutes.

Postpartum haemorrhage

Primary postpartum haemorrhage consists of blood loss from the vagina in excess of 500 ml and occurring within 24 hours of delivery (Fig. 13.23).

Secondary postpartum haemorrhage consists of excessive vaginal blood loss occurring at any subsequent time in the puerperium up to 6 weeks after delivery.

Atonic uterine haemorrhage

Haemorrhage may occur from any part of the genital tract, but most commonly from the placental site as a result of (see Fig. 14.17):

- Uterine atony – if the uterus does not contract, then the decussation of myometrial fibres does not exert the usual haemostatic compression of the uterine vessels
- Retention of the placenta or placental fragments.

A contracted empty uterus never bleeds.

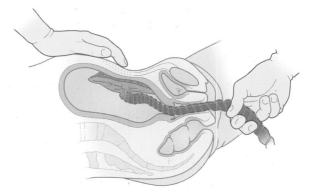

Fig. 13.23 Primary postpartum haemorrhage may occur in the presence of a retained placenta.

Traumatic uterine haemorrhage

This may occur from cervical laceration, which commonly occurs at '3 o'clock' or '9 o'clock' positions, not anteriorly or posteriorly. It may also arise from uterine rupture and, in particular, from rupture of a previous caesarean scar.

Vaginal lacerations

Haemorrhage occurs from vaginal and perineal lacerations and this bleeding may be profuse – particularly when it involves vaginal or vulval varicosities.

Predisposing factors

Various factors predispose to postpartum haemorrhage, including:

- Overdistension of the uterus, e.g. in multiple pregnancy, hydramnios
- Uterine hypotonia associated with prolonged labour
- Antepartum haemorrhage – placenta praevia
- Multiple fibroids
- Grand multiparity
- General anaesthesia where agents such as halothane are employed.

Low implantation of the placenta appears to be associated with difficulties in efficient constriction of uterine blood vessels at the site of the implantation. Placental abruption is associated with an increased incidence of postpartum haemorrhage, partly because blood entrapped behind the placenta is expelled during the third stage but also because there may be difficulty with contractility in myometrium damaged by an antepartum haemorrhage. Occasionally, haemorrhage may occur because of coagulation disorders.

Management

Postpartum bleeding may be sudden and profound and may rapidly lead to cardiovascular collapse. Treatment is directed towards controlling the bleeding and replacing the blood loss (Fig. 13.24).

Controlling the haemorrhage

A brief visual inspection will suffice to ascertain:

- The amount of blood loss
- Whether the placenta has been expelled.

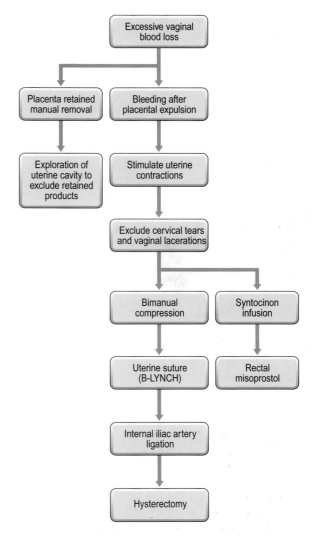

Fig. 13.24 Flow chart showing management of postpartum haemorrhage.

If the placenta has been expelled, the following actions are taken:

- Palpate the uterine fundus. If the uterus is soft, then massage of the uterus will immediately stimulate a contraction and expel any retained clot.
- Inject ergometrine maleate 0.5 mg intravenously and start an oxytocin infusion consisting of 40 units of Syntocinon in 500 ml of Hartmann's solution.

Although ergometrine has become less popular because of induced vomiting and raised blood pressure, it is still the most potent oxytocic agent available and should therefore be used as first choice in this situation.

- Check that the placenta and membranes are complete. If they are not, then manual exploration of the uterine cavity is indicated.
- If the bleeding continues despite the presence of a well-contracted uterus, the vagina and cervix should be examined with a speculum under good illumination and any laceration should be sutured to ensure haemostasis.

If the placenta is retained:

- Massage the uterus to ensure it is well contracted
- Apply cord traction and counter-pressure against the uterine fundus – the placenta is partially separated and will often deliver with gentle but sustained cord traction, as it may be trapped in the cervix
- If this manoeuvre fails, then proceed to manual removal of the placenta – with either regional or general anaesthesia.

Treatment of persistent postpartum haemorrhage

If bleeding continues after removal of the placenta, the following steps should be taken:

- The uterine cavity should be re-explored to be sure that no placental cotyledons have been left behind
- Intramuscular or intramyometrial injection of carboprost (prostaglandin 15-methyl-$F_{2\alpha}$) should be administered
- Rectal misoprostol (synthetic prostaglandin E_2) should be administered
- Check for coagulation disorders.

If medical treatment fails, there are a number of surgical treatments that can be implemented:

- Bimanual compression of the uterus
- The B-Lynch suture involves placement of a purse string suture to compress the uterus
- Tamponade of uterus using Foley catheter balloon or Sengstaken-Blakemore tube
- Internal iliac ligation
- Hysterectomy.

Replacement of blood loss and resuscitation

It is essential to replace blood loss throughout attempts to control the uterine bleeding. Blood substitutes such as Hemacel can be safely used to replace up to 1500 ml of blood loss but on occasions, massive blood transfusions are necessary to save life.

Vaginal wall haematomas

Profuse haemorrhage does at times occur from vaginal and perineal lacerations and it is important to control this bleeding as soon as possible. The practice of leaving a perineal or vaginal tear unsutured for long periods of time is inadvisable, both from the point of view of blood loss and as a potential source of infection.

Venous bleeding can be controlled by compression but arterial bleeding necessitates ligation of the vessel. If control is not achieved, then formation of a haematoma is likely to occur and this may occur in one of two sites (Fig. 13.25).

- **Superficial:** Bleeding occurs below the insertion of the levator ani and the accumulation of blood will be seen to distend the perineum, accompanied by acute pain. The previous sutures must be removed, the haematoma drained and haemostasis secured. This may not always be easy at this stage because of tissue damage, so a drain should be inserted before the wound is re-sutured.
- **Deep:** Bleeding may occur deep to the insertion of the levator ani and a large haematoma may develop. This is more difficult to diagnose and, while it is most likely to arise after forceps or ventouse delivery,

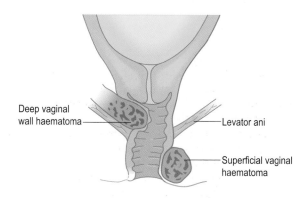

Deep vaginal wall haematoma

Levator ani

Superficial vaginal haematoma

Fig. 13.25 The sites of vaginal wall haematomas.

it can occur after a spontaneous vaginal delivery. The haematoma is not visible externally but presents with symptoms of continuous pelvic pain, unexplained anaemia and retention of urine. It can be readily diagnosed by vaginal examination as the swelling bulges into the upper part of the vaginal wall. The haematoma is drained by an incision over and into the haematoma. It is very difficult to identify any bleeding point at this stage because of extensive tissue damage, although any obvious bleeding points should be ligated.

A large corrugated drain should be inserted into the cavity and the vagina is firmly packed. A catheter should be left indwelling and adequate blood transfusion and antibiotic therapy should be instituted.

Bleeding usually arises from a branch of the pudendal artery.

Perineal wound breakdown

Breakdown of perineal wounds is a common complication and results from infection and haematomas in the perineal wound.

The wound edges gape and the underlying tissues become exposed. The wound should be regularly cleaned and any slough should be removed. Most of these wounds can be left to granulate from the bottom up but, if they are deep and the wound is clean, resuturing may speed up the recovery process. If the sphincter is damaged, it should be repaired at the time but, on occasions, repair may need to be deferred until the tissues are healed.

Amniotic fluid embolism

This is a condition that occurs around the time of delivery and results in cardiovascular and respiratory collapse. It is a rare condition, occurring in about 1/80 000 pregnancies, but it has a high mortality rate. Amniotic fluid enters the maternal circulation and causes sudden intravascular coagulation, resulting in pulmonary insufficiency and a haemorrhagic diathesis.

The patient suddenly collapses with dyspnoea, cyanosis and hypotension. Treatment requires immediate oxygenation, monitoring of central venous pressure and adequate restoration of the circulating blood volume. Fresh frozen plasma is given if the fibrinogen level is low.

ESSENTIAL INFORMATION

Preterm labour

- Labour occurring prior to 37 weeks
- Occurs in 6% of pregnancies
- Causes are
  - Antepartum haemorrhage
  - Multiple pregnancy
  - Infection
  - Polyhydramnios
  - Socioeconomic
- Chances of survival same as at term by 34 weeks
- Prevention is by treatment of infection
- Treatment is by administration of corticosteroids and tocolysis which
  - Is contraindicated after 34 weeks, APH, infection, cervix more than 5 cm
  - Delays delivery by 48 hours
  - Allows time to transfer or give steroids
  - May cause pulmonary oedema

- Is associated with an increased chance of breech presentation
- Delivery should be by caesarean section if breech presentation

Premature rupture of membranes

- Rupture of membranes before 37 weeks
- Causes are
  - Infection
  - Multiple pregnancy
  - Polyhydramnios
  - Smoking
- Usually followed by labour within 48 hours
- May be treated conservatively by monitoring for signs of infection before 36 weeks
- May lead to chorioamnionitis

Prolonged pregnancy

- Occurs in 10% of pregnancies
- Is associated with increase in perinatal mortality after 42 weeks
- Is associated with increased incidence of meconium
- Management options are
  - Routine induction after 41 weeks
  - Increased monitoring

Breech presentation

- Occurs in 3% pregnancies at term
- Associated with
  - Preterm delivery
  - Multiple pregnancy
  - Fetal abnormality
  - Placenta praevia
  - Uterine abnormalities
- External cephalic version at 38 weeks
- Elective caesarean section
- Criteria for vaginal delivery are
  - Fetal weight less than 4 kg, more than 1.5 kg
  - Flexed or frank breech

Rare presentations

- Face presentation 1/500
- Brow presentation 1/1500
- Unstable lie associated with
  - High parity
  - Polyhydramnios
  - Uterine anomalies
  - Low-lying placenta

Cord prolapse

- Predisposing factors
  - Multiple pregnancy
  - Malpresentation
  - Polyhydramnios
- Anticipation where pp high
- Treatment
  - Head–knee position
  - Urgent caesarean section

Occipitoposterior position

- 10–20% cephalic presentation
- Associated with backache, prolonged labour
- Treatment
  - Adequate analgesia
  - Syntocinon
  - Caesarean section
  - Rotational forceps

Abnormalities of uterine action

- 90% of primigravidae deliver within 16 hours
- Diagnosis partogram
- Management
  - Pain relief
  - Fluid replacement
  - Mobilize if hypotonic uterus
  - Stimulate with oxytocin
  - Rupture membranes
  - Operative delivery if lack of progress or fetal distress

MANAGEMENT OF TWIN PREGNANCY

Multiple pregnancies exhibit every type of pregnancy complication at a greater frequency than occurs in singleton pregnancy. Early diagnosis is therefore essential and provides a convincing argument for routine early pregnancy ultrasound scanning (Fig. 14.2).

The commonest clinical sign of twin pregnancy is the greater size of the uterus, which is easier to detect in early, rather than late, pregnancy. There are, of course, other reasons why the uterus may be abnormally enlarged, such as hydramnios and uterine fibroids.

Treatment of any antenatal complication is the same as in singleton pregnancies, but remember that the onset of complications tends to be earlier and of greater severity. Routine hospital admission from 28 weeks gestation for bed rest has been advocated in the past, but clinical trials have failed to demonstrate efficacy. However, careful antenatal supervision and more frequent antenatal visits are indicated. It is important that women with multiple pregnancies are booked for confinement in hospitals where there are suitable special-care baby units.

Intrauterine growth restriction is common and, therefore, serial ultrasound measurements to assess fetal growth are important. If there is evidence of growth restriction in one or both fetuses, early induction of labour should be considered. The overall incidence of IUGR in twins is 29%, involving 42% of monochorionic twins and 25% of dichorionic twins. Thus, frequent assessment using ultrasound scans every 4 weeks from 24 weeks is advised.

MANAGEMENT OF LABOUR AND DELIVERY

Delivery poses many complexities in twin pregnancy because of the variety and complexity of presentations and because the second twin is at significantly greater risk from asphyxia due to placental separation and cord prolapse.

Presentation at delivery

There are a number of permutations for presentation in twin pregnancy at delivery, which are partly influenced by the management of the second twin. Rounded-up figures for these presentations are shown in Figure 14.3.

By far the commonest presentation is cephalic/cephalic (50%), followed by cephalic/breech (25%), breech/cephalic (10%) and breech/breech (10%). The remaining 5% consist of cephalic/transverse, transverse/cephalic, breech/transverse, transverse/breech and transverse/transverse.

Method of delivery

A decision about the method of delivery should preferably be made before the onset of labour.

Caesarean section

Delivery by elective caesarean section is indicated for the same reasons that exist for singleton pregnancies. However, the threshold for intervention is generally lower. Where an additional complication exists, such as a previous caesarean scar, a long history of subfertility, severe pre-eclampsia or diabetes mellitus, most obstetricians will opt for elective section. Premature labour between 28 and 34 weeks gestation is an indication for caesarean delivery, as also is malpresentation of the first twin. Furthermore, the presentation does have an important part to play in deciding the best method of delivery. Caesarean section rates have increased in the UK from 28% in 1980–85 to 42% in 1995–96 and, in

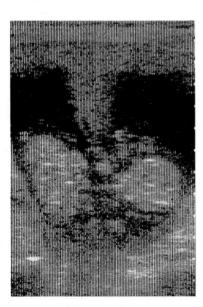

Fig. 14.2 Ultrasound scan of twins early in pregnancy.

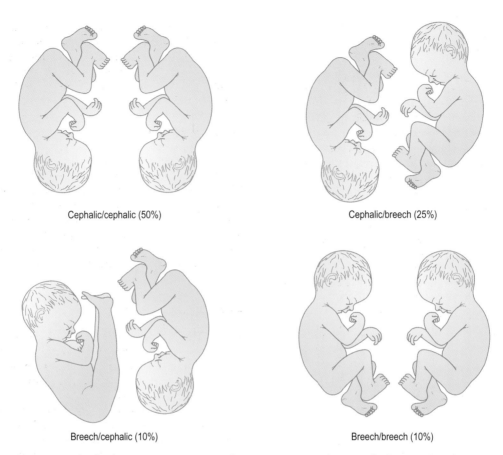

Cephalic/cephalic (50%)   Cephalic/breech (25%)

Breech/cephalic (10%)   Breech/breech (10%)

Fig. 14.3 The four major presentations of twin pregnancy. The 5% of other variations are not listed in these major groups.

general, very few obstetricians now advise vaginal delivery for twin breech presentation or for a breech presentation of the first twin, for fear of locked twins.

Vaginal delivery

When labour is allowed to proceed normally, it is advisable to establish an intravenous line at an early stage. Labour normally lasts the same time as a singleton labour.

The first twin can be monitored with a scalp electrode or by abdominal ultrasound and, if possible, both infants should be monitored. When the first twin is delivered, the lie and presentation of the second twin must be immediately checked and the fetal heart rate recorded.

For delivery of the second twin, the membranes should be left intact until the presenting part is well into the pelvis and cord prolapse excluded. If the uterus does not contract within a few minutes, an oxytocin infusion should be started. If fetal distress occurs, then delivery should be expedited by forceps delivery or breech extraction. Under very exceptional circumstances, it may be necessary to deliver the second twin by caesarean section. It is important to use oxytocic agents with delivery of the second twin as there is an increased risk of postpartum haemorrhage.

Not all obstetricians advocate immediate stimulation of the uterus after delivery of the first twin. It is reasonable to await the spontaneous onset of further contractions without further intervention if the fetal heart rate is normal. However, because of the ever-

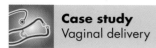

Case study
Vaginal delivery

A 22-year-old woman in her first pregnancy with twins presented at 37 weeks gestation in spontaneous labour. The presentation of both babies was cephalic. An epidural catheter was sited for analgesia and labour progressed uneventfully, with the first twin delivering spontaneously. The presentation of the second twin was confirmed as cephalic with a longitudinal lie. As the presenting part was still above the pelvic brim, a Syntocinon infusion was commenced to maintain uterine contractions, and the membranes were left intact awaiting descent of the presenting part. Shortly afterwards, external monitoring of the fetal heartbeat showed a bradycardia of 60 beats/minute. Delivery of the second twin was expedited by reaching inside the uterus with the membranes still intact (internal podalic version), locating the feet of the fetus and rotating the fetus to the breech position before rupturing the membranes and delivering the infant by breech extraction.

present risk of placental separation and intrauterine asphyxia in the second twin, an upper limit of 30 minutes between the two deliveries is generally accepted as reasonable practice. The delivery of a brain-damaged second twin after a long birth interval will always lead to the question as to why intervention did not take place at an earlier stage.

Higher-order multiple births such as triplets or quadruplets are now delivered by caesarean section. Under these circumstances, the onset of labour is often premature, the birthweights are low and the presentations uncertain.

COMPLICATIONS OF LABOUR

There are several complications of labour, some of which are associated with malpresentation. Babies may become obstructed, particularly where there is a transverse lie presenting and that is, in fact, an indication for delivery by caesarean section. If caesarean section is performed in the presence of an obstructed transverse lie, it may on occasions be preferable to make a vertical incision in the lower and upper segment rather than a transverse incision because of the possibility of extension of the lower segment incision into the uterine vessels and the broad ligaments, resulting in uncontrollable haemorrhage.

Locked twins

This is a very rare complication, where the first twin is a breech presentation and the second is cephalic. Clinically, the twins lock chin to chin. The condition is usually not recognized until delivery of part of the first twin has occurred and its survival is unlikely. It may sometimes be possible to disimpact the locked twins, but if this fails a destructive operation to the first twin may be necessary to stand any chance of saving the second child.

Conjoined twins

The union of twins results from the incomplete division of the embryo after formation. It is a rare complication, with a calculated frequency of 1/546 twin pregnancies. Union may occur at any site but commonly is head to head or thorax to thorax.

If the union is recognized by ultrasound before the onset of labour, then the twins should be delivered by caesarean section, as a significant number of these infants can be surgically separated. If the abnormality is not recognized before the onset of labour, then the labour will usually obstruct.

Perinatal mortality

The perinatal death rate is significantly higher for multiple pregnancies. In general, the mortality rate increases with the number of fetuses. The mortality rate for twins is approximately four times higher than for singleton pregnancies and the mortality rate for the second twin is 50% higher than for the first twin.

The commonest cause of death in both twins is prematurity. Second-born twins are more likely to die from intrapartum asphyxia with separation of the placenta following delivery of the first twin, or where cord prolapse occurs in association with a malpresentation or a high presenting part when the membranes are ruptured.

Overall, perinatal mortality rates are 37, 52 and 231/1000 live and stillbirths for twins, triplets and higher multiple births respectively. In comparison with singleton births of like gestational age, twins and triplets have a relative risk for low-birthweight infants (< 2.5 kg) of 10 and 19 and for very low birthweights (< 1.5 kg) of 10 and 33.

Perhaps of greater concern is the fact that the risk of producing a child with cerebral palsy is eight times greater in twins and 47 times greater in triplets than in singleton pregnancies.

ESSENTIAL INFORMATION

Prevalence of multiple pregnancy

- Monozygous twin rates constant
- Dizygous rates increasing

Determination of chorionicity

- Monochorionic – always same sex
- Dichorionic – same or different sex
- Familial factors – dizygotic twins
- Increasing age and parity – dizygotic twins
- Ovulation induction and in-vitro fertilization

Complications

- Miscarriage
- Antepartum haemorrhage
- Polyhydramnios
- Pre-eclampsia
- Increased perinatal mortality

- Fetofetal transfusion
- Conjoined twins
- Other congenital abnormalities

Management

- Treatment of complications
- Management of IUGR

Management of labour and delivery

- Dependent on presentation
- Previous obstetric history
- High caesarean section rates

Complications of labour

- Locked and conjoined twins
- Cerebral palsy rates increased

15 The puerperium

The puerperium is defined as the 6-week period commencing after the completion of the third stage of labour. During this time major physiological changes occur, with the adaption of the mother to breastfeeding and the return to the non-pregnant state of the various body systems.

PHYSIOLOGICAL CHANGES

Genital tract

The uterus undergoes rapid and massive change by a process of catabolism of muscle fibres. The fibres undergo autolysis and atrophy. Within 10 days the uterus has involuted from a size where it is palpable at the umbilicus to one where it is no longer palpable as an abdominal organ (Fig. 15.1). By 6 weeks the uterus has returned to the non-pregnant size. Where breastfeeding is established over a long period, uterine involution may proceed to a level where the size of the uterus is actually less than is found in the normal non-pregnant state.

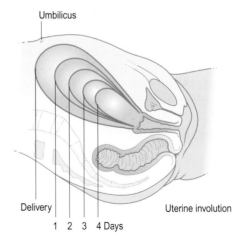

Fig. 15.1 Uterine involution in the puerperium results in a rapid reduction in size.

The endometrium regenerates within 6 weeks and menstruation occurs within this time if lactation has ceased. It lactation continues, the return of menstruation may be deferred for 6 months or more.

Discharge from the uterus is known as *lochia*. At first this consists of blood, either fresh or altered, is called *lochia rubra* and lasts 2–14 days. It then changes to a serous discharge, *lochia serosa*, and finally becomes a slight white discharge, *lochia alba*. These changes may continue for up to 4–8 weeks after delivery. Abnormal persistence of lochia rubra may indicate the presence of retained placental tissue or fetal membranes.

Cardiovascular system

Cardiac output and plasma volume return to normal within approximately 1 week. There is a fluid loss of 2 litres during the first week and a further loss of 1.5 litres over the next 5 weeks. This loss is associated with an apparent increase in haematocrit and haemoglobin concentration. There is an increase of serum sodium and plasma bicarbonate as well as plasma osmolality. An increase in clotting factors during the first 10 days after delivery is associated with a higher risk of deep vein thrombosis and pulmonary embolism. There is also a rise in platelet count and greater platelet adhesiveness. Fibrinogen levels decrease during labour but increase in the puerperium.

Endocrine changes

There are rapid changes in the endocrine system in all facets. There is a rapid fall in the serum levels of oestrogens and progesterone and they reach non-pregnant levels by the seventh postnatal day. This is associated with an increase in serum prolactin levels in those women who breastfeed. By the 10th postnatal day, hCG is no longer detectable.

LACTATION AND BREASTFEEDING

Breastfeeding is the preferred method of infant feeding because, in addition to fulfilling nutritional requirements, it also provides antibodies against infection and protection against various forms of gastroenteritis associated with unhygienic preparation of artificial feeds. Women tend to avoid breastfeeding for social and emotional reasons and often for reasons of convenience. In a relatively small percentage of cases, there are physical reasons why lactation is either not possible or inappropriate, such as inverted nipples, previous breast surgery, breast implants or cracked and painful nipples that do not respond to treatment.

While breastfeeding is desirable and women should be encouraged, it must be remembered that the majority of infants who are artificially fed also thrive. In other words, the enthusiasm of the attendants should not be allowed to override the mother's wishes. Encouragement and education in antenatal classes are important factors, but many women simply do not like the idea of breastfeeding.

Breast preparation

The breasts and nipples should be washed regularly. The breasts should be comfortably supported and the nipples cleared of colostrum. Aqueous-based emollient creams may be used to soften the nipple and thus avoid cracking during suckling. Occasional expression of colostrum in the third trimester helps with subsequent milk secretion. Inverted nipples may present an insuperable barrier to breastfeeding.

Breastfeeding

The child should be put to the breast as soon after delivery as possible. Suckling is initially limited to 2–3 minutes on each side but subsequently this period may be increased. Once the mother is comfortably seated, the whole nipple is placed in the infant's mouth, taking care to maintain a clear airway (Fig. 15.2). Correct attachment of the baby to the breast is essential to the success of breastfeeding. The common problems such as sore nipples, breast engorgement and mastitis usually occur because the baby is poorly attached to the breast or is not fed often enough. Most breastfeeding is given on demand and the milk flow will meet the demand stimulated by suckling. Once the baby is attached correctly to the nipple, the sucking pattern changes from short sucks to long deep sucks with pauses.

Colostrum is the first fluid secreted from the breasts and is rich in proteins and, in particular, immunoglobulins. It is less rich in fats and carbohydrates. Within 3 days, full milk flow becomes established and provides the complete food for the child for the first 3–4 months. There is normally some weight loss in the first week of life. The mother should be reassured that this is normal. After suckling, the child is held upright to enable swallowed air to be regurgitated.

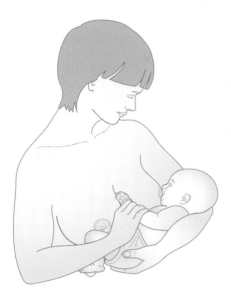

Fig. 15.2 The mother should be comfortable and the child placed well on to the breast to ensure adequate suckling.

It may on occasions be necessary to express milk and store it, either because of breast discomfort or cracked nipples or because the baby is sick. Milk can be expressed manually or by using hand or electric pumps. Breast milk can be safely stored in a refrigerator at 2–4°C for 3–5 days or frozen and stored for up to 3 months in the freezer.

Full milk flow supervenes by the third or fourth day after delivery and may be accompanied by painful vascular engorgement.

Suppression of lactation

Many women elect not to breastfeed. Firm support of the breasts, restriction of fluid intake, avoidance of expression of milk and analgesia may be sufficient to suppress lactation. The administration of oestrogens will effectively suppress lactation but carries some risk of thromboembolic disease. It should, however, be noted that the original description of 'risk' was based on observation of doses of oestrogens far in excess of the quantities necessary to suppress lactation. There is, therefore, a case to be made for administering oral oestrogens to suppress lactation.

Bromocriptine will inhibit prolactin release and hence suppress lactation, but the dosage necessary to produce this effect tends to create considerable side effects. It should, however, be emphasized that it is preferable to avoid all drug therapy if suppression can be achieved by conservative management.

PSYCHOLOGICAL CHANGES AND DISORDERS IN THE PUERPERIUM

Mild degrees of depression and emotional lability are almost the 'norm' in the puerperium but may become severe in some cases and require psychiatric support. Psychiatric illness may present as severe, incapacitating depression but the more florid forms of puerperal psychosis involve confusion and delirium with disorientation in time and space and a complete loss of interest in the child. In some women, frank mania may occur. Early recognition of these symptoms is important if danger to mother and child is to be avoided, and early psychiatric support must be sought. These problems are discussed in greater detail in Chapter 16.

COMPLICATIONS OF THE PUERPERIUM (Box 15.1)
Puerperal pyrexia

The commonest problem of the puerperium is the development of a pyrexia, i.e. a rise of temperature in excess of 38°C on more than one occasion.

 Box 15.1
Complications of the puerperium

- Genital tract infections
- Urinary infection
- Wound infection
- Mastitis
- Thromboembolism
- Incontinence/urinary retention
- Anal sphincter dysfunction
- Breakdown of episiotomy wound

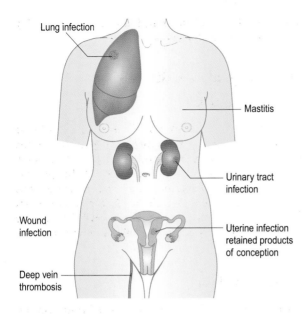

Fig. 15.3 The pathogenesis of puerperal pyrexia.

Aetiology

Puerperal pyrexia must be assumed to be due to infection until proved otherwise. A systematic investigation is undertaken to elucidate the cause and site of the infection (Fig. 15.3).

Genital tract infection

The genital tract is particularly vulnerable to infection. The commonest site is within the uterine cavity. Infection may be introduced via external sources or arise from contamination from endogenous sources. Infection is particularly common following prolonged labour or prolonged rupture of the membranes.

The clinical signs include subinvolution of the uterus, which remains bulky and larger than would normally be anticipated. It is often tender to palpation. The lochia may be offensive or purulent but is often apparently normal. Retained products of conception predispose to infection and will also result in excessive and persistent bloodstained lochia. A cervical swab should be taken for culture as a routine procedure in any women with puerperal pyrexia. The common organisms isolated from this site include *Escherichia coli*, *Staphylococcus pyogenes*, *Streptococcus faecalis* and haemolytic streptococci.

Infection may also occur in episiotomy wounds or perineal tears, although these infections are relatively uncommon because the vascularity of the perineum provides a higher resistance to infection. The perineum becomes tender and reddened and may be seen to exude purulent discharge. Where genital tract infection is suspected, swabs should be taken for culture and antibiotic therapy should be started before the culture results are available.

Urinary tract infection

The postpartum woman is particularly vulnerable to urinary tract infection. This is due to a combination of trauma to the bladder, incomplete emptying, particularly related to perineal pain, and the introduction of bacterial organisms by catheterization.

Urinary tract infection is often unaccompanied by any symptoms, with the exception of a low-grade pyrexia, but, if ascending infection supervenes, acute pyelonephritis may develop. This will produce bilateral loin pain, frequency of micturition and dysuria and lower abdominal pain after voiding. In cases of puerperal pyrexia, a midstream specimen of urine should be sent for culture.

Breast infection

Mastitis most often occurs in the second week after delivery and may therefore develop after discharge from hospital. Infection may be introduced through a cracked nipple and often originates from the mother's skin or nasopharynx or from the infant's nasopharynx. The development of pyrexia is accompanied by pain and local tenderness. The breast develops a reddened, tender area and, if abscess formation occurs, the skin becomes oedematous and develops the classic '*peau d'orange*' appearance.

Early recognition of infection enables early introduction of antibiotic therapy. If abscess formation occurs, surgical drainage is necessary.

If the mother is still lactating, feeding is discontinued from the affected breast. In most cases, lactation should be suppressed unless there is strong motivation to continue.

Other sites of infection

Following caesarean section, infection may occur in the skin wound or in the peritoneal cavity. Where general anaesthesia is used, lung infection may occur, although with modern anaesthesia this is an uncommon complication.

Perineal discomfort

Most women who have had a perineal tear or an episiotomy will need some form of analgesia during the first week after delivery. It is important that the perineal wounds are kept clean and, traditionally, the use of ice packs sometimes brings relief, particularly where there is vulval oedema. The healing process usually progresses rapidly, although the discomfort may persist for some weeks after delivery. Over-vigorous suturing of the perineum may result in narrowing of the introitus and dyspareunia and every effort should be made to ensure that this does not occur, by checking that the introitus admits at least two fingers at the time of the primary suturing. Where wound breakdown occurs, the wound should be kept clean and allowed to heal from the bottom up. Resuturing should not be performed unless the wound is clean and there is no residual inflammation around the wound margins.

Postpartum anal sphincter dysfunction

In recent years, it has become increasingly apparent that impaired faecal continence occurs in up to 25% of primiparous women after vaginal delivery. In the majority of women, the symptoms are minor and transient but in some women, incontinence of flatus or faeces or urgency of defaecation persist and may be socially and emotionally inhibiting. The symptoms are often not admitted unless the mother is specifically questioned.

The injury to the anal canal occurs during vaginal delivery and may result from direct anal sphincter muscle disruption, traction neuropathy of the pudendal nerves or a combination of both mechanical and neurological trauma.

The nature of the injury can be elucidated by anal manometry, endoanal ultrasound and neurophysiological assessment.

Conservative management involves dietary manipulation, the use of antidiarrhoeal agents such as codeine phosphate or loperamide, pelvic floor exercises, sensory biofeedback therapy and augmented biofeedback.

Where the anal sphincter is completely disrupted, as from a recognized third-degree tear, it should be immediate repaired in the delivery ward. If the disruption is only recognized at a later date, it may be better to delay the repair for several months.

Thromboembolic disease

Thrombophlebitis

This is the commonest form of thromboembolic disease and tends to arise within the first 3–4 days after delivery. Localized inflammation, tenderness and thickening occur in the superficial leg veins. Although the condition is painful and may spread along the leg veins, it rarely leads to serious embolic disease and does not require anticoagulant treatment. Anti-inflammatory drugs and local applications of glycerine and ichthyol should be used.

Phlebothrombosis

Deep vein thrombosis is a much more serious complication that tends to arise 7–10 days after delivery and is particularly likely to occur after operative delivery or prolonged immobilization. Clotting occurring in deep veins may be silent and presents only when the clot breaks loose and lodges in the lung as a pulmonary embolus, with consequent chest pain and haemoptysis. Massive pulmonary embolus results in sudden death unless treated by prompt surgical management.

Management

Deep vein thrombosis commonly presents in the third trimester or within 6 weeks postpartum. The clinical symptoms and signs include leg pain, swelling and erythema of the affected leg and, where there is embolism, chest pain and haemoptysis.

The diagnosis of femoral vein thrombosis can be confirmed by Doppler flow ultrasound and limited venography and, where chest pain occurs, a perfusion lung scan should confirm the diagnosis of pulmonary embolus.

As soon as the diagnosis is suspected, anticoagulant treatment should be started with intravenous or subcutaneous heparin. The limb should be rested until anticoagulant therapy produces pain relief; then gradual mobilization may be introduced. When the acute process has been controlled, the anticoagulant therapy can be changed to warfarin and should be continued for 3 months. Specialized leg supports such as TED stockings are used to provide support for the affected leg.

Deep vein thrombosis arising during pregnancy should be treated with either unfractionated or low-molecular-weight heparin given intravenously for acute control and subcutaneously for longer-term therapy. Either form of heparin does not cross the placenta, so there is no risk to the fetus. However, long-term heparin use may cause maternal osteoporosis and thrombocytopenia. The treatment should be discontinued during labour and recommenced shortly after delivery. Fresh frozen plasma should be available to treat any excessive maternal blood loss at the time of delivery.

Oral anticoagulants such as warfarin must be avoided in the first 12 weeks of pregnancy as these drugs cross the placenta and can produce a characteristic embryopathy with agenesis of the corpus callosum, optic atrophy, blindness and midline cerebellar atrophy. About 30% of all infants born to mothers where the drug is given between 6–12 weeks gestation are affected. Central nervous system abnormalities may occur as the result of warfarin therapy at any stage of pregnancy and the therapy may also result in fetal haemorrhage. These drugs are therefore best avoided during pregnancy but where, for practical reasons, it is considered best to continue oral anticoagulants, the mother should certainly be switched to heparin well before the onset of labour, as fetal haemorrhage may be a significant complication. Heparin does not cross into breast milk and warfarin does so only in very low concentration so that it is safe to use either treatment in the lactating and breastfeeding mother.

Other complications

Urinary retention is a common problem in the immediate puerperium and may result in overflow incontinence. The major cause of retention is pain from the perineum. Traditional methods of encouraging micturition include hot baths, relief of perineal pain by analgesic drugs and local applications of ice-packs. If these procedures fail, then the bladder should be

Case study
Deep vein thrombosis

Mrs Angela G developed a painful right calf at 16 weeks gestation with a swollen lower leg. A diagnosis of deep vein thrombosis was established and she was started on an intravenous heparin infusion. Within the week, the pain subsided and the swelling diminished. She was mobilized and given a support stocking and her treatment was changed to subcutaneous heparin. At 38 weeks gestation, Angela complained of lower back pain and was treated symptomatically. She went into labour at term and had a normal vaginal delivery. However, the lumbar back pain now became severe and an X-ray of her lumbar spine revealed collapse of an osteoporotic L4 vertebra. This was associated with the long-term heparin treatment.

catheterized on an intermittent basis until the residual urine is less than 50 ml.

True incontinence is a rare complication and is usually associated with a vesicovaginal fistula resulting from pressure necrosis during obstructed labour, or following direct injury to the bladder. Injection of a coloured dye into the bladder will establish the diagnosis. A catheter is left indwelling until there is evidence of closure of the fistula or surgical repair is undertaken.

Stress incontinence and urgency of micturition are also common problems following delivery. Stress incontinence is associated with some degree of prolapse of the bladder neck and can often be improved by the use of pelvic floor exercises. It is advisable to avoid any surgical intervention for at least 3 months after delivery as spontaneous improvement is likely to occur.

ESSENTIAL INFORMATION

Physiological changes

- Uterine involution
- Lochial loss
- Endometrial regeneration
- Reduction of cardiac output
- Fluid loss 2 litres first week

Endocrine changes

- Oestrogen/progesterone
- hCG undetectable 10 days

Lactation and breastfeeding

- Colostrum
- Milk flow 2–3 days
- Suckling process, lactation suppression

Psychological changes

- Puerperal depression

Puerperal pyrexia

- Genital tract infection
- Urinary tract infection
- Breast infection
- Wound infection

Perineal damage

- Anal sphincter dysfunction
- Urinary incontinence

Thromboembolic disease

effects, particularly in postpartum women, both parkinsonism and acute dystonias. These can be prevented or treated by using an anti-parkinsonian agent such as procyclidine 10 mg twice a day. Alternatively the new 'atypical' antipsychotics such as risperidone or olanzapine may be used. Lithium carbonate can also be used to treat acute episodes of mania, as well as in its more familiar use as a prophylactic against recurrence of manic depressive illness. For severe depressive psychoses, electroconvulsive therapy (ECT) may be used.

Antidepressants take between 10 and 14 days to begin their effect. Puerperal psychosis usually responds very quickly to treatment. There should be substantial improvement within days, with recovery taking place within 2 weeks for mania and 4–6 weeks for the depressive psychoses. In the latter, antidepressants will need to be used to maintain recovery after the cessation of ECT.

Risk of relapse

Early-onset puerperal psychosis, although responding to treatment very well, frequently relapses after recovery. Continuation of medication is, therefore, very important for 6 months following recovery. A patient who has presented with a manic psychosis may relapse with a depressive psychosis or a further episode of mania. If this happens on more than one occasion, the clinician may well think of using lithium carbonate in order to stabilize the mood for up to 6 months to 1 year postpartum. If the patient has suffered from a previous episode of non-postpartum manic depressive illness, prophylaxis should be continued for 2 years following delivery.

Risk of recurrence

The risk is now estimated to be 1/2 following any subsequent childbirth. The risk is likely to be highest if the woman has a baby within 2 years of recovery from her illness. Such patients should therefore be advised to delay their next pregnancy until they have been well for at least 2 years.

> ! All women should be asked at booking whether they have had a previous serious mental illness.

Severe major postnatal depression

(Box 16.3)

This affects between 3% and 5% of all women delivered. It too develops in the early weeks following delivery but does not show the abrupt onset of puerperal psychosis, developing more slowly. A third of the patients present within the first 3 weeks after delivery, and they are the most severely disturbed. However, two-thirds present later, between 10 and 12 weeks post-partum. Most of these women would have been diagnosable at the 6-week postnatal check. This latter group are often missed and go untreated.

Women with severe postnatal depression have the classic biological syndrome of early-morning wakening, a mood that is worse in the morning and impaired appetite, concentration and interests. They are often

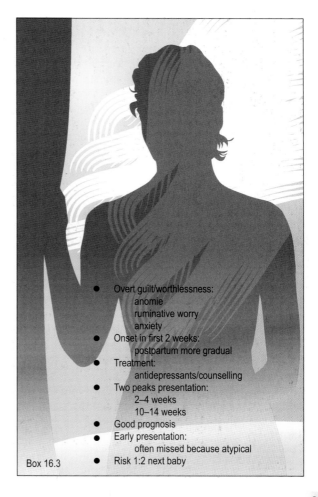

- Overt guilt/worthlessness:
  anomie
  ruminative worry
  anxiety
- Onset in first 2 weeks:
  postpartum more gradual
- Treatment:
  antidepressants/counselling
- Two peaks presentation:
  2–4 weeks
  10–14 weeks
- Good prognosis
- Early presentation:
  often missed because atypical
- Risk 1:2 next baby

Box 16.3

indecisive and find it uncharacteristically difficult to cope with everyday life. Their mood is profoundly lowered. They feel flat, empty and weary, there is a loss of zest and interest in life and a loss of the ability to feel pleasure or enjoyment (anhedonia). They feel guilty and incompetent, and about one-third have intrusive obsessional thoughts of harm coming to their children. They are often frightened that they are bad mothers. Severe anxiety and panic attacks are also common.

Management

Antidepressants

Severely depressed mood and biological symptoms predict a response to antidepressants, which will be needed to ensure the earliest and complete recovery. A wide variety of antidepressants are now available. There are two large groups, the tricyclic antidepressants (e.g. imipramine and dothiepin) and the selective serotonin-reuptake inhibitors (SSRIs; e.g. fluoxetine and paroxetine). Theoretically they are all equally effective but have different side effect profiles. Tricyclic antidepressants can cause drowsiness and dry mouth. The SSRIs can cause insomnia and increased agitation. If a woman has a previous experience of responding to a particular antidepressant it is sensible to use the same antidepressant again. Otherwise the choice is determined by the particular symptoms of the woman and whether she is breastfeeding.

If she is breastfeeding, if anxiety and insomnia is a major problem or if she is profoundly depressed, a tricyclic antidepressant can be chosen. However it should be remembered that these are fatal in overdose and great caution needs to be exercised if the woman is at risk of deliberate self-harm. A suggested initial regime would be dothiepin or imipramine starting at 75 mg at night increasing over a few days to 150 mg at night.

If the woman has prominent symptoms of anxiety, panic and intrusive obsessional thoughts, an SSRI can be used. Fluoxetine, because of its long half-life, should be avoided in breastfeeding. A suggested initial regime would be 20 mg of fluoxetine or paroxetine or 50 mg of sertraline.

All antidepressants take 7–14 days to begin working and must be continued for at least 6 months.

Hormones

Although progesterone therapy has had much popular support there is no evidence to support its use either as a prophylactic against postnatal depression or as treatment for postnatal depression. There is some evidence to suggest that the use of progesterone, both as a treatment and in the form of a progesterone-only contraceptive, may increase the likelihood of suffering from a depressive illness, particularly in those women who are at risk.

There is some clinical and theoretical evidence to support the use of oestrogens in the treatment of postnatal depression. They are likely to have an antidepressant effect on the central nervous system. However the work needs to be replicated on a large scale before it can be recommended as a first line of treatment for postnatal depression, particularly in view of the current concerns about the use of hormone replacement therapy.

Risk of relapse

Providing medication is continued for 6 months, the majority of women can expect to recover fully. However, some will need to continue their medication for longer. The risk following future pregnancies is 1/2 for those women who have postpartum-only illnesses. The risk of recurrence outside childbirth is low. However, for those women who have had episodes not associated with childbirth, the risk following subsequent births is lower than this but the risk of non-postpartum episodes is increased.

Mild postnatal depression (Box 16.4)

This is the most common condition following childbirth. At least 7% of women will reach the criteria for mild major depressive illness and many more would meet the criteria for minor depressive illness. This form of depression tends to affect a vulnerable population, and usually presents later in the postpartum year, often via the health visitor, with problems coping, particularly with the infant. The symptoms are variable and the patient is often tearful, having difficulty in coping, complaints of irritability and lack of satisfaction with motherhood. Symptoms of anxiety, initial insomnia and a sense of loneliness and isolation are common. The patient is often distractible and better in company. She frequently has social and marital problems. The full biological syndrome of major depressive illness is absent.

effects on the child. Social and psychological interventions are particularly important but are likely to take place in primary care. Preventive strategies, using modified antenatal classes, could possibly reduce morbidity in this group in their next pregnancy.

AETIOLOGY OF POSTPARTUM MOOD DISORDERS

It is generally assumed that biological factors are the most important aetiological factors for the severe illnesses, i.e. postpartum psychosis and severe depressive illness, and that psychosocial factors the most important for mild postnatal depressive illness.

Neuroendocrine factors

The constancy of incidence across cultures and over time, the close temporal relationship of the onset to childbirth and the more recent findings of a high risk of subsequent postpartum illness and a lowered risk of non-postpartum episodes would tend to suggest a neuroendocrine basis for the severe conditions. Changes in cortisol, oxytocin, endorphins, thyroxine, progesterone and oestrogen have all been implicated in the causation of this condition. Comparable dramatic changes in steroidal hormones outside the postpartum period have a well-known association with affective psychoses and mood disorders. A plausible recent theory is that the sudden fall in oestrogen triggers a hypersensitivity of D_2 receptors in a predisposed group of women and may be responsible for the very severe mood disturbance that follows. The occurrence and severity of the postnatal 'blues' has been shown to be related to both the absolute level of progesterone and the relative drop from the prepartum level. However, there is no known association between the postpartum 'blues' and affective psychoses and no evidence as yet to implicate progesterone in the aetiology of these conditions.

Obstetric factors

Emergency caesarean section has been shown to be associated with postpartum psychosis in first-time mothers. Previous obstetric loss has been associated with severe postnatal depressive illness, as has infertility and an adverse experience of childbirth. However, there is no direct evidence to suggest that other obstetric complications predispose to severe psychiatric illness.

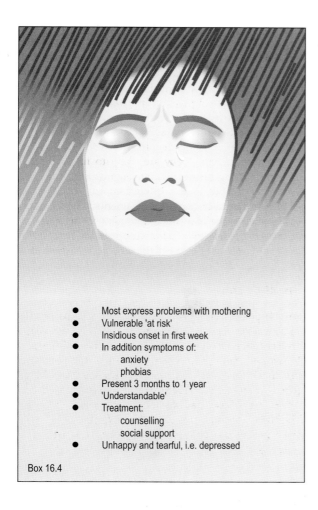

- Most express problems with mothering
- Vulnerable 'at risk'
- Insidious onset in first week
- In addition symptoms of:
    anxiety
    phobias
- Present 3 months to 1 year
- 'Understandable'
- Treatment:
    counselling
    social support
- Unhappy and tearful, i.e. depressed

Box 16.4

Management

Psychological treatments are as effective as antidepressants and more effective than standard care for this group of patients. Six weekly sessions of specific counselling by a trained health visitor are effective treatment, as is a similar course of cognitive psychotherapy. The latter form of treatment would appear to be particularly popular with patients and confers some benefit on those patients who are suffering from depression only within the context of childbirth, and on their children. Social support and practical help from a female confidante improves the mental health and wellbeing of the mother and the child both as a preventative and treatment strategy. This form of common depression, often associated with social adversity and marital conflict, may become chronic and have adverse

Social factors

Severe postpartum illness can affect women with much-wanted babies from happy and stable marriages, who live in comfortable economic circumstances. Apart from a family history and personal history of psychiatric disorder, there is little to distinguish women suffering from severe mental illness from other postpartum women.

However, women suffering from minor postnatal depression do show significant differences both from well women and from women suffering from severe postnatal depression or puerperal psychosis. The risk factors for mild postnatal depression appear to be predominately psychosocial. They include being young, either single or only recently married, lack of a female confidante, chronic social adversity, marital discord, previous psychiatric history, prior social services involvement and antenatal admission in the last trimester of pregnancy. They are significantly more likely than other women to have been admitted on multiple occasions, but for non-serious conditions, usually abdominal pain with no explanation or unfounded concerns about retarded uterine growth.

 Family history of serious illness in maternal relatives also increases risk.

BREASTFEEDING AND MEDICATION

Many women who present with mental illness early in the puerperium are breastfeeding, and its continuation is usually very important to them. Depressed women are often advised to stop breastfeeding, partly because it is commonly believed that psychotropic medication adversely affects the infant and partly because it is commonly believed that the mother's mood will improve. There is no evidence that stopping breastfeeding in itself improves the mother's mental state. In reality it often adds to the burden of guilt she feels. Continuing breastfeeding, particularly when depressed, often helps to maintain a relationship with the baby and a feeling of usefulness, and may protect the infant from the effects of maternal depression.

Continuing breastfeeding requires a great deal of skill on the part of the psychiatric nurse when women are so very disturbed. Totally breastfeeding the infant may not

be possible in the first few days of a severe puerperal psychosis. Nonetheless, it should be possible to maintain lactation with a combination of expressing the milk and frequent suckling of the infant.

When it is clearly important to continue breastfeeding, the choice of psychotropic medication becomes very important (Box 16.5). Lithium should not be given to breastfeeding women. The available evidence suggests that tricyclic antidepressants in full dosage are safe for breastfeeding. They are present in only very small amounts in breast milk, and significant quantities are not detectable in the infant's serum. The use of neuroleptics is more contentious. Phenothiazines, such as chlorpromazine in a single dosage of 50 mg and not more than 200 mg a day, or trifluoperazine in a single dosage of 5 mg and not more than 15 mg a day, are also probably safe for breastfeeding mothers. However, the

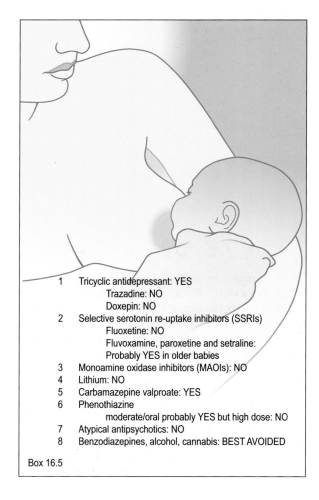

1   Tricyclic antidepressant: YES
       Trazadine: NO
       Doxepin: NO
2   Selective serotonin re-uptake inhibitors (SSRIs)
       Fluoxetine: NO
       Fluvoxamine, paroxetine and setraline:
       Probably YES in older babies
3   Monoamine oxidase inhibitors (MAOIs): NO
4   Lithium: NO
5   Carbamazepine valproate: YES
6   Phenothiazine
       moderate/oral probably YES but high dose: NO
7   Atypical antipsychotics: NO
8   Benzodiazepines, alcohol, cannabis: BEST AVOIDED

Box 16.5

long-term effects on the developing child and adult are unknown. The infant should be closely monitored, and breastfeeding should be suspended if the baby is drowsy, does not wake and cry for its feeds or does not suckle strongly.

If the severity of the mental state requires the use of parenteral medication or a single dose of more than the equivalent of 100 mg of chlorpromazine, it is probably safer to suspend breastfeeding for a period of 12–24 hours and express the milk. Paediatric advice should be sought if the baby is premature, of low birthweight or jaundiced.

There is no evidence on the safety of atypical antipsychotics in breastfeeding and their use can not be recommended.

Summary

Although few psychotropic drugs are known to be teratogenic or to have adverse effects on the developing fetus or neonate, no psychotropic drug is of proven safety. It is therefore very important that psychotropic medication should not be prescribed lightly during pregnancy or lactation and that such drugs should be prescribed only where there are positive indications for their use. Close collaboration between the obstetrician and psychiatrist is recommended before treatment of a mental illness with psychotropic medication. Breast-feeding should not routinely be suspended in mothers who require psychotropic medication. There is an adequate range of psychotropic drugs available to safely treat the mentally ill pregnant or lactating woman.

MENTAL ILLNESS IN PREGNANCY

There is probably a slightly increased risk of minor (neurotic) mental illness during the first trimester of pregnancy, with about 15% of pregnant women suffering from such conditions having been previously well prior to conception. These illnesses usually resolve spontaneously as the pregnancy progresses. The incidence of psychiatric disorder in the second trimester of pregnancy is 8%, and in the third 5%. Women who develop a minor illness (usually anxiety or reactive depression) in the first trimester of pregnancy are not thought to be at increased risk of developing postnatal depression after delivery. However, those very few women who develop such an illness in the last trimester of pregnancy may be at increased risk of postnatal

depression and should be followed up. Psychotropic medication is not usually required for women who develop minor mental illness in pregnancy. Counselling and improving social support is the preferred and effective treatment.

The risk of developing a new episode of major mental illness (manic–depressive illness or schizophrenia) is low during pregnancy and probably lower than at other times in a woman's life. This is in contrast to the dramatic increase in risk following childbirth. Similarly, women with a past history of major psychiatric disorders are probably not at increased risk of relapsing during pregnancy. However, on the rare occasion that they do, or when such an illness develops for the first time in pregnancy, it requires treatment.

For severe depressive illnesses, tricyclic antidepressants, e.g. dothiepin 150 mg daily, can be used but they will need to be reduced by 25 mg every 2 weeks so that the mother is receiving less than 75 mg or, preferably, has stopped taking the antidepressant before delivery. This is because there have been some reports of babies born to mothers receiving a full therapeutic dose of tricyclic antidepressants suffering from neonatal jitteriness and anticholinergic side effects. After delivery, the antidepressant can be gradually increased back to a therapeutic level. This is to mitigate the substantial risk of the mother developing a postpartum relapse.

In clinical practice, SSRIs are now more widely used than tricyclic antidepressants. It is therefore common-place for women to conceive while taking SSRIs and for them to be prescribed during pregnancy. There is no evidence to suggest that SSRIs are teratogenic and there is no rationale for abruptly stopping them upon conception. However they too should be tapered and stopped before delivery. Babies born to mothers receiving SSRIs may experience neonatal complications, including hypoglycaemia, hypothermia and jitteriness. SSRIs can be re-instituted immediately after delivery but fluoxetine should not be used if the mother is breast-feeding.

Very rarely, a new episode of mania can occur during pregnancy. This can be treated, as is usual, with chlorpromazine or another neuroleptic in the smallest possible dose that effects resolution of the symptoms. Again, this will need to be reduced to the minimum possible dose before delivery. There have been some reports of mothers suffering from hypotensive episodes following delivery on large doses of neuroleptics. There have also been reports of babies suffering from hypotonia and extrapyramidal side effects. Once delivered, the neuroleptic should be increased again to mitigate the substantial risk of a manic relapse following delivery.

There is insufficient evidence on the safety of the new atypical antipsychotics (risperidone, olanzapine and clozapine) in pregnancy to recommend their use. If it is known that a woman who is taking one of these medications is trying to conceive, they should be changed to a traditional antipsychotic drug if at all possible. If a woman conceives on these atypical antipsychotics, wherever possible she should be changed to a traditional antipsychotic drug. However, if there is a major concern about a relapse of her condition, they should be reduced to the minimum possible dose and paediatric advice should be sought at delivery.

Lithium should not be used in pregnancy as it is teratogenic in the first trimester and may cause cardiac defects, and in the last trimester has been associated with fetal hypothyroidism. However, if the mother is not breastfeeding, lithium may be reintroduced after delivery, aiming at a therapeutic serum level by day 5. This has been shown in non-randomized clinical studies to be very effective at preventing a postpartum manic relapse.

Anticonvulsants, particularly carbamazepine and sodium valproate, are widely used as mood stabilizers for women with manic depressive illness. They are known to be teratogenic in the first trimester. Current advice is that these anticonvulsant mood stabilizers should not be used in women who are intending to conceive. They should therefore be withdrawn before conception if at all possible. If a woman conceives on these drugs, there is no rationale for their abrupt cessation and no evidence that they cause problems with the developing fetus later in pregnancy. Unlike lithium, they are safe for use in breastfeeding.

The risk to the fetus from receiving psychotropic medication in utero has to be balanced against the risk posed by maternal disturbance.

Chronic mental illness and pregnancy

With the exception of anorexia nervosa, no psychiatric condition is associated with a reduction in biological fertility. Therefore, all forms of psychiatric disorder may present associated with pregnancy. A particular problem for the psychiatrist and obstetrician is posed by those women whose stability of mental health and social functioning depends upon taking regular medication.

Manic–depressive illness

If a woman has a history of multiple episodes of manic–depressive illness, she may be receiving a combination of one or more of the following groups of drugs: antidepressants, neuroleptics and lithium. She may often be given advice to stop taking these drugs before conceiving, and may therefore face not only a dramatic increase in the risk of relapse following delivery (1/2) but also a risk of relapsing during pregnancy in the weeks following cessation of medication. If at all possible, such women should discuss with their psychiatrist before conception the likely effects on their mental health of stopping their medication and of childbirth. If the patient, family and psychiatrist have every reason to believe that, given a stable mental state, the woman can meet the needs of the developing child, she will need assistance to manage her condition. She should be advised to gradually reduce her dosage of lithium before conception. If necessary, her mental state will need to be stabilized with antidepressants if she becomes depressed, or with a small dose of neuroleptic if she becomes hypomanic. Her mental health should then improve as the pregnancy progresses. Once delivered, she should be restarted on her normal regime. If she wishes to breastfeed, this should include a neuroleptic. If she does not wish to breastfeed, then lithium can be started on the first postpartum day.

Chronic schizophrenia

These women will usually be maintained either on an oral neuroleptic or, commonly, an intramuscular depot injection of a neuroleptic such as fluphenazine decanoate or flupenthixol. If this medication is stopped they run a substantial risk of a relapse in their schizophrenic illness within 3 months. Again, ideally these women should discuss with their psychiatrist their capacity to parent as well as the effects on their mental health of pregnancy and the postpartum period. If, when well and stable, even on medication, they have the resources to effectively parent a child, they should be advised not to stop their medication in order to conceive or during pregnancy. However, as they approach delivery their medication should be reduced to the minimum level compatible with mental health and then increased on the day of delivery to the normal regime. Women with chronic schizophrenia may benefit from a period of inpatient admission to a mother and baby unit to help them get off to the best possible start with their infant and provide an opportunity to assess their capacity to care for the child.

Providing medication is continued, the risk of relapse in the immediate postpartum period is not high. However, such women may remain vulnerable to the stresses and strains of child-rearing for some months and years to come.

PREVENTION

Secondary prevention

The identification of vulnerable women and those at high risk, vigilance in the first 2 weeks, early detection and vigorous treatment will reduce maternal morbidity and adverse affects on the child. The inclusion of routine questions designed to detect postnatal depression or the use of a simple screening schedule such as the Edinburgh Postnatal Depression Scale would allow for the detection of the 10% of women who are suffering from major depressive illness and their treatment with either antidepressant or psychological therapies as indicated.

Primary prevention

Hormonal strategies have yet to be confirmed by clinical trials. For those women at high risk of a bipolar illness by virtue of a previous postpartum episode or past psychiatric history, the use of lithium carbonate has been shown in non-randomized clinical studies to be effective. Such a strategy will involve a high degree of co-operation between the psychiatrist and obstetrician. Lithium should be started at 400 mg at night on the first postpartum day, increasing to a dose that produces a therapeutic level (0.6–0.8 mmol/l) by day 3–5 postpartum. Breastfeeding is not possible on this regime. For those women who wish to breastfeed, a small dose of a neuroleptic such as 1.5 mg of haloperidol at night may be equally effective.

Women with a past history of severe depressive illness may wish to start antidepressants on the day of delivery. They should start their previously effective antidepressant at half-dosage on the day of delivery (e.g. 75 mg of dothiepin) and gradually increase it by 25 mg every 3–4 days until they are taking a therapeutic dose (150 mg of dothiepin) by 2 weeks post-partum.

Psychosocial interventions

Mothers with chronic life difficulties, poor marriages, lack of a female confidante and a past history of maternal deprivation and previous depressive episodes are at risk of developing mild postnatal depression following delivery. However, just as important is the risk that they will not enjoy their children. Providing specially modified antenatal classes for this vulnerable group with an emphasis on social support and anticipatory learning of the likely difficulties that face new mothers has been shown to be effective in reducing the rates of postnatal depression. Also effective is the providing of a social confidante, practical assistance and advice-giving through linking such women with an experienced volunteer mother.

THE 'BLUES'

The majority of women experience some alteration in their emotional state between the third and 10th day post-partum. This is known as the 'baby blues'. The most common day of onset is day 5. The 'blues' is probably associated with both the absolute level of progesterone and the relative drop of progesterone from the predelivery to postpartum level. However, despite its probable hormonal basis, it should be remembered that bouts of low mood and tearfulness are very common 3–5 days after an exciting event and also after many surgical events.

The 'blues' is characterized by a low, tearful and labile mood, irritability, insomnia and a tendency to be oversensitive to criticism and transient bouts of despair and catastrophizing – 'blowing things out of proportion'. The severity of the 'blues' varies from being relatively mild to quite distressing, but it is an essentially normal and probably inevitable consequence of childbirth and should not be confused with mental illness. Unlike mental illness it usually only lasts 48 hours, it responds to kindness and reassurance and does not deteriorate over the following days as postnatal depression does. However, tearful and anxious episodes may occur on occasion for a number of weeks following childbirth, particularly when the mother is tired or the baby is difficult to settle.

It is important that all professionals involved with the care of newly delivered mothers know of the timing, characteristics and essentially benign nature of the 'blues'. It is also important that women themselves and their partners are made aware of this phenomenon during antenatal classes.

CONCLUSION

Postpartum mood disorder of all severities is a common complication of childbirth. In many cases it is pre-dictable and perhaps avoidable. In all cases awareness by the obstetrician of risk factors and the clinical syndromes will allow for early detection, prompt treatment and a reduction in morbidity, with subsequent benefits to the woman, her infant and her family (Table 16.1).

Table 16.1
Psychiatry and obstetrics

Time	Action	Risk factors
Booking clinic	Take family and personal history	Severe postnatal depression
	Psychiatric disorder	Puerperal psychosis
	Refer to past history	Previous serious psychiatric disorder
Antenatal care	Vigilance	Previous baby, previous loss, infertility
		Multiple antenatal admissions
		High anxiety
Delivery	Vigilance	Caesarean section
		Maternal danger
Postnatal	Vigilance	Baby admitted to special care baby unit
		Maternal readmission
		Early maternal disturbance
Postnatal examination	6 weeks	Screen for postnatal depression

ESSENTIAL INFORMATION

Importance of psychiatric disorders

- Substantial morbidity
- Effective treatment
- Adverse consequences
- Predict risk
- Regular health contact
- Prevention

Risk factors for mild postnatal depression

- Single
- Young
- Short interval
- Early deprivation
- Chronic life difficulties
- Society adversity trend
- Lack of confidante

- Past psychiatric history
- Question TOP index pregnancy
- Antenatal admission, non-serious conditions
- Life events
- Prior social services involvement

Adverse sequelae of postnatal depression

- Immediate:
  - Physical morbidity
  - Suicide/infanticide
  - Prolonged psychiatric morbidity
  - Social attachments mother–infant
  - Emotional development
- Later:
  - Social–cognitive affects in the child
  - Psychiatric morbidity in the child
  - Marital breakdown

Risk factors for serious mental illness

- Primiparity
- Past psychiatric history
- Family psychiatric history

Prevention of mental illness

- Counsel women with chronic severe mental illness about pregnancy
- Manic–depressive illness: consider restarting treatment after delivery
- Maintain chronic schizophrenic medication throughout pregnancy
- Previous history of puerperal psychosis/severe postnatal depression: close contact first week
- Consider prophylaxis after delivery
- Assess all women at 6 weeks postnatal check for postnatal depression

Psychotropic medication in pregnancy

- Balance risk to the fetus of maternal medication against risk to the fetus of maternal relapse
- Mood stabilizers, lithium, carbamazepine and sodium valproate are teratogenic
- All antidepressants should be tapered and preferably stopped before delivery
- More information on older drugs
- Only use medication in pregnancy when absolutely necessary
- Close psychiatric and obstetric liaison

SECTION 3
Essential gynaecology

17

History taking and examination in gynaecology

The term 'gynaecology' describes the study of diseases of the female genital tract and reproductive system. There is a continuum between gynaecology and obstetrics so that the division is somewhat arbitrary. Complications of early pregnancy such as miscarriage and ectopic pregnancy are generally considered under the title of gynaecology.

HISTORY

When taking a history, start by introducing yourself and explaining who you are. Details of the patient's name, age and occupation should always be recorded at the beginning of a consultation. The age of the patient will influence the likely diagnosis for a number of presenting problems. Occupation may be relevant both to the level of understanding that can be assumed and the impact of different gynaecological problems on the patient's life. The history should be comprehensive, but not intrusive in a manner that is not relevant to the patient's problem. For example, while it is essential to obtain a detailed sexual history from a young couple presenting with subfertility, it would be both irrelevant and distressing to ask the same questions of an 80-year-old widow with a prolapse. The history must, therefore, be geared to the presenting symptom.

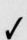 Remember; the presenting symptom may not always be related to the main anxiety of the patient and that some time and patience may be required to uncover the various problems that bring the patient to seek medical advice.

The presenting complaint

The patient should be asked to describe the nature of her problem, and a simple statement of the presenting symptoms should be made in the case notes. A great deal can be learned by using the actual words employed by the patient. It is important to ascertain the timescale of the problem and, where appropriate, the circumstances surrounding the onset of symptoms and their relationship to the menstrual cycle. It is also important to discover the degree of disability experienced for any given symptom. In many situations, reassurance that there is no serious underlying pathology will provide sufficient 'treatment' because the actual disability may be minimal.

More detailed questions will depend on the nature of the presenting complaint. Disorders of menstruation are the commonest reason for gynaecological referral and a full menstrual history should be taken from all women of reproductive age (see below). Another common presenting symptom is abdominal pain and the history must include details of the time of onset, the distribution and radiation of the pain, and its relationship to the periods.

If vaginal discharge is the presenting symptom the colour, odour and relationship to the periods should be noted. It may also be associated with vulval pruritus, particularly in the presence of specific infections. The presence of an abdominal mass may be noted by the patient or may be detected during the course of a routine examination. Symptoms may also result from pressure of the mass on adjacent pelvic organs, such as the bladder and bowel.

Vaginal and uterine prolapse are associated with symptoms of a mass protruding through the vaginal introitus or difficulties with micturition and defecation. Common urinary symptoms include frequency of micturition, pain or dysuria, incontinence and the passage of blood in the urine (haematuria).

Where appropriate a sexual history should include reference to the frequency of coitus, the occurrence of pain during intercourse – *dyspareunia* – and functional details relating to libido, sexual satisfaction and sexual problems.

Menstrual history

The first question that should be asked in relation to the menstrual history is the date of the last menstrual period.

The time of onset of the first period, the *menarche*, commonly occurs at 12 years of age and can be considered to be abnormally delayed at more than 16 years or abnormally early at 9 years. The absence of menstruation at the age of 16 in a girl with otherwise normal development is known as *primary amenorrhoea*. The menarche should be distinguished from the *pubarche*, which is the onset of the first signs of sexual maturation. Characteristically, the development of

breasts and nipple enlargement predates the onset of menstruation by approximately 2 years.

 Failure to check the date of the last period may lead to serious errors in subsequent management.

The length of the menstrual cycle is the time between the first day of one period and the first day of the following period. While there is usually an interval of 28 days, the cycle length may vary between 21 and 42 days in normal women and may only be significant where there is a change in menstrual pattern. It is important to be sure that the patient does not describe the time between the last day of one period and the first day of the next period, as this may give a false impression of the frequency of menstruation. Absence of menstruation for more than 6 months in a woman who has previously had periods is known as *secondary amenorrhoea*. Menstruation occurring at intervals of less than 21 days is known as *polymenorrhoea* or *epimenorrhoea*. *Oligomenorrhoea* is the term used to describe menstruation that occurs at intervals of between 6 weeks and 6 months.

The amount and duration of the period may change with age but may also provide a useful indication of a disease process. Normal menstruation lasts 4–7 days, and normal blood loss varies between 30 and 80 ml. A change in pattern is often more noticeable and significant than the actual time and volume of loss. In practical terms, excessive menstrual loss is best assessed on the history of the number of pads or tampons used during a period and the presence or absence of clots. Excessively prolonged or heavy regular periods are described by the term *menorrhagia*, and irregular acyclic heavy bleeding is known as *metrorrhagia*. Periods that are both frequent and excessive are known as *menometrorrhagia* or *polymenorrhagia*.

The cessation of periods at the end of menstrual life is known as the *menopause* and bleeding that occurs more than 12 months after this is described as *postmenopausal bleeding*. A history of irregular vaginal bleeding or blood loss that occurs after coitus or between periods should be noted.

Previous gynaecological history

A detailed history of any previous gynaecological problems and treatments must be recorded. It is also important, where possible, to obtain any records of previous gynaecological surgery. Many women are uncertain of the precise nature of their operations. The amount of detail needed about previous pregnancies will depend on the presenting problem. In most cases the number of previous pregnancies and their outcome (miscarriage, ectopic, or delivery after 24 weeks) is all that is required.

For all women of reproductive age who are sexually active it is essential to ask about contraception. This is important not only to determine the possibility of pregnancy but because the method of contraception used may itself be relevant to the presenting complaint (e.g. irregular bleeding may occur on the contraceptive pill or when an intrauterine device is present). For women over the age of 20, ask about the date and result of the last cervical smear.

Previous medical history

This description should take particular account of any history of chronic lung disease and disorders of the cardiovascular system as these are highly relevant where any surgical procedure is likely to be necessary. A record of all current medications and any known drug allergies should be made.

Family and social history

A family history of diabetes, tuberculosis and carcinoma of the genital tract should be noted.

A social history is important with all problems but is particularly relevant where the presenting difficulties relate to abortion or sterilization. For example, a 15-year-old girl requesting a termination of pregnancy may

be being put under substantial pressure by her parents to have an abortion and yet may not really be happy about doing this.

EXAMINATION

A general examination should always be performed at the first consultation, including assessment of blood pressure and routine urine analysis. Careful note should be taken of any signs of anaemia. The distribution of facial and body hair is often important, as hirsutism may be a presenting symptom of various endocrine disorders. Body weight and height should also be recorded.

The intimate nature of gynaecological examination makes it especially important to ensure that every effort is made to ensure privacy. The examination should ideally take place in a separate area to the consultation. The patient should be allowed to undress in privacy and, if necessary, to empty her bladder first. Before starting the examination explain what will be involved in vaginal examination and that she can ask for the examination to be stopped at any stage. A chaperone should generally be present, although the patient has a right to refuse.

Breast examination

Breast examination should be performed if there are symptoms or at the first consultation in women over the age of 45. The presence of the secretion of milk at times not associated with pregnancy, known as *galactorrhoea*, may indicate abnormal endocrine status. Systematic palpation with the flat of the hand should be undertaken to exclude the presence of any nodules in the breast or axillae (Fig. 17.1).

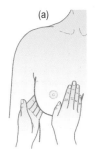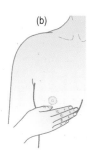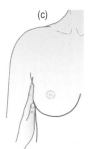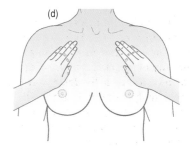

Fig. 17.1 Systematic examination of the four quadrants of the breasts.

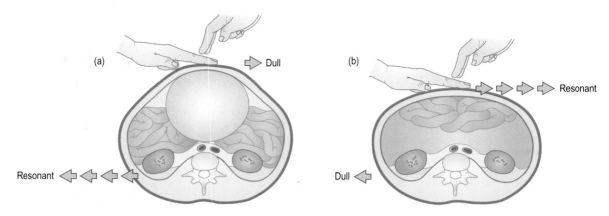

Fig. 17.2 (a) Percussion over a large ovarian cyst – central dullness and resonance in the flanks. (b) Percussion in the presence of ascites – dullness in the flanks and central resonance.

Examination of the abdomen

Inspection of the abdomen may reveal the presence of a mass. The distribution of body hair should be noted, and the presence of scars, striae and hernias. Palpation of the abdomen should take account of any guarding and rebound tenderness. It is important to ask the patient to outline the site and radiation of any pain in the abdomen, and palpation for enlargement of the liver, spleen and kidneys should be carried out. If there is a mass try to determine if it is fixed or mobile, smooth or regular, and if it arises from the pelvis (you shouldn't be able to palpate the lower edge above the pubic bone). Check the hernial orifices and feel for any enlarged lymph nodes in the groin. Percussion of the abdomen may be used to outline the limits of a tumour, to detect the presence of a full bladder or to recognize the presence of tympanitic loops of bowel. Free fluid in the peritoneal cavity will be recognized by the presence of dullness to percussion in the flanks and resonance over the central abdomen (Fig. 17.2).

Auscultation of bowel sounds is indicated in patients with postoperative abdominal distension or acute abdominal pain where obstruction or an ileus is suspected.

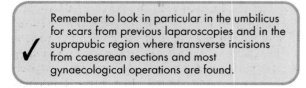
✓ Remember to look in particular in the umbilicus for scars from previous laparoscopies and in the suprapubic region where transverse incisions from caesarean sections and most gynaecological operations are found.

Pelvic examination

The patient should be examined resting supine with the knees drawn up and separated or in stirrups in the lithotomy position (Fig. 17.3). Parting the lips of the labia minora with the left hand, look at the external urethral meatus and inspect the vulva for any discharge, redness, ulceration and old scars. Speculum examination should be performed before digital examination to avoid any contamination with lubricant. A bivalve or Cusco's speculum is most commonly used and enables a clear view of the cervix to be obtained.

Holding the lips of the labia minora open with the left hand insert the speculum into the introitus with the

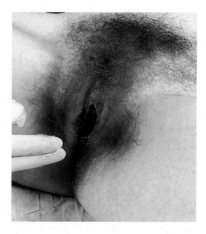

Fig. 17.3 Inspection of the external genitalia.

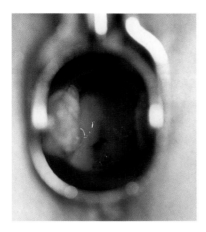

Fig. 17.4 View of normal cervix on speculum examination.

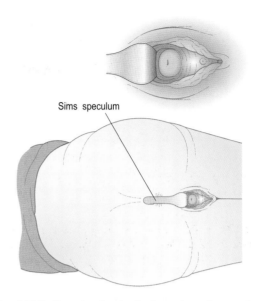

Sims speculum

Fig. 17.5 Examination in the lateral semiprone position with a Sims' speculum enables inspection of the vaginal walls.

widest dimension of the instrument in the transverse position, as the vagina is widest in this direction. When the speculum reaches the top of the vagina gently open the blades and visualize the cervix (Fig. 17.4). Make a note of the presence of any discharge or bleeding from the cervix and of any polyps or areas of ulceration. Remember that the appearance of the cervix is changed after childbirth, with the external os more irregular and slit-like.

The commonest finding is of a so-called *erosion* or *ectropion*. This is an area of cervical epithelium around the cervical os that appears a darker red colour than the smooth pink of the rest of the cervix. It is not an erosion at all but normal columnar epithelium extending from the endocervical canal on to the ectocervix. If the clinical history suggests possible infection, take swabs from the vaginal fornices and cervical os and place in transport medium to look for *Candida, Trichomonas* and *Neisseria* spp. and take a separate swab from the endocervix for *Chlamydia*.

Where vaginal wall prolapse is suspected, a Sims' speculum should be used, as it provides a clearer view of the vaginal walls. Where the Sims' speculum is used, it is preferable to examine the patient in the semiprone or Sims' position (Fig. 17.5).

Taking a cervical smear

This should be done at least 3 months after pregnancy and not during menstruation. Explain the purpose of the test and warn the patient that she may notice some spotting afterwards.

Record the patient's name and hospital number on a suitable slide. After inserting a speculum as above, wipe away any discharge or blood. Note the appearance of the cervix (Fig. 17.6). A 360° sweep should be taken with a suitable spatula pressed firmly against the cervix at the junction of the columnar epithelium of the endocervical canal and the squamous epithelium of the ectocervix. The specimen is spread immediately on to a clear glass slide in a thin, even layer. The slide is fixed with 95% alcohol alone or in combination with 3% glacial acetic acid. Fixation requires 30 minutes in solution. Finally, complete the cytology request form with details of previous smears, last period, contraception and results of previous smears.

Bimanual examination

Bimanual examination (Box 17.1) is performed by introducing the middle finger of the examining hand into the vaginal introitus and applying pressure towards the rectum (Fig. 17.7). As the introitus opens, the index finger is introduced as well. The cervix is palpated and has the consistency of the cartilage of the tip of the nose. It must be remembered that the abdominal hand is used to compress the pelvic organs on to the examining vaginal hand. The size, shape, consistency and position of the uterus must be noted. The uterus is commonly

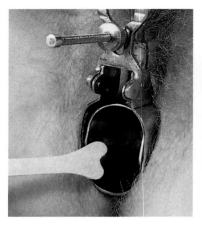
(a)

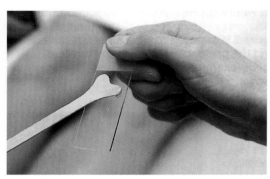
(b)

Fig. 17.6 (a) A cervical smear is taken using an Ayres spatula. (b) The material obtained is plated on to a glass slide and fixed.

ℹ️ **Box 17.1**

When conducting a vaginal examination you should:
- Explain that an intimate examination is needed and why
- Explain what the examination will involve
- Obtain the patient's permission
- Offer a chaperone or invite the patient to bring a relative or friend
- Allow the patient to undress in privacy
- Keep discussion relevant and avoid unnecessary personal comments
- Explain findings and encourage questions and discussion

---

preaxial or anteverted, but will be postaxial or retroverted in some 10% of women. Provided the retroverted uterus is mobile, the position is rarely significant. It is important to feel in the pouch of Douglas for the presence of thickening or nodules, and then to palpate laterally in both fornices for the presence of any ovarian or tubal masses. An attempt should be made to differentiate between adnexal and uterine masses, although this is often not possible. For example, a pedunculated fibroid may mimic an ovarian tumour, whereas a solid ovarian tumour, if adherent to the uterus, may be impossible to distinguish from a uterine fibroid. The ovaries may be palpable in the normal pelvis if the patient is thin, but the fallopian tubes are only palpable if they are significantly enlarged.

In a child or in a woman with an intact hymen, it may be necessary to perform a single-finger vaginal examination or a rectal examination. It should always be remembered that a rough or painful examination rarely produces any useful information and, in certain situations such as tubal ectopic pregnancy, may be dangerous.

PRESENTING YOUR FINDINGS

Start by introducing the patient by name and age and give the main reason for admission. If there are several problems deal with each in turn. If the history consists of a long narrative of events, try to summarize these rather than recap each event. Present the remainder of the history in a logical structured way, not skipping back and forward between items. At the end of your history give a summary in no more than one or two sentences.

Unless you are asked only to discuss one particular part of the examination, always start by commenting on the patient's general condition, including pulse and blood pressure. For abdominal examination list the findings on inspection first followed by those on palpation and percussion (if there is abdominal distension or a mass). If there is a mass arising from the pelvis describe it in terms of a pregnant uterus (e.g. a mass reaching the umbilicus would be a 20-week-size pelvic mass). If there are areas of tenderness specify whether they are associated with signs of peritonism (guarding

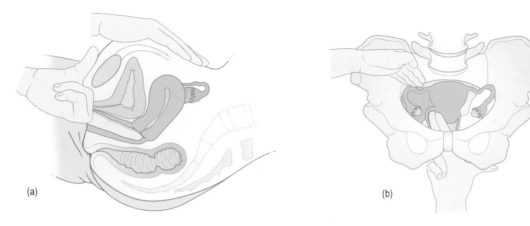

(a)

(b)

Fig. 17.7 (a) Bimanual examination of the pelvis. (b) Examination of the lateral fornix.

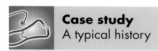

Case study
A typical history

This is Ms Smith, a 29-year-old housewife who has been referred by her general practitioner to the clinic because of bleeding and a positive pregnancy test. Ms Smith has had three episodes of painless vaginal bleeding over the last 3 days. Her last menstrual period was 7 weeks ago and prior to this she had a regular 28-day menstrual cycle. She has no previous gynaecological history of note and her last cervical smear was 2 years ago and was negative. This is a planned pregnancy and before conceiving she was using the combined oral contraceptive pill until 3 months ago. She has had two previous pregnancies with uncomplicated normal vaginal deliveries at term. She underwent a appendicectomy at the age of 14 and had no problems with the general anaesthetic at the time. She is currently taking folic acid and has no known allergies. She lives with her partner and two children. She does not smoke or drink.

In summary, Ms Smith is a 29-year-old woman with a history of painless vaginal bleeding at 7 weeks in her third pregnancy.

and rebound). On pelvic examination describe the findings on inspection of the vulva and then of the cervix (if a speculum examination was carried out). Describe the size, position and mobility of the uterus and any tenderness. Finally, say whether there were any palpable masses or tenderness in the adnexae.

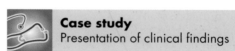

Case study
Presentation of clinical findings

On general examination Ms Smith looked well. She was not clinically anaemic and her body mass index was 31. Her blood pressure was 110/70 and her pulse 88 and regular. Examination of the chest and heart was unremarkable. On abdominal examination there was a scar in the right lower quadrant consistent with a previous appendicectomy. On palpation the abdomen was soft and non-tender with no palpable masses and no organomegaly. On pelvic examination the external genitalia were normal apart from an old scar on the perineum consistent with a previous tear or episiotomy. On speculum examination the cervix was closed and there was a small amount of free blood in the vagina. She had an 8-week-size mobile, anteverted uterus and there were no palpable adnexal masses.

ESSENTIAL INFORMATION

History

- Presenting complaint
  - Onset and duration of main complaint
  - Associated symptoms, relationship to menstrual cycle
  - Previous treatment and response
  - Specific closed questions
- Previous gynaecological history
  - Previous investigations or treatment
  - Contraceptive history
  - Sexual history
  - Cervical smear
  - Menstrual history
- Previous pregnancies
  - How many (gravidity)
  - Outcome (parity)
  - Surgical deliveries (birth weight)
- Past surgical and medical history
  - Previous abdominal surgery
  - Major cardiovascular/respiratory disease
  - Endocrine disease
  - Thromboembolic disease
  - Breast disease
- Drug history and allergies

- Social and family history details
  - Home circumstances
  - Support
  - Smoking
  - Family history

Examination

- General examination
  - General condition, weight, height
  - Pulse, blood pressure
  - Anaemia
  - Goitre
  - Breast examination (if indicated)
  - Secondary sex characteristics, body hair
- Abdominal examination
  - Inspection – distension, scars
  - Palpation – masses, organomegaly, tenderness, peritonism, nodes, hernial orifices
  - Percussion – ascites
- Pelvic examination
  - Explanation, comfort, privacy, chaperone
  - Inspection of external genitalia
  - Speculum examination, smear, swabs
  - Bimanual examination
  - Rectal examination if indicated

18 Disorders of menstruation and the menopause

PUBERTY AND MENARCHE

The nature of the menstrual cycle has been described in Chapter 2. Menstruation is the periodic change occurring in primates which results in the flow of blood and endometrium from the uterine cavity, and which may be associated with various constitutional disturbances.

Puberty is the process of sexual maturation beginning with the maturation of the hypothalamus. This results in an increased release of pituitary gonadotrophins and, hence, stimulation of the ovary with the production of sex hormones. Other trophic hormones such as adreno-corticotrophic hormone (ACTH), thyroid-stimulating hormone (TSH) and growth hormone also gradually increase over a period of 3–4 years. The sexual changes of puberty can be divided into three phases.

Thelarche

The first of the sexual changes to occur is the development of the breast (Fig. 18.1). Nipple enlargement begins between 9 and 11 years of age with thickening of the duct system as a result of increasing oestrogen production. At the same time, the vaginal epithelium increases in thickness and vaginal pH decreases.

Adrenarche

The growth of pubic hair occurs at about 11–12 years of age and is followed by the development of axillary hair (Fig. 18.2). Both phenomena are dependent on adrenal development.

Menarche

The final manifestation of sexual maturity in the female is the onset of menstruation. The average age of the menarche in the UK is between 12 and 13 years, and it occurs in 95% of girls between the ages of 11 and 15. There has been no significant change in the age of the menarche in western Europe over the last 30 years

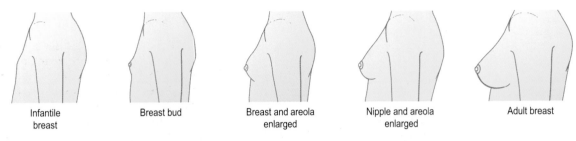

Fig. 18.1 Development of the female breast during thelarche.

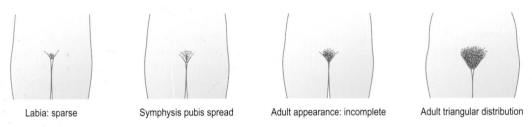

Fig. 18.2 Pubic hair distribution leading up to full sexual maturation during the adrenarche.

although there is some variation among different ethnic groups. The menstrual cycle is often irregular in the first 2 years and may show intervals of 4–6 months between periods. The cycles are frequently anovulatory, and prolonged bleeding may occur.

The growth spurt

Throughout the period of sexual maturation, marked changes occur in growth (Fig. 18.3). A rapid increase in growth occurs between 11 and 14 years. The legs lengthen first, and this is followed by increases in shoulder breadth and in trunk length. The pelvis enlarges and changes in shape. Maximal height is reached at between 17 and 18 years, and growth is terminated by the fusion of femoral epiphyses.

Precocious puberty

The development of physical signs of sexual maturation before the age of 8 years and the onset of menstruation before the age of 10 years are indications of precocious puberty. The majority of cases carry no pathological connotation.

Aetiology

Precocious puberty may occur at any point in the hypothalamic–pituitary–ovarian axis or as a result of abnormalities in the adrenal or thyroid glands. Causes may be:

- Constitutional
- Neurological
- Ovarian tumours
- Adrenal tumours
- Gonadotrophin-secreting tumours
- Others – hypothyroidism; exogenous oestrogens.

The majority of cases of precocious puberty are constitutional in origin. It is, however, important to exclude other organic causes before classifying the problem as constitutional. There are a group of cases where the activity of the hypothalamic–pituitary axis is stimulated by intracranial lesions such as meningitis, encephalitis, hydrocephalus or cerebral tumours. Of the ovarian lesions, the commonest are the granulosa cell tumours. These must be differentiated from follicular cysts, which may be associated with hypothalamic causes.

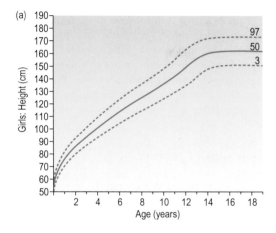

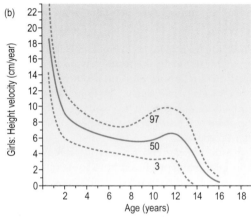

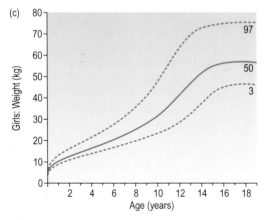

Fig. 18.3 (a) Centile change for height in the female. (b) Height velocity indicates the slowing down of the rate of growth with a secondary acceleration around the time of puberty. (c) Changes in weight show a wider scatter than with height.

Investigation

All children exhibiting precocious sexual development must be investigated to exclude any underlying pathology. General and pelvic examination may reveal evidence of ovarian lesions. A skeletal survey should be undertaken for any bony abnormalities. Skull radiography and computed axial tomography (CT) scanning may reveal the presence of abnormalities of the sella turcica, suprasellar calcification and lesions involving the floor of the fourth ventricle. Ultrasound scanning of the pelvis should reveal any ovarian tumours.

Management

In children where there is a specific lesion causing precocious sexual maturation, the management depends on the treatment of the condition. In constitutional precocious puberty, management is concerned with the abnormal bone growth and the emotional and psychological problems contingent on early sexual maturation. Advanced bone growth results in the girl initially being much taller than her classmates, but the early fusion of the epiphyses means that her ultimate stature is smaller than normal. It is sometimes possible to inhibit hypothalamic activity by the administration of medroxyprogesterone acetate 100–200 mg intramuscularly every 2–4 weeks or by giving the anti-androgenic agent cyproterone acetate by the oral route.

These children may need protection from sexual assault as they may conceive if coitus occurs. The youngest recorded pregnancy and confinement occurred in a 6-year-old child with precocious sexual development.

Delayed puberty

Delayed puberty commonly presents as *primary amenorrhoea*. This is defined as the failure to menstruate by the age of 16 years in the presence of normal development of secondary sex characteristics or 14 in the absence of the other features of puberty. However, delayed puberty is also revealed by failure in development of secondary sexual characteristics.

If the secondary sexual characteristics are normal apart from amenorrhoea, the diagnosis is likely to be:

- Haematocolpos – the retention of menstrual fluid because of an imperforate hymen (Fig. 18.4)
- Vaginal agenesis – congenital absence of the vagina
- Resistant ovary syndrome (see below)

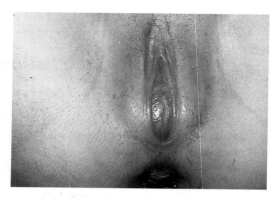

Fig. 18.4 Imperforate hymen. Menstrual loss has accumulated in the vagina and can be seen bulging the hymen.

- Testicular feminization or other chromosomal abnormalities.

If the secondary sexual characteristics are poor, then the amenorrhoea may be due to:

- Constitutional delay in puberty
- Gonadal dysgenesis – primitive streak ovaries or the congenital absence of ovarian tissue
- Hypothalamic–pituitary failure.

If there are signs of virilization in the female, then the following diagnoses should be considered:

- Congenital adrenal hyperplasia
- Virilizing adrenal tumours
- Virilizing ovarian tumours
- Cushing's syndrome
- Chromosomal abnormalities such as the 46 XY female.

General examination should take account of the age, height, weight and arm span of the individual and also features of abnormal somatic structures such as neck webbing and short metatarsal bones. Pelvic examination will reveal whether there are any abnormalities of the genital tract.

The resistant ovary syndrome

This is a rare but important cause of primary amenorrhoea. Secondary sexual characteristics are usually normal. Follicle-stimulating hormone (FSH) and luteinizing hormone (LH) levels are raised to the menopausal range but, unlike true ovarian failure, the ovaries con-

tain numerous ova. Stimulation with human menopausal gonadotrophin or with human chorionic gonadotrophin meets with little success. It must be remembered that these women are able to conceive and may sometimes ovulate spontaneously. Prognosis for childbearing must be guarded, but, unlike true ovarian failure, ovulation and spontaneous menstruation may occur.

Intersexuality

Ambiguous genital development is a rare, but disturbing problem and successful management at a physical and psychological level should be started as soon after birth as possible.

Causes of ambiguous genitalia may include the following.

- Where the fetus has a Y chromosome and so is karyotypically male, the testes may not form, or they may function abnormally and produce oestrogens, as in *testicular feminization*. The failure of androgen production or androgen insensitivity at the target organ site will result in development of female external genitalia.
- Virilization may occur in a karyotypic female with androgens being produced from some outside source, such as occurs in congenital adrenal hyperplasia.
- Mosaicism – on occasions, true hermaphroditism does occur, and testicular and ovarian tissues form in the same fetus.

The appearance of the hermaphrodite, the undermasculinized male and the masculinized female are all similar. Differential diagnosis is dependent on establishing the karyotype, and measuring 17-oxosteroids and the intermediate products of cortisol metabolism as well as electrolyte levels.

> **!** Congenital adrenal hyperplasia needs early recognition if the child is to survive. Salt loss may be a major factor in this condition and the infant should be treated with cortisone acetate and prednisolone or bromohydrocortisone.

Sexual assignment is particularly important in all intersex cases and should be allocated on the basis of phenotypic sex.

SECONDARY AMENORRHOEA AND OLIGOMENORRHOEA

Normal menstruation requires the pulsatile release of gonadotrophin-releasing hormone (GnRH) from the hypothalamus to stimulate the release of the gonado-trophins, FSH and LH, from a functioning anterior pituitary. The ovaries must be able to respond to these signals and to produce oestrogen and progesterone. Finally the endometrial cavity must be intact and the lower genital tract must be patent to allow shedding of the endometrium if conception does not occur.

Secondary amenorrhoea is defined as the cessation of menses for 6 or more months in a woman who has previously menstruated. Oligomenorrhoea is the occurrence of five or fewer menstrual periods over 12 months. In practice, the distinction between the two can be somewhat arbitrary as they share many of the same causes.

Aetiology

There are numerous causes of amenorrhoea although the commonest are physiological. Amenorrhoea may result from any disorder of the endocrine or central nervous system or abnormalities of the target organ.

Physiological causes include pregnancy, the puerperium, lactation and the menopause.

Pathological causes can be divided into disorders of the hypothalamus, anterior pituitary, ovary and genital tract (Fig. 18.5).

Hypothalamic disorders

Hypothalamic amenorrhoea (hypogonadotrophic hypogonadism) occurs when there is a deficiency of GnRH pulsatile secretion. It is characterized by low or normal levels of FSH and LH, normal prolactin levels, normal imaging of the pituitary fossa and hypo-oestrogenism. This form of amenorrhoea is often associated with excessive weight loss or exercise, stress and chronic renal failure.

There is a critical relationship between body weight and menstruation. A loss of body weight of 10–15% of normal weight for height is likely to cause abnormal menstruation. This may result from vigorous dieting or it may be a manifestation of *anorexia nervosa*. This condition is characterized by an extreme neurotic aversion to food. There is usually an underlying emotional

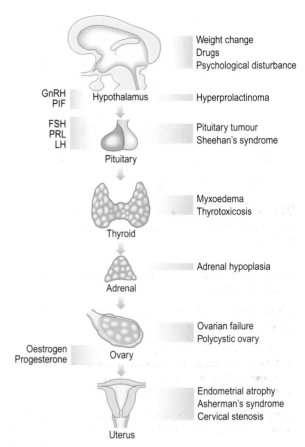

Fig. 18.5 Causes of secondary amenorrhoea. GnRH, gonadotrophin-releasing hormone; PIF, prolactin-inhibiting factor; FSH, follicle-stimulating hormone; LH, luteinizing hormone; PRL, prolactin.

problem with conflicts over sexuality, obsession with weight loss associated with a persistent refusal to eat adequately, and self-induced vomiting or purgation. Gonadotrophin and oestrogen levels are low but, unlike panhypopituitarism, other hormone levels are normal. This is a serious condition, which results in death in 10–15% of the subjects involved. Early recognition is important because it is essential to supplement dietary replacement with long-term psychiatric therapy.

Emotional stress is a common cause of amenorrhoea. It often occurs where the environment is changed, as for example when a woman changes her occupation or leaves her home environment for institutional life. This problem usually resolves itself but may persist for some years.

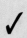

✓ Although the combined oral contraceptive pill causes suppression of the hypothalamic pituitary axis there is no evidence that this is prolonged when it is discontinued.

Pituitary disorders

Pituitary disorders are associated with hyperprolactinaemia and hypo-oestrogenism as a result of the inhibition of GnRH release. Secretion of breast milk (*galactorrhoea*) occurs in about a third of patients. Around 40% of cases are associated with a prolactin-secreting tumour of the anterior pituitary (micro- or macroadenoma). All patients with secondary amenorrhoea should have a prolactin estimation and, if the levels are abnormally raised, imaging of the pituitary fossa with CT or magnetic resonance imaging. Growth of a macroadenoma may cause bitemporal hemianopia as a result of compression of the optic chiasm.

Apart from the presence of pituitary adenomas, pituitary amenorrhoea may occur where there is destruction from postpartum necrosis, as in *Sheehan's syndrome*, or where there is surgically inflicted damage.

The release of prolactin from the anterior pituitary is inhibited by the neurotransmitter dopamine. Drugs with antidopaminergic effects (Box 18.1) will result in iatrogenic elevated prolactin levels and amenorrhoea.

Ovarian disorders

Ovarian failure

Premature ovarian failure occurs in approximately 1% of women under the age of 40. Autoimmune disease of the ovaries is a rare condition that sometimes presents as a premature menopause. Surgical removal of the ovaries or destruction by radiation or infection results in secondary amenorrhoea. All these conditions are characterized by high levels of gonadotrophins and hypo-oestrogenism (*hypergonadotrophic hypogonadism*). Ovarian neoplasms, particularly those associated with excessive production of oestrogen or testosterone, may cause amenorrhoea but constitute only a very small percentage of known causes.

Polycystic ovarian syndrome

Polycystic ovarian syndrome (PCOS) accounts for 80% of cases of oligomenorrhoea. It is associated with the *Stein–Leventhal syndrome*, in which multiple cysts occur in the ovaries (Fig. 18.6) and are associated with hirsutism, oligomenorrhoea or amenorrhoea, subfertility and changes in body habitus, with obesity (Box 18.2). The ovaries are clinically enlarged and are palpable vaginally.

On direct inspection, the ovaries have smooth, white surfaces. There is sometimes luteinization of the theca interna cells and focal stromal luteinization.

Biochemical investigations (Fig. 18.7) indicate abnormally raised luteinizing hormone (LH) levels and absence of the LH surge. Oestrogen and follicle-stimulating hormone (FSH) levels are normal, and as a result there is an increase in the LH:FSH ratio. There may be increased secretion of testosterone and of D4-androstenedione and dehydroepiandrosterone. Prolactin levels are increased in 15% of cases.

Pathogenesis. Although the cause of PCOS remains obscure, theories include an underlying disorder in androgen biosynthesis and insulin resistance. Inappropriate exposure of antral follicles to excessive concentrations of androgens results in inhibition of FSH release and may result in polycystic changes in the ovaries. The primary source of androgen may be the ovary or the adrenals. The excretion of dehydroepiandrosterone – an exclusively adrenal steroid – is elevated in up to 50% of all women with PCOS. The principal androgens raised in PCOS in the ovary include testosterone and androstenedione, and the production will not be suppressed by adrenal steroids but can be suppressed by GnRH agonists. Insulin and insulin-like growth factor significantly increase the production of testosterone and androstenedione from ovarian theca cells. About 20% of women with PCOS develop non-insulin-dependent diabetes by the age of 30 years.

Diagnosis. The diagnosis of PCOS is based on ultrasound scan of the ovaries using a vaginal probe and a

Box 18.1
Drugs that may cause hyperprolactinaemia

- Phenothiazines
- Antihistamines
- Butyrophenones
- Metoclopramide
- Cimetidine
- Methyldopa

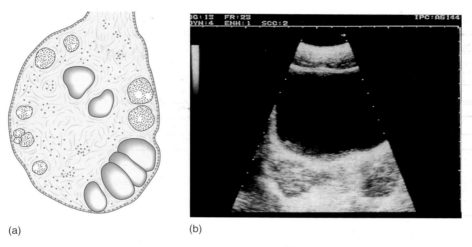

(a)   (b)

Fig. 18.6 Polycystic ovaries. (a) The capsule of the ovary is thickened and there are numerous small cysts in the ovarian cortex. (b) Ultrasound appearances showing mottled appearance of both ovaries characteristic of multiple small cysts.

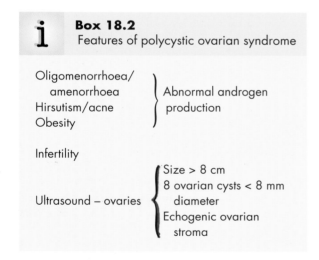

Box 18.2
Features of polycystic ovarian syndrome

Oligomenorrhoea/
    amenorrhoea   ⎫ Abnormal androgen
Hirsutism/acne   ⎬ production
Obesity   ⎭

Infertility

                      ⎧ Size > 8 cm
                      ⎪ 8 ovarian cysts < 8 mm
Ultrasound – ovaries ⎨   diameter
                      ⎪ Echogenic ovarian
                      ⎩   stroma

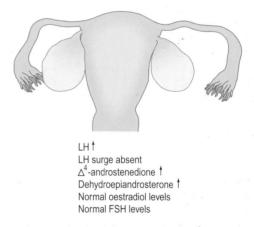

LH ↑
LH surge absent
Δ^4-androstenedione ↑
Dehydroepiandrosterone ↑
Normal oestradiol levels
Normal FSH levels

Fig. 18.7 Biochemical features of the Stein–Leventhal syndrome.

hormone profile including measurement of FSH/LH, testosterone and androstenedione (Fig. 18.6b).

Failure of uterine response

Damage to the target organ may result in secondary amenorrhoea. This includes surgical removal of the uterus or damage to the endometrium as with *Asherman's syndrome*. In this condition, over-vigorous curettage, particularly when performed in the presence of endometritis, results in the formation of intrauterine adhesions or synechiae. Destruction of the endometrium may also result from tuberculous infection.

Cryptomenorrhoea

Secondary amenorrhoea may be due to retention of menstrual products because of cervical stenosis, as a result of surgical trauma or infection. This may occur in the presence of malignant disease of the cervix.

Investigations

The possibility of pregnancy should always be considered and if necessary excluded by pregnancy test. The history should include details of recent emotional stress, changes in weight, menopausal symptoms and current medication. In the majority of cases nothing abnormal is found on clinical examination, although a body mass index of less than 19 kg/m^2 is likely to be associated with amenorrhoea. In the absence of clinical evidence of thyroid or adrenal diseases it is unusual to find biochemical evidence. The differential diagnosis is established by the measurement of FSH and LH, prolactin and thyroid function tests. A pelvic ultrasound can provide additional evidence of polycystic ovarian syndrome, ovarian tumours and abnormalities of the lower genital tract.

The administration of medroxyprogesterone acetate 10 mg daily for 5 days should produce withdrawal bleeding 2–7 days after completing the course (*progestogen challenge test*). A positive test indicates a functional uterus with an intact endometrium and a patent outflow tract where circulating levels of oestrogen are adequate.

Management

The treatment depends on the cause. Outside the physiological group, the vast majority of cases are hypothalamic in origin. Most of these will eventually resolve spontaneously and, where weight loss is the main underlying factor, the emphasis should be on restoring normal body mass. However, oestradiol levels are low and in some cases it is useful to administer cyclical oestrogen therapy. Hyperprolactinaemia will usually respond to stopping any dopamine-inhibiting drugs or to treatment with dopamine agonists such as bromocriptine or cabergoline. Treatment for PCOS depends on which of the presenting symptoms predominate. If the problem is primarily one of subfertility, then clomiphene citrate or human menopausal gonadotrophin can be used to stimulate ovulation. Prolonged unopposed oestrogen action may result in the development of hyperplastic endometrium, which may undergo malignant change. Hyperplasia will often regress following the administration of a pro-gestational agent such as medroxyprogesterone acetate or megestrol acetate.

Weight reduction needs to be emphasized where there is a problem with obesity, as there is evidence to show that weight reduction alone can improve the menstrual pattern, endocrine profile and fertility. Hirsutism can be treated by the use of depilatory aids and electrolysis but the presence of hirsutism, acne and alopecia may also respond to antiandrogens such as cyproterone acetate combined with an oestrogen such as ethinylestradiol given on a cyclical basis. Surgical management of PCOS includes resection of a wedge of ovarian tissue or drilling of the ovary with laparoscopic needle-point diathermy or laser puncture of the ovarian surface. These procedures appear to restore normal ovarian function, although the mechanism remains unclear. Medical management with the oral hypoglycaemic metformin also appears to be effective in some cases.

MENORRHAGIA

The median blood loss per month in menstruation is 40 ml. Blood loss of more than 80 ml per month is considered abnormal but in practice menorrhagia is usually defined as a subjective increase in menstrual loss. Fewer than 50% of women complaining of heavy periods actually have a loss of more than 80 ml per month when this is objectively measured. Menorrhagia is the commonest reason for gynaecological referral and 5% of women aged 30–49 will see their GP about it each year.

Causes

Menorrhagia may be due to underlying pelvic pathology or dysfunctional uterine bleeding.

Fibroids are the commonest structural lesion to cause heavy regular bleeding, although not all women with fibroids have objective evidence of abnormal loss. Endometrial carcinoma is rare under the age of 40 and is more likely to cause irregular bleeding. Adenomyosis (implantation of endometrial glands in the myometrium) is associated with a uniformly enlarged tender uterus and is normally diagnosed following hysterectomy. Inert or copper-containing intrauterine contraceptive devices are associated with increased blood loss.

Dysfunctional bleeding is the term used to describe abnormally heavy or prolonged menstrual bleeding where there is no uterine or systemic cause. It accounts for more than 80% of cases of menorrhagia and can be either ovulatory or anovulatory. Anovulatory bleeding tends to occur at the extremes of reproductive life and is associated with a shortening of the luteal phase of the cycle. The majority of cycles associated with heavy periods are ovulatory.

The pathophysiology of dysfunctional uterine bleeding is poorly understood, and therefore classification is generally unsatisfactory. There is some evidence of an imbalance of prostaglandin levels in the myometrium with a deficiency in prostaglandin F.

Metropathia haemorrhagica

This condition most commonly occurs around the time of the menopause but may also occur in the adolescent female. The history classically involves a period of amenorrhoea followed by prolonged, heavy and irregular bleeding of such severity that it may occasionally be life-threatening. The persistence of an unruptured follicular cyst in one ovary results in extended and excessive oestrogen production, causing cystic or adenomatous endometrial hyperplasia. The endometrium becomes greatly thickened and when it can no longer be sustained by the continuing high levels of oestrogen it eventually breaks down in a patchy fashion. The haemorrhage commonly follows a period of 6–8 weeks of amenorrhoea. Myometrial hyperplasia also occurs so that the uterus is often bulky, the endometrium being up to 1 cm thick and having the characteristic 'Swiss cheese' appearance.

History and examination

An accurate history is essential to establish the pattern of bleeding and the duration of symptoms. Estimating the degree of blood loss is very subjective although the presence of clots, the need to change sanitary protection at night and 'flooding' (the soiling of bedclothes or underwear during menstruation) are more likely to indicate significant bleeding. A recent change in the pattern of menstruation and associated pain are more likely to be associated with the development of pelvic pathology. Pain is associated with adenomyosis and chronic pelvic inflammatory disease. Structural lesions of the uterus and cervix are more likely in the presence of intermenstrual bleeding. The commonest iatrogenic cause of heavy bleeding is the presence of an IUD. Malignancy is extremely rare under the age of 40 but women with a history of diabetes, hypertension, PCOS and obesity are at increased risk of endometrial carcinoma.

Women with heavy periods should have a general examination for signs of anaemia and thyroid disease and a pelvic examination including a cervical smear if indicated. The finding of a pelvic mass on pelvic examination is most likely to indicate the presence of uterine leiomyomata (fibroids) but may indicate a uterine malignancy or ovarian tumour.

Investigations

A full blood count is the only investigation needed before starting treatment provided that examination is normal.

Patients should be referred for further investigation if:

- There is a history of irregular or intermenstrual bleeding or of risk factors for endometrial carcinoma
- Their cervical smear is abnormal
- Pelvic examination is abnormal
- They do not respond to first-line treatment after 6 months.

Additional investigation is mainly to confirm or exclude the presence of pelvic pathology and in particular of endometrial malignancy. The main methods of investigation are endometrial biopsy, hysteroscopy and transvaginal ultrasound. Investigations for systemic causes of abnormal menstruation such as thyroid disease are only indicated if there are other features on examination or the history.

Endometrial biopsy can be performed as an outpatient procedure either alone or in conjunction with hysteroscopy.

Hysteroscopy is visualization of the uterine cavity using an endoscope introduced through the cervix. It can be performed under general anaesthetic or as an outpatient investigation. Hysteroscopy with endometrial biopsy has largely replaced the traditional dilation and curettage (D&C), which is a blind procedure and misses a proportion of localized lesions.

Pelvic ultrasound may be of value in distinguishing fibroids from other causes of a pelvic mass, such as ovarian tumours. In premenopausal women the thickness of the endometrium will vary at different times of the cycle but it may be possible to visualize structural lesions such as polyps in the endometrial cavity.

Medical treatment

In the absence of malignancy the treatment chosen will depend on whether contraception is required, whether irregularity of the cycle is a problem and the possible contraindications to certain treatments. Where a conventional IUD is in place, mefenamic or tranexamic acid can be used or the device may be replaced by a levonorgestrel intrauterine system (Mirena®).

Non-hormonal

Non-steroidal anti-inflammatory drugs such as mefenamic acid inhibit prostaglandin synthetase. They reduce blood loss by 30% and their analgesic properties may be an advantage if there is associated dysmenorrhoea. The principal side effect is gastrointestinal irritation.

Tranexamic acid is an antifibrinolytic agent that reduces blood loss by about 50%. It increases the risk of thrombosis so is contraindicated in patients with a previous history of thromboembolic disease.

Both groups of drugs have the advantage of only needing to be taken during menstruation.

Hormonal treatments

Use of the combined oral contraceptive pill or the levonorgestrel intrauterine system is associated with a 30% and 90% reduction in average monthly blood loss respectively. Hormone replacement therapy (HRT) may be useful in perimenopausal women to control ovulatory dysfunctional bleeding.

Synthetic progestogens such as norethisterone and medroxyprogesterone acetate given in the second half of the cycle have not been shown to reduce blood loss although they may have a role in establishing a more predictable cycle in patients with irregular bleeding. Given in higher doses over a longer time they are associated with significant reduction in blood loss and are sometimes used in an acute situation to control heavy menstrual bleeding (oral medroxyprogesterone acetate 10 mg daily for 10 days)

Danazol is a synthetic androgen derivative that acts on the hypothalamic–pituitary axis and endometrium. Given at high doses it will normally cause amenorrhoea but is associated with significant side effects in 50% of patients and is normally limited to 6 months use. However, at a lower dose (200 mg) given continuously, it reduces menstrual loss by up to 60% and is better tolerated. It is normally used as second-line treatment in women where other medical treatment has failed.

Surgical treatment

Endometrial resection or ablation

The endometrium can be removed or destroyed using an operating hysteroscope. The most widely used techniques are laser ablation and endoscopic resection with a diathermy wire loop (Fig. 18.8). The endometrium is prepared by treatment with danazol or GnRH analogues for 4–8 weeks prior to surgery. The uterine cavity is distended with an irrigation fluid such as glycine or normal saline. The procedure takes a similar amount of operation time as a hysterectomy but the subsequent hospital stay and recovery time following discharge are considerably less. There is a risk of intraoperative uterine perforation and, possibly, damage to other organs requiring laparotomy and repair. The other potential complication is fluid overload from excessive absorption of the irrigation fluid, resulting in cerebral or pulmonary oedema. Approximately 40% of patients will become amenorrhoeic, with a further 30–40% achieving a significant reduction in their symptoms.

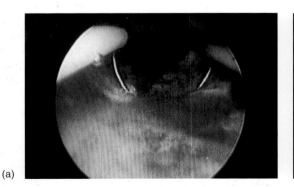
(a)

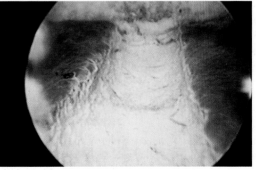
(b)

Fig. 18.8 Endometrial resection. View of the uterine cavity before (a) and after (b) excision using a resectoscope.

A minority of patients will eventually need further surgery and hysterectomy.

Hysterectomy

This remains the definitive treatment, and is more likely to be appropriate for those women with pelvic pathology such as adenomyosis and fibroids than medical treatment or endoscopic surgery. It is associated with a mortality of 1/2000. Significant complications occur in 25–43% of patients and are more common in patients undergoing abdominal hysterectomy.

The majority of operations are carried out through a transverse lower abdominal or midline incision, *total abdominal hysterectomy*. The round ligaments, Fallopian tubes and ovarian vessels are cut and ligated on each side either medial or distal to the ovaries, depending on whether these are to be conserved (see below). The uterovesical peritoneum is opened and the bladder is reflected off the lower part of the uterus and cervix so as to displace the ureters away from the uterine vessels, which are then cut and ligated. Finally, the cervical ligaments are cut and the vagina opened around the cervix, allowing removal of the uterus. If there has been no history of cervical disease the cervix can be conserved by removing the uterine corpus above the internal os after the uterine vessels have been ligated (*subtotal hysterectomy*). This may be indicated if other pelvic disease makes dissection of the cervix difficult, in order to reduce the risk of ureteric damage, or because of patient preference.

In *vaginal hysterectomy* the vaginal skin is opened around the cervix and the bladder and reflected up into the pelvis. The peritoneum over the uterovesical and rectovaginal space is opened, and the cervical ligaments are cut and ligated. The uterine and ovarian vessels are ligated, the uterus is removed and the peritoneum and vaginal skin are closed. Removal of the ovaries is possible but is less commonly carried out by this route. The absence of an abdominal wound substantially reduces postoperative morbidity, making this the method of choice for hysterectomy. It is contraindicated where malignancy is suspected. Other relative contraindications include a uterine size of over 14 weeks, endometriosis and lack of uterine descent.

In *laparoscopically assisted vaginal hysterectomy* the ovarian and uterine pedicles are cut under laparoscopic control though the abdomen and the remainder of the operation is completed vaginally. This may enable oophorectomy or a vaginal operation to be carried out where a full abdominal procedure might otherwise have been required.

Conservation of the ovaries, if normal, is usually recommended for women under the age of 45 years undergoing hysterectomy for menorrhagia to avoid the onset of a surgically induced early menopause. For women near the menopause this advantage has to be offset against the risk of later ovarian malignancy, and the option of oophorectomy should be discussed.

DYSMENORRHOEA

Dysmenorrhoea or painful menstruation is the commonest of all gynaecological symptoms.

Primary dysmenorrhoea occurs in the absence of any significant pelvic pathology. It usually develops within the first 2 years of the menarche and is often familial, with a strong likelihood that the attitude of the mother may influence the response of the daughter. Nevertheless, it would be a mistake to underestimate the severity of dysmenorrhoea in some women. The pain is often intense and cramping and can be crippling and severely incapacitating so that it causes a major disruption of social activities. It is usually associated with the onset of menstrual blood loss but may begin on the day preceding menstruation. It tends not to be associated with menorrhagia. The pain only occurs in ovulatory cycles, is lower abdominal in nature but sometime radiates down the anterior aspect of the thighs. The pain often disappears or improves after the birth of the first child. Dysmenorrhoea may be associated with vomiting and diarrhoea. Pelvic examination reveals no abnormality of the pelvic organs.

Secondary or *acquired dysmenorrhoea* is caused by organic pelvic pathology and it usually has its onset many years after the menarche. Any woman who develops secondary dysmenorrhoea should be considered to have organic pathology in the pelvis until proved otherwise. Common associated pathologies include endometriosis, adenomyosis, pelvic infections and intrauterine lesions such as submucous fibroid polyps. The diagnosis and management of these conditions are discussed in Chapters 22 and 23.

Investigations

A careful history is of great importance in this condition. Pelvic examination may not be helpful in primary dysmenorrhoea but it is advisable to perform either a vaginal or rectal examination to exclude any obvious pelvic pathology. However, in secondary dysmenorrhoea a pelvic examination is essential and, if pelvic pathology is not palpable, laparoscopy is advisable. This is only performed in cases with primary dysmenorrhoea if the condition is particularly resistant to therapy.

Management

Discussion and reassurance are an essential part of management. Primary dysmenorrhoea tends to present some months after the menarche and is associated with ovulatory cycles, early cycles frequently being anovulatory. The intensity of pain may be aggravated by apprehension and fear, and reassurance that the pain does not indicate any serious disorder may lessen the symptoms. It is also common for the pain to either disappear or substantially lessen after the birth of the first child.

Drug therapy

Dysmenorrhoea can be effectively treated by drugs that inhibit prostaglandin synthesis and hence uterine contractility. These drugs include aspirin, mefenamic acid, naproxen or ibuprofen. As dysmenorrhoea is often associated with vomiting, headache and dizziness, it may be advisable to start therapy either on the day before the period is expected, or as soon as the menstrual flow commences.

If these drugs are inadequate, suppression of ovulation with the contraceptive pill is highly effective in reducing the severity of dysmenorrhoea. Where it is ineffective, then careful consideration should be given to the possibility of underlying pathology.

If all conservative medical therapy fails, then relief may sometimes be achieved by mechanical dilatation of the cervix or by the surgical removal of the pain fibres to the uterus in an operation known as presacral neurectomy, but these methods of treatment should be approached with considerable caution.

In cases of secondary dysmenorrhoea, the treatment is dependent on the nature of the underlying pathology. If the pathology is not amenable to medical therapy, the symptoms may only be relieved by hysterectomy.

PREMENSTRUAL SYNDROME

Premenstrual syndrome (PMS) is defined as the occurrence of one or more non-specific somatic, psychological and behavioural symptoms severe enough to disrupt social, family or occupational life occurring in at least 4 of the last 6 months during the pre-menstrual phase which resolve completely (primary) or improve markedly (secondary) by the end of menstruation.

Symptoms and signs

The condition is commonly precipitated by stress and tension, either at home or at work, and particularly afflicts women during the third decade of life. The common symptoms include:

- **Behavioural changes:** there are symptoms of depression and tension often associated with unreasonable outbursts of temper. Suicide occurs more often in the premenstrual week, and minor crimes are also more frequent in the second half of the cycle.
- **Symptoms of bloatedness:** many women experience these symptoms. Their clothing feels uncomfortably tight, and this symptom does not subside until the onset of menstruation. Although there is a cyclical increase in weight in both symptomatic and asymptomatic women in the premenstrual week, weight gain is not usually excessive in those with premenstrual syndrome. The exception is the small group of women who suffer from cyclical oedema, where generalized oedema and oliguria occur in the second half of the cycle.
- **Breast symptoms:** breast tenderness, enlargement of the breasts and heaviness and pain are features of the syndrome in most women.
- **Gastrointestinal symptoms:** nausea and vomiting and constipation or diarrhoea occur occasionally but are not major symptoms.

Pathogenesis

Premenstrual syndrome is related to the ovarian cycle but the exact mechanism is unknown. There is no clear evidence of progesterone deficiency or an abnormal ratio in the levels of oestrogen and progesterone. Possible explanations include beta-endorphin deficiency, prolactin excess and abnormalities in fatty acid and prostaglandin synthesis.

Management

Treatment depends on establishing the correct diagnosis and the menstrual calendar may help both the patient and her doctor to gain insight into which symptoms are likely to respond to treatment. The main principles of treatment are a combination of increasing the ability to cope with symptoms and alteration of hormone status. Reassurance and support must be an important and continuing requirement in the treatment of premenstrual syndrome, and it may be necessary to try a variety of therapies before a satisfactory response can be obtained.

The assessment of any form of therapy is particularly difficult because of a 70–80% placebo response. It is inadvisable to accept the validity of any form of drug therapy that has not been subjected to a placebo-controlled, double-blind trial, as virtually any form of therapy will produce an improvement in symptoms in some women.

Dietary changes involve eating little and often and taking plenty of carbohydrates to keep blood sugar levels up while reducing salt and alcohol intake during the premenstrual phase. Psychotherapy, counselling, discussion in self-help groups and education augmented by exercise help by increasing tolerance to premenstrual symptoms and reducing mild underlying psychological problems.

Vitamin B_6 and evening primrose oil are frequently self-prescribed for PMS. Vitamin B_6 (pyridoxine) is a cofactor in neurotransmitter synthesis. Although there is no evidence of any actual deficit in PMS the largest controlled study showed an 82% response rate to vitamin B_6 compared to 70% on placebo. Peripheral neuropathy has been reported at high doses but a dose of 100 mg is probably safe. Evening primrose oil contains the unsaturated fatty acid precursors of prostaglandins. There is some evidence of improvement in selected symptoms but the recommended dose of 8 capsules a day is difficult to sustain. Antiprostaglandin painkillers such as ibuprofen may be useful for breast pain and headaches. Diuretics such as spironolactone may be of benefit in the small group of women who experience true water retention but should only be used for symptoms of bloating where there is measurable weight gain. The dry extract of the *Agnus castus* fruit (20 mg daily) may also be effective in reducing symptoms of irritability, mood change, headache and breast fullness.

Users of the combined contraceptive pill report lower levels of PMS than those using barrier contraception but individual response varies and is unpredictable. There is no evidence to suggest that progestogens and progesterone supplements (given as pessaries or injections) are any more effective than placebo.

The most effective treatments are those that suppress normal ovulation but these are also the treatments associated with the most significant side effects. Danazol is effective in reducing breast symptoms and some psychological symptoms but is associated with significant androgen and hypo-oestrogenic side effects.

Gonadotrophin-releasing hormone agonists suppress symptoms during treatment but these recur when treatment is stopped. They are unsuitable for long-term use because of osteoporosis. As a last resort bilateral oophorectomy (usually with hysterectomy) will provide a surgical cure for symptoms if these are true PMS. This should only be undertaken after treatment with GnRH agonists has shown that the symptoms are abolished by suppression of ovulation.

MENOPAUSE

The *climacteric* is that part of the ageing process which embraces the transition from the reproductive to the non-reproductive phase of life. The *menopause* marks the end of menstruation but, as with the menarche in relation to puberty, it reflects only one manifestation of a series of changes. The age of the physiological menopause varies with race and socioeconomic conditions, but in western Europe and the USA the average age of onset is 51 years.

Spontaneous cessation of the periods before the age of 40 years is defined as premature menopause. The menopause may be physiological or artificial, when it is associated with removal of the ovaries or the uterus.

Hormonal and menstrual changes in the climacteric

The menstrual cycle shortens in women over the age of 40 years, and the change in the cycle length is related to shortening of the follicular phase. FSH levels are higher at all stages of the cycle than levels seen in younger women, whilst oestradiol levels are lower.

The transition from menstruation to amenorrhoea is often characterized by menstrual irregularity. Prolonged episodes of bleeding following a period of amenorrhoea may be associated with anovulatory cycles and with hyperplastic endometrium. Persistent irregular bleeding in the premenopausal phase should never be considered normal, because it may be associated with uterine neoplasms.

Vaginal bleeding which occurs more than 1 year after the menopause is known as *postmenopausal bleeding*. The possibility of carcinoma of the body of the uterus should be considered, and diagnostic hysteroscopy and endometrial biopsy should be performed in all cases. Ultrasound measurement of endometrial thickness can also be used, as significant endometrial pathology is unlikely where this is less than 3 mm.

Other causes of postmenopausal bleeding include other benign and malignant tumours of the lower genital tract, stimulation of the endometrium by exogenous oestrogen (e.g. HRT and oestrogens from ovarian tumours), infection and senile atrophic vaginitis.

Hormone changes after the menopause

There is a marked reduction in ovarian production of oestrogen and, in particular, of oestradiol. Some oestrogen production occurs in the adrenal gland but the major source of oestradiol appears to be the 'fat' organ with peripheral conversion of both oestrone and testosterone. Thus, heavy women have higher circulating oestrogen levels than slender women. There is considerable variation in the circulating levels of oestradiol in the menopause, and this may account for the variation in severity of menopausal symptoms. The absence of any significant oestrogen production results in excessive release of FSH and LH, with the major increases occurring in FSH. The levels of gonadotrophins continue to show random oscillations similar to the pattern seen in the premenopausal phase. Androgens produced in the ovary and adrenal gland are mainly androstenedione and testosterone and these levels fall in menopausal women. There is also a reduction in adrenal androgen secretion, including that of dehydroepiandrosterone (DHEA) and DHEA sulphate. Oestrogen production by the ovary is reduced but the production of testosterone persists.

Symptoms and signs of the climacteric

Vascular disturbances

The commonest symptom of the menopause is the development of hot flushes. These episodes consist of flushes and perspiration, occur in about 80% of the female population and may persist for up to 5 years after the menopause. The flushes are associated with an increase in skin temperature and conductance. They are also associated in some way with high gonadotrophin levels, but this relationships is not as clear as might at first appear. There are other women where oestrogen levels are low and gonadotrophin levels are high, but who do not develop hot flushes. There is no doubt that the administration of oestrogens relieves these symptoms, but they return when the oestrogen therapy is discontinued.

Changes in target organ response

The reduction in ovarian oestrogen production results in involution and regression of target organs (Fig. 18.9).

The most obvious response is the cessation of menstruation. Periods generally exhibit a gradual reduction in both amount and duration, with occasional delays in menstruation. The vaginal walls lose their rugosity and become smooth and atrophic. In severe cases, this may also be associated with chronic infection and atrophic vaginitis. The cervix diminishes in size, and there is a reduction in cervical mucus production. The uterus also shrinks in size, and the endometrium becomes atrophic.

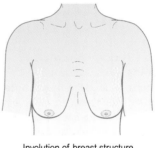

Involution of breast structure

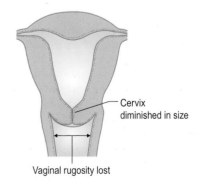

Cervix diminished in size

Vaginal rugosity lost

Fig. 18.9 Characteristic changes in the breasts and genitalia following the menopause.

The breasts exhibit parallel changes with involution of breast structure and the disappearance of cyclical breast changes, which may bring considerable relief to some women.

Although it is not in any proper sense an endocrine target organ, the bladder epithelium may also become atrophic with the development of frequency, dysuria and urge incontinence in the absence of any overt urinary tract infection. It is important to recognize these symptoms because they can be relieved by oestrogen replacement therapy.

Epidermal appendages

The skin tends to become thinned and wrinkled after the menopause as a result of oestrogen deprivation; these changes can be reversed by the use of local oestrogen creams or by HRT. There is loss of scalp hair and of pubic and axillary hair. There is an androgen-based increase in the growth of coarse terminal hair so that a slight moustache may develop, and loss of scalp hair sometimes results in partial or complete baldness, but this is uncommon.

Bone changes

Osteoporosis is an important health hazard in the menopausal woman. The loss of trabecular bone is the major disorder. Bone loss occurs at a rate of about 2.5% per year for the first 4 years after the menopause so that fractures become a major source of morbidity in the menopausal female. Thus, by the age of 65 years, vertebral fractures occur in 25% of all women.

Bone loss is most severe in women who have an artificial menopause. Hip fractures increase in incidence from 0.3/1000 at an age of 45 years to 20/1000 at age 85 years, and there is also a 10-fold increase in Colles fractures.

Osteoporosis is associated with increased bone re-sorption with normal bone formation. There is no doubt that there is a net loss of calcium. These changes are associated with oestrogen deficiency and there is little doubt that prolonged and early HRT can prevent the development of osteoporosis. The means by which these effects are achieved remains uncertain. Fractures late in life carry serious implications in relation to life expectation because of the immobilization of the elderly woman.

Cardiovascular complications

There is evidence of an increase in coronary heart disease following the menopause that is not simply an age-related phenomenon. Serum cholesterol levels rise at the time of the menopause. There is an increase in all lipoprotein fractions, with a decrease in the ratio of the high- to low-density fractions. There is no specific association between the menopause and hypertension.

Psychological and emotional symptoms

Many women experience severe emotional disorders at the time of the menopause with depression and anxiety states. The emotional disturbances of the menopause are often associated with feelings of inadequacy and uncertainty about the woman's role with the departure of children from the home. However, there is no doubt that in many women these symptoms are related to oestrogen deficiency and that HRT can return such women to a normal state. The severity of the symptoms should not be underestimated. The depression may be acute and can sometimes result in a successful suicidal attempt. There are many other symptoms ascribed to the menopause, including anorexia, excessive fatigue, nausea and vomiting and bowel disorders.

Treatment of the menopause

Many women pass through the menopause without any symptoms, and there is considerable variation in serum oestradiol levels between individuals after the menopause. Oestrogen therapy is the most effective treatment for symptomatic relief but is associated with significant adverse effects in a minority of women. The decision to use HRT is made on an individual basis taking into account each woman's history, risk factors and personal preferences (Table 18.1). This should be done in a way that can be understood so that each woman can make an informed choice.

Hormone replacement therapy

Oestrogen therapy may be given on its own or as a combined or sequential therapy with a progestogen. The type of therapy recommended will depend on whether the uterus has been removed and whether the therapy planned is to be short- or long-term. There

Table 18.1
Relative risks and benefits seen in women taking combined oestrogen and progestogen HRT (Adapted from the Women's Health Initiative Study. JAMA 2002; 288: 321–333)

	Relative risk vs placebo group at 5 years
Heart attacks	1.29
Stroke	1.41
Breast cancer	1.26
Venous thrombosis	2.11
Fractured neck of femur	0.63
Colorectal cancer	0.66

should be regular reappraisal of the risk and benefits on any woman taking long-term HRT.

Oral therapy

Ethinylestradiol or conjugated equine oestrogen (Premarin) is given continuously with concomitant administration of a progestogen in women with an intact uterus to prevent the development of endometrial hyperplasia or malignancy. Progestogens are commonly given for 10–12 days every 4 weeks, to produce a monthly withdrawal bleed, but there is no loss of protective effect when this is reduced to 12-weekly intervals. Those women who have previously stopped their periods and wish to avoid further bleeds can be offered combination therapy which includes continuous progestogen administration with an oestrogen or a compound such as Tibolone.

Parenteral therapy

Oestrogen can also be administered by injection or by subcutaneous implants. This is best achieved with oestradiol benzoate, 100 mg, in a pellet that is inserted in the subcutaneous tissue of the anterior abdominal wall. This is often combined with testosterone, which has the advantage of a mild anabolic effect and of enhancing libido. The pellets usually last for anything up to 6 months and are particularly useful in women who have experienced a surgical menopause. Tachyphylaxis with progressively shorter intervals between implants and the return of symptoms even in the presence of normal or high oestradiol levels can be a problem.

If the implants are given to a woman with an intact uterus, then it is important to give a progestogen, such as norethisterone acetate 5mg, for the first 7 days of each month. This will provoke withdrawal bleeding as long as active oestrogen absorption occurs.

Topical therapy

Oestradiol can be given percutaneously by self-adhesive patches or gel. Patches are applied to any area of clear, dry skin other than the face or breast, and changed twice a week. The gel is rubbed into the skin once a day. A progestogen can be given either orally or transdermally. This route has the advantage of bypassing liver metabolism, and gives more stable serum hormone levels than with implants. The major complication is one of skin irritation.

Contraindications

Hormone replacement therapy is contraindicated in the presence of endometrial and breast carcinoma, thromboembolic disease, acute liver disease and ischaemic heart disease. Other conditions such as fibrocystic disease of the breast, uterine fibroids, familial hyperlipidaemia, diabetes and gall bladder disease provide a relative contraindication but relief of symptoms may sometimes be more important than other considerations.

Risks. The potential complications of hormone replacement therapy include an increased incidence of carcinoma of the endometrium, breast and possibly ovary. The risks of these cancers increase the longer that HRT is taken. Although previous observational studies had suggested a protective effect against heart disease and stroke this is no longer felt to be the case and indeed the risk of these conditions may be increased in patients taking some types of combined therapy. The risk of venous thrombosis is increased but the overall incidence is low. Some women develop hypertension on oestrogen therapy and periodic checks on blood pressure are therefore important. Caution should be taken when there is a history of gall bladder disease. The development of irregular uterine bleeding after more than 6 months on HRT is an indication for endometrial biopsy.

> **!** Hormone replacement therapy should no longer be prescribed for the prevention of coronary heart disease.

Benefits. The principal benefits of HRT use are in the relief of menopausal symptoms and the prevention of osteoporosis. HRT use is associated with a reduction in the risk of fracture of the neck of femur and in the incidence of colorectal cancer.

Alternatives to oestrogen-containing HRT

As the principal indication for long-term use of HRT is the prevention of osteoporosis, patients need to be aware of the increased risk of some conditions with long-term use and the alternative treatment options available to prevent osteoporosis.

Tibilone is a synthetic androgen with oestrogenic properties. It does not cause endometrial proliferation so there is no withdrawal bleed but it is only suitable for women more than a year after the menopause. It is effective at reducing vasomotor symptoms and osteoporosis.

Selective oestrogen receptor modulators (SERMs) act on oestrogen receptors in bone without affecting the breast or endometrium. Those currently available are effective at doing this but do not relieve vasomotor symptoms and are associated with the same increased risk of thrombosis as conventional oestrogen therapy.

Clonidine is an antihypertensive that has some effect on vasomotor symptoms but no effect on other symptoms or long-term health. Biofeedback techniques, acupuncture and selected use of anxiolytics or sedatives may help to control psychological symptoms of insomnia and anxiety. Cyclical bisphosphonate therapy increases bone mass and reduces the rate of fracture and provides an effective alternative for women at risk of osteoporosis who are unwilling or unable to take hormone replacement therapy. Calcium supplements alone do not appear to prevent bone loss.

ESSENTIAL INFORMATION

Puberty

- Normal sequence is thelarche, adrenarche, growth spurt, menarche
- Menarche normal between 11 and 15
- Early cycles anovulatory
- Most cases of precocious puberty are constitutional
- Primary amenorrhoea not always synonymous with delayed puberty

Secondary amenorrhoea

- Absence of menstruation for more than 6 months
- Physiological causes – pregnancy, breastfeeding
- Pathological causes – hypothalamic dysfunction, hyperprolactinaemia, polycystic ovarian syndrome
- Ask about – weight, stress, chronic illness, medication, contraception
- Investigations – pregnancy test, FSH, LH, prolactin, ultrasound

Menorrhagia

- Prolonged or heavy regular bleeding
- Commonest diagnosis is dysfunctional uterine bleeding
- Only routine investigation needed is full blood count
- Mainstay of treatment is medical

Premenstrual syndrome

- Cyclical changes occurring in the luteal phase of the cycle and ceasing at the onset of menstruation
- Commonest symptoms mood changes, breast tenderness, bloating and gastrointestinal symptoms
- Treatment options are pyridoxine, evening primrose oil, suppression of ovulation
- High placebo response rate

Menopause

- Part of climacteric
- Onset 50–51 years
- Hypergonadotrophic, hypogonadic
- Associated with vasomotor instability, atrophic changes in genital tract and breast, cardiovascular changes and osteoporosis
- Hormone replacement therapy effective in symptom relief and osteoporosis
- Increased risks of breast cancer, venous thrombosis, stroke and heart attacks with HRT

19 Infertility and disorders of sexual function

INFERTILITY

The incidence of infertility varies in different countries and has been recorded to be as high as 50% in some west African communities compared with values of around 12% in western European societies.

It is important to differentiate between infertility, which is diminished fertility, and sterility, which is absolute infertility. *Primary infertility* is defined as diminished fertility throughout the reproductive years and *secondary infertility* implies failure to conceive after one or more successful pregnancies.

If conception does not occur after 12 months of normal sexual activity without contraception, the couple should be considered to be potentially infertile, as 80% of couples normally conceive within 1 year. It is therefore reasonable to proceed with investigations at this time.

Such a definition has to be modified by circumstances. For example, if a woman has had secondary amenorrhoea for 2 years, it would be pointless to wait for 12 months of regular sexual exposure before investigating her subfertility. At the other extreme, if her partner was away for a substantial part of the year, it would be sensible to defer intensive investigations until regular sexual exposure could be established. Both partners must be investigated, as infertility may result from male or female factors and is often associated with a combination of both factors. At the completion of all investigations, about a third will exhibit no identifiable cause for their infertility, and long-term follow-up studies on these couples have shown that only 30–40% will conceive over a 7-year period after investigation.

Changes in the socioeconomic status of women in Western society has resulted in the deferment of childbearing. Age undoubtedly affects fertility. Studies on various racial groups show consistently that natural fertility progressively declines from the age of 25 years. Evidence suggests that women who marry at 40 years of age have a 60% chance of not having children, and after the age of 44 years the chances of conception are very poor. This reduction in fertility may be partly ascribed to a reduction in the frequency of coitus, a reduction in

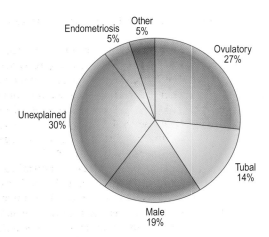

Fig. 19.1 Causes of primary infertility in western European couples.

the frequency of ovulation, a reduction in male fertility associated with an increased production of defective sperm and, finally, an increased propensity to miscarry in older women.

The relative incidence of causative factors will vary according to country and whether the problem is primary or secondary. Furthermore, in many couples, there are multiple reasons for the infertility. Figure 19.1 shows the pattern of causative factors of primary infertility in a Western population.

History and examination

Both partners should be requested to attend at the initial interview. On occasions, the male partner may be reluctant to attend and this should not be considered as a basis for refusing investigation. It should, however, be apparent to the woman that the value of investigation will be seriously limited without the cooperation of her partner.

The initial interview

The initial interview should take into account the following factors:

- Age, occupation and educational background
- Number of years that conception has been attempted and the previous history of contraception
- Previous marriages and pregnancies of either partner

- Whether the infertility is primary or secondary and, if necessary, the details of any complications associated with previous pregnancies
- Coital history, including frequency of intercourse – any history of dyspareunia, of impotence or difficulty in ejaculation may be important
- Previous history of sexually transmitted disease
- General medical history of any concurrent or previous serious illness and of any surgery, particularly in relation to appendicitis in the female or herniorrhaphy in the male; a history of undescended testes or of orchidopexy may be particularly important.

Female causes of infertility

General factors such as the age of both partners, a history of serious systemic illness, inadequate nutrition and emotional stress may all be factors that contribute to infertility but the major defined problems are found in defects of ovulation, tubal disease and cervical hostility.

Disorders of ovulation

Disorders of ovulation are divided into five categories:

- Primary amenorrhoea – the failure of onset of menstruation by the age of 16 years – is rarely a presenting symptom in relation to subfertility, and has been considered separately
- Secondary amenorrhoea – no menstruation for 6 months or more in a woman with a previous history of menstruation
- Oligomenorrhoea (infrequent periods) – periods occur between 6 weeks and 6 months and may be ovulatory or anovulatory; however, even if the cycles are ovulatory, ovulation is so infrequent that fertility becomes impaired
- Anovulatory cycles – cycle length may be within normal limits but ovulation does not occur
- Ovulation appears to occur but the ovum is entrapped in the follicle; the corpus luteum may be defective and implantation does not occur.

Endocrine causes of oligomenorrhoea and secondary amenorrhoea

Anovulation is commonly, although not invariably, associated with amenorrhoea or oligomenorrhoea and these conditions may occur as the result of any one of a series of changes in the hypothalamic–pituitary–ovarian axis. Alterations in the menstrual cycle are commonly associated with periods of stress and also with excessive weight gain or obesity and, at the other extreme, with anorexia nervosa or self-inflicted starvation.

Pituitary failure, as in Sheehan's syndrome, is now a rare condition but pituitary tumours in the form of pituitary microadenomas, which are prolactin-secreting, are a relatively common cause of secondary amenorrhoea.

Ovarian failure may occur as a result of premature menopause and the presence of streak ovaries. Polycystic ovary syndrome is the most common cause of anovulation. It is associated with hirsutism, obesity and oligomenorrhoea. The aetiology, investigation and management of polycystic ovarian syndrome is discussed in Chapter 18.

Anovulatory 'normal cycles'

The presence of a normal menstrual cycle does not necessarily imply that ovulation is occurring. The oocyte may not be released from the follicle while luteinization of the unruptured follicle may still occur. This is known as the *luteinized unruptured follicle (LUF) syndrome,* and is commonly associated with endometriosis. The diagnosis can only really be made by laparoscopic inspection of the ovary to establish whether there is any evidence of an ovulation stigma.

Abnormalities of implantation and the luteal phase

Implantation requires the presence of adequate development of the secretory phase of the endometrium. Luteal phase inadequacy results in either failure of implantation or early miscarriage. Diagnosis may be difficult and the aetiology is not understood, but there is no doubt that the problem arises in the first half of the cycle with defective follicular development.

Tubal factors

The function of the Fallopian tubes involves both ovum pick-up and transport of the fertilized gamete. Ovum pick-up is dependent on the action of the tubal fimbriae in pulling the ostium of the tube over the follicle. The action of the tubal cilia also serves to aspirate the ovum. Subsequent progress and nutrition of the zygote by the tube is determined by the muscular action of the tubal

wall, by the ciliated action and secretion of the tubal epithelium.

It is estimated that tubal factors account for about 14% of cases of infertility, although this figure varies considerably according to the population involved. Occasionally, congenital anomalies occur but the commonest cause of tubal damage is infection. Infection may cause occlusion of the fimbrial end of the tube, with the collection of fluid (hydrosalpinx) or pus (pyosalpinx) within the tubal lumen (Fig. 19.2).

Acute salpingitis results from sexually transmitted diseases. In the developed world it is caused mainly by chlamydial infection but it may also result from infection with other organisms such as *Neisseria gonorrhoeae,* *Escherichia coli,* anaerobic and haemolytic streptococci, staphylococci and *Clostridium welchii.* The incidence of tubal damage is approximately 8% after the first episode of pelvic infection, 16% after two and 40% after three episodes. Tuberculosis of the tubes may occur in women with pulmonary tuberculosis but has become increasingly rare as a cause of subfertility.

Infections arising from intrauterine contraceptive devices and following miscarriage or termination of pregnancy, and infections in the puerperium, commonly result in cornual blockage – often without any other significant change in the remainder of the tube. Pelvic infection from appendicitis associated with peritonitis results in peritubal adhesions and leaves the tubal lining unaffected.

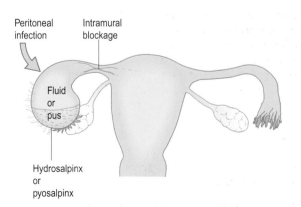

Fig. 19.2 The pathogenesis of tubal obstruction and subfertility: intramural tubal obstruction results from intrauterine infection.

Infections that affect the lumen of the tube result in loss of the ciliated epithelium and damage and fibrosis within the tubal wall, thus impairing the peristaltic function of the tube in promoting movement of the gamete.

> **!** Even in the presence of a patent tube, damage to the wall and lumen may result in severe impairment of tubal function.

Lesions of the uterine cavity

The effect of uterine abnormalities on fertility is controversial. Conditions that impinge on the uterine cavity may interfere with implantation. Intramural and submucous fibroids do not appear to interfere with implantation unless they distort the uterine cavity. Severe intrauterine infections following pregnancy associated with retained products of conception and where uterine curettage is performed may result in complete ablation of the uterine cavity by adhesion of the walls, or partial occlusion of the cavity by the formation of intrauterine adhesions or synechiae. This condition is known as *Asherman's syndrome.*

Congenital abnormalities of the uterus do not interfere with conception as a rule but may be associated with recurrent miscarriage.

Cervical factors

Ejaculation occurs into the vagina, and semen is deposited around the cervix. However, the cervix is effectively closed with cervical mucus, and sperm migration occurs by penetration of sperm into the cervical mucus. At the time of ovulation, endocervical cells secrete copious, clear, watery mucus, which has a high water content and consists of long chains of polypeptide macromolecules with occasional side chains of carbohydrate. The chains of molecules contain channels that allow a direct passage of the spermatozoa into the uterine cavity. Sperm penetration occurs within 2–3 minutes of deposition. Between 100 000 and 200 000 sperm colonize the cervical mucus and remain at this level for approximately 24 hours after coitus. Approximately 200 sperm eventually reach the fallopian tube. The vagina is generally hostile to sperm survival, and sperm remaining in

the vagina soon become immobilized. Mucus produced by the cervix under the influence of progesterone is hostile to sperm penetration.

Thus, poor penetration of sperm may result from cervical infection, from antisperm antibody activity in either cervical mucus or seminal plasma, from production of abnormal mucus by the cervix or from the effect of progestational agents on the mucus.

INVESTIGATION OF INFERTILITY

Investigation of the female

The investigation of the female involves determination of three basic issues:

- Does ovulation occur on a regular basis?
- Is there any impairment of tubal function and of implantation?
- Is there a cervical factor preventing sperm invasion?

In addition all women presenting with infertility should have their immunity to rubella checked and, if seronegative be offered, vaccination before undertaking further treatment for their infertility.

Detection of ovulation

The assessment of ovulation depends on the menstrual history. In the presence of a regular menstrual cycle ovulatory status can be investigated by changes in basal body temperature, cervical mucus or hormone levels, by endometrial biopsy or by ultrasound.

Basal temperature

An increase of 0.5 °C occurs in basal body temperature in the luteal phase of the menstrual cycle. The temperature should be recorded sublingually before rising each morning, and provides a useful indication of the regularity of ovulation (Fig. 19.3).

> **!** Ovulation may occur in the absence of any temperature shift and use of basal body temperature charts (BBTC) can cause emotional stress and interfere with the sexual relationship of the couple. Therefore, BBTC should not be used to time intercourse.

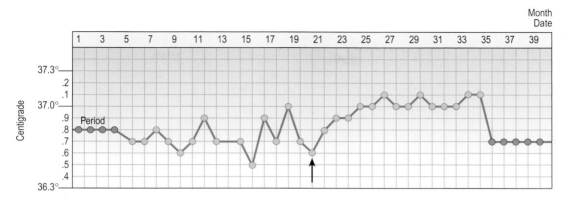

Fig. 19.3 Ovulatory chart in a 35-day cycle. The temperature falls immediately prior to ovulation and rises during the luteal phase of the cycle.

Cervical mucus

The production of mucus increases during the follicular phase to reach a peak at the time of ovulation, with profuse production of clear, acellular mucus with low viscosity and high 'stretchability' (*Spinnbarkeit*; Fig. 19.4). Although these changes can be recognized by the woman herself, they can be unreliable as an indicator of ovulation. Some women experience pain in the mid-cycle (*Mittelschmerz*) associated with ovulation and can therefore estimate the timing of their ovulation. Mid-cycle mucus also dries on a glass slide with a characteristic fern pattern. This pattern presents a granular amorphous appearance that disappears with the influence of progesterone.

Hormonal tests

Serial measurement of FSH and LH in either blood or urine shows a well-defined peak that occurs approxi-

mately 20 hours before ovulation and can therefore be used as a technique for timing ovulation. However, commercially available detection kits for LH are expensive and monitoring ovulation in this way can be as stressful as using temperature charts.

The best hormonal evidence that ovulation has occurred is the measurement of serum progesterone in the luteal phase of the cycle. The interpretation of the results depends on the day of the cycle, and values in excess of 32 nmol/l indicate that ovulation has occurred. However, none of these tests is infallible.

> ✔ There is no need to measure thyroid function or prolactin levels in women with regular periods unless they have symptoms of galactorrhoea or thyroid disease.

Endometrial biopsy and vaginal cytology

Biopsy of the endometrium can be performed without anaesthesia or formal dilatation and curettage. The presence of secretory-phase endometrium is taken as evidence of ovulation. However, it should be remembered that a luteal phase defect occurs in 30% of cycles in normal women without any apparent effect on fertility.

Ultrasonography

Ultrasound examination of the ovaries can be used to identify follicular growth. Follicular diameter increases from 11.5 mm 5 days before ovulation to 20 mm on the

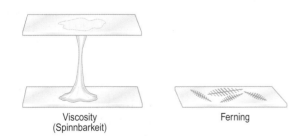

Fig. 19.4 Characteristics of cervical mucus: the 'stretchability' can be evaluated between two glass slides (left); mid-cycle mucus shows ferning (right).

day before ovulation and decreases to approximately half this size on the day after ovulation. This is a useful and practical way of monitoring the time of ovulation. Ultrasound may be of value in evaluation of the ovaries for conditions such as polycystic ovarian syndrome.

Investigation of non-ovulation

If there is evidence of non-ovulation, then further investigation should include measurement of:

- Serum prolactin – to exclude hyperprolactinaemia
- FSH and LH levels in secondary amenorrhoea – high levels of gonadotrophins in the presence of low levels of oestrogen indicate ovarian failure
- Tomography of the sella turcica if prolactin levels are raised, to search for evidence of a pituitary prolactinoma.

Investigation of tubal function

It is essential to establish tubal patency before embarking on prolonged drug therapy in either partner. Tubal patency is assessed by the following.

Hysterosalpingography(HSG)

A radio-opaque dye is injected into the uterine cavity and fallopian tubes. This technique can be performed without anaesthesia, provided the approach is gentle and the dye is injected slowly. The dye outlines the uterine cavity and will demonstrate any filling defects. It will also show whether there is evidence of tubal obstruction and the site of the obstruction (Fig. 19.5). The examination is performed 3–5 days after the end of menstruation. Patients should be screened for *Chlamydia* or given appropriate antibiotic prophylaxis to reduce the risk of infection.

Laparoscopy and dye insufflation

Laparoscopy enables direct visualization of the pelvic organs and, in particular, enables the diagnosis of endometriosis (Fig. 19.6). Methylene blue is injected through the uterine cavity to demonstrate tubal patency. It is not always possible to be certain of the site of tubal obstruction. This technique may be combined with hysteroscopy to assess the uterine cavity. Antibiotic prophylaxis should be used if pelvic infection is detected, to prevent any flare-up of the disease.

Assessment of tubal patency with ultrasound

Tubal patency can be assessed using ultrasound by injecting normal saline or contrast medium in the same way as for HSG. The procedure is less widely available but avoids the risk of irradiation and allows assessment of the ovaries at the same time.

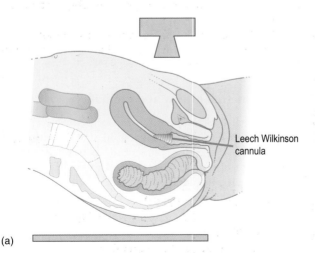

Leech Wilkinson cannula

(a)

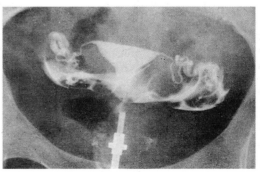

(b)

Fig. 19.5 (a) Hysterosalpingography enables assessment of the site of tubal obstruction and the presence of pathology in the uterine cavity. (b) The triangular outline of the uterine cavity can be seen and the spill of dye on both sides from the fimbrial ends of the fallopian tubes. The dye spreads over the adjacent bowel.

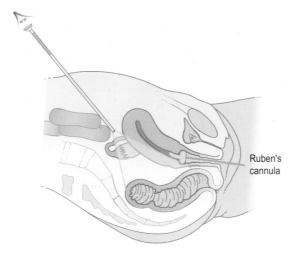

Ruben's cannula

Fig. 19.6 Dye laparoscopy for evaluation of tubal patency.

Investigation of the cervical factor

A series of tests has been developed to examine this factor. However, they are not recommended in the routine investigation of the infertile couple because of the lack of established normal criteria for these tests and poor correlation between findings and fertility.

The postcoital test

This is the most widely used method of assessment and involves asking the couple to have intercourse and examining the cervical mucus some 2–6 hours later. The test is best performed at the time of ovulation. The mucus is examined microscopically for the presence of progressive motile sperm. The presence of pus cells in the mucus is also noted, as well as evidence of clumped or abnormal sperm.

In vitro sperm penetration tests

A series of in vitro tests has been developed that essentially examines the reaction between cervical mucus and semen from the partners on a slide or in a glass capillary and also the rate of sperm migration and sperm clumping or abnormal motility. Where there is a specific interaction with clumping of sperm, the mucus is tested against donor semen to see if the same effect is obtained.

Investigation of the male partner

The simplest and most important investigation of the male partner is semen analysis (Box 19.1). Semen should be collected by masturbation into a sterile container after a period of 2 days abstinence and examined within 2 hours of collection. Special note should be made of:

- **Volume:** 80% of fertile males ejaculate between 1 and 4 ml of semen. Low volumes may indicate androgen deficiency and high volumes abnormal accessory gland function.
- **Sperm concentration:** The absence of all sperm (azoospermia) indicates sterility. However, the lower limit of normality is more difficult to define. It is generally accepted that the lower limit is probably between 15 million and 20 million sperm/ml, but the findings should not be accepted on a single sample. Furthermore, abnormally high values, in excess of 200 million sperm/ml, may be associated with subfertility.
- **Total sperm count** is sometimes used as an alternative to sperm concentration. The lower limit of normal is accepted as 50 million per ejaculate.
- **Sperm motility** is an important measurement of fertility and normal semen should show good motility in 60% of sperm within 1 hour of collection. The characteristic of forward progression is equally important. The World Health Organization now grades sperm motility according to the following criteria:
  Grade 1 – rapid and linear progressive motility
  Grade 2 – slow or sluggish linear or non-linear motility

Box 19.1
Normal semen analysis (WHO reference values)

- Volume: 2–5 ml
- Count: $> 20 \times 10^6$/ml
- Motility: > 50% progressive motility at 1 h (25% linear)
- Morphology: > 30% normal
- Liquefaction time: within 30 min
- White blood cells in sample: $< 10^6$/ml

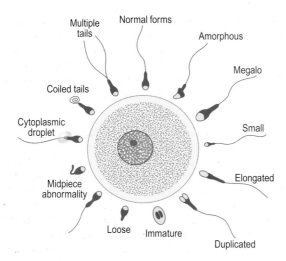

Fig. 19.7 Abnormal forms of spermatozoa.

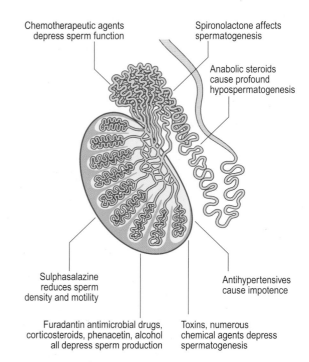

Fig. 19.8 Influence of chemical agents on spermatogenesis.

Grade 3 – non-progressive motility
Grade 4 – immotile.
- **Sperm morphology** shows great variability even in normal fertile males. It is unusual to see a count with more than 80% normal forms. It is important to look for leukocytes as they may indicate the presence of infection. If pus cells are present, the semen should be cultured for bacteriological growth. In general terms, fertility relates poorly to abnormal sperm morphology. The wide variety of forms that can be demonstrated in the seminal fluid is shown in Figure 19.7.

Spermatogenesis and sperm function may be affected by a wide range of toxins and therapeutic agents. Various toxins and drugs may act on the seminiferous tubules and the epididymis to inhibit spermatogenesis. Chemotherapeutic agents depress sperm function and sulfasalazine (sulphasalazine) reduces sperm motility and density (Fig. 19.8). Otherwise, drugs such as anti-hypertensive agents cause impotence, and anabolic steroids may produce profound hypospermatogenesis.

In the presence of a normal semen analysis, further tests on the male are unlikely to contribute to subsequent management. In the presence of oligospermia or azoospermia, further studies should include the following.

Hormone measurements

High levels of FSH indicate severe testicular damage whereas normal levels may indicate obstructive disease. Low or undetectable levels are found in males with hypopituitarism. The presence of high FSH levels and azoospermia obviates the need for further investigation as these findings indicate irreversible failure of spermatogenesis.

Levels of LH and testosterone are of limited value, although low values of both hormones may indicate a pituitary or hypothalamic disorder and high levels of LH with low levels of testosterone are characteristic of Klinefelter's syndrome.

Hyperprolactinaemia may occur in the male in association with a pituitary adenoma and may cause impotence or oligospermia.

Cytogenetic studies

Chromosome analysis in males with azoospermia may indicate the presence of a karyotype of XXY or XYY and, occasionally, autosomal translocation in the presence of oligospermia. About 2% of infertile males exhibit an abnormal karyotype.

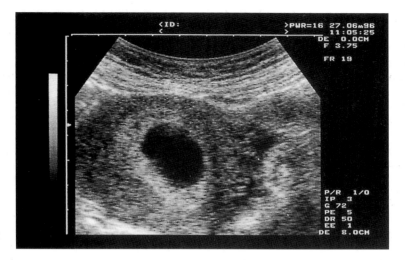

Fig. 20.3 The empty gestation sac of anembryonic pregnancy seen on ultrasound scan.

number that would be expected by chance alone. Most women who have had two or more consecutive miscarriages are anxious to be investigated and reassured that there is no underlying cause for the miscarriage. However, it is important to remember that after two consecutive miscarriages the likelihood of a successful third pregnancy is still around 80%. Even after three consecutive miscarriages, there is still a 55–75% chance of success. This implies that recurrent miscarriage is unlikely to be a random event and that it is necessary to seek a cause.

Aetiology

In many cases no definite cause can be found for miscarriage. It is important to identify this group as the prognosis for future pregnancy is generally better than average.

Genetic abnormalities

Chromosomal abnormalities are a common cause of early miscarriage and may result in failure of development of the embryo with formation of a blighted ovum or with later expulsion of an abnormal fetus. In any form of spontaneous miscarriage up to 55% of products of conception will have an abnormal karyotype. The most common chromosomal defects are autosomal trisomies, which account for half the abnormalities,

while polyploidy and monosomy X account for a further 20% each. Although chromosome abnormalities are common in sporadic miscarriage, parental chromosomal abnormalities are present in only 3–5% of partners presenting with recurrent pregnancy loss. These are most commonly balanced reciprocal or Robertsonian translocations or mosaicisms.

Endocrine factors

Progesterone production is predominately dependent on the corpus luteum for the first 8 weeks of pregnancy, and the function is then assumed by the placenta. Progesterone is essential for the maintenance of a pregnancy, and early failure of the corpus luteum may lead to miscarriage. However, it is difficult to be certain when falling plasma progesterone levels represent a primary cause of miscarriage and when they are the index of a failing pregnancy. The prevalence of polycystic ovarian syndrome is significantly higher in women with recurrent miscarriage than in the general population. Women with poorly controlled diabetes and untreated thyroid disease are at higher risk of miscarriage and fetal malformation.

Maternal illness and infection

Severe maternal febrile illnesses associated with infections, such as influenza, pyelitis and malaria, predispose to miscarriage. Specific infections such as syphilis, *Listeria monocytogenes*, *Mycoplasma* spp. and *Toxoplasma gondii* also cause miscarriage but there is no evidence that these organisms cause recurrent miscarriage, particularly in the second trimester. The presence of bacterial vaginosis has been reported as a risk factor for preterm delivery and second trimester, but not first trimester, miscarriage. Other severe illnesses involving the cardiovascular, hepatic and renal systems may also result in miscarriage.

Abnormalities of the uterus

Congenital abnormalities of the uterine cavity, such as a bicornuate uterus or subseptate uterus, may result in miscarriage (Fig. 20.4). Uterine anomalies can be demonstrated in 15–30% of women experiencing recurrent miscarriage. The impact of the abnormality depends on the nature of the anomaly. The fetal survival rate is 86% where the uterus is septate and worst when the uterus is unicornuate. It must also be remembered that over 20% of all women with congenital uterine anomalies also have renal tract anomalies. Following damage to the endometrium and inner uterine walls, the surfaces may become adherent, thus partly obliterating the uterine cavity. The presence of these synechiae may lead to recurrent miscarriage.

Cervical incompetence

Cervical incompetence clinically results in midtrimester spontaneous miscarriage or early preterm delivery. The miscarriage tends to be rapid, painless and bloodless. The diagnosis is established by the passage of a Hegar 8 dilator without difficulty in the non-pregnant woman or by ultrasound examination or a premenstrual hysterogram. Cervical incompetence may be congenital but most commonly results from physical damage caused by mechanical dilatation of the cervix or by damage inflicted during childbirth.

Autoimmune factors

Antiphospholipid antibodies – lupus anticoagulant (LA) and anticardiolipin antibodies (aCL) – are present in 15% of women with recurrent miscarriage but only 2% of women with normal reproductive histories. Without treatment the rate of live births in women with primary antiphospholipid syndrome may be as low as 10%. Pregnancy loss is thought to be due to thrombosis of the uteroplacental vasculature and impaired trophoblast function. In addition to miscarriage there is an increased risk of intrauterine growth restriction, preeclampsia and venous thrombosis.

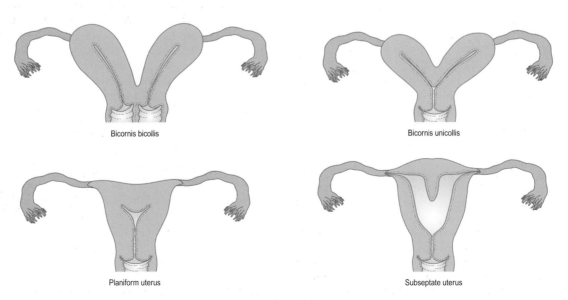

Bicornis bicollis

Bicornis unicollis

Planiform uterus

Subseptate uterus

Fig. 20.4 Anomalies of the genital tract.

Thrombophilic defects

Defects in the natural inhibitors of coagulations – antithrombin III, protein C and protein S – are more common in women with recurrent miscarriage. The majority of cases of activated protein C deficiency are secondary to a mutation in the factor V (Leiden) gene.

Alloimmune factors

Research into the possibility of an immunological basis of recurrent miscarriage has generally explored the hypothesis that there is a failure to mount the normal protective immune response or that the expression of relatively non-immunogenic antigens by the cytotrophoblast may result in rejection of the fetal allograft. There is evidence that unexplained spontaneous miscarriage is associated with couples who share an abnormal number of HLA antigens of the A, B, C and DR loci. Despite attempts to treat women with paternal lymphocytes, which initially appeared to reduce the incidence of recurrent miscarriage, subsequent studies have failed to confirm the initial findings.

Management

Examination of the patient should include gentle vaginal and speculum examination to ascertain cervical dilatation. Some women may prefer not to be examined because of apprehension that the examination may promote miscarriage, and their wishes should be respected. An ultrasound scan is valuable in deciding whether the fetus is alive and normal, and urinary hCG estimation will also provide additional useful information. If there is pyrexia, a high vaginal swab should be taken for bacteriological culture.

Miscarriage may be complicated by haemorrhage and severe pain, and may necessitate blood transfusion and relief of pain with opiates. If there is evidence of infection, antibiotic therapy should be started immediately and adjusted subsequently if the organism identified in culture is not sensitive to the prescribed antibiotic.

Septic miscarriage complicated by endotoxic shock is treated by massive antibiotic therapy and adequate, carefully controlled fluid replacement. Non-sensitized Rhesus-negative women should be given anti-immunoglobulin if miscarriage has occurred after 12 weeks, or if they undergo surgical evacuation of the uterus.

 There is no evidence that bed-rest improves the prognosis in cases of threatened miscarriage.

Surgical management

Surgical evacuation of retained products of conception involves dilatation of the cervix and suction curettage to remove the products (Fig. 20.5). This is the modality of choice when there is heavy bleeding or there is a very bulky uterus suggesting a large residuum of retained products of conception. Some women will choose this option for missed miscarriages, because it is a self-limiting procedure that allows women to put the emotional trauma of the miscarriage quickly behind them. Complications of surgical treatment include perforation of the uterus and continuing bleeding associated with incomplete evacuation of the uterus. Intrauterine infection may result in tubal infection and tubal obstruction with subsequent infertility. If uterine perforation is suspected and there is evidence of intraperitoneal haemorrhage or damage to the bowel, then laparotomy should be performed.

Medical management

When the uterine contents have not begun to be expelled naturally, the process can be expedited by the use of a prostaglandin analogue such as misoprostol or

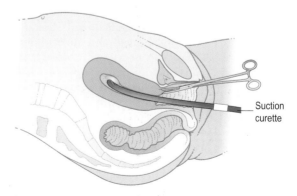

Fig. 20.5 Evacuation of retained products of conception.

Suction curette

dinoprostone with or without the antiprogesterone mifepristone. Passage of the products will normally be accomplished in approximately 48–72 hours, but many women find the uncertainty, and the fact that they miscarry at home, disturbing. The major problem is persistent bleeding in a small number, necessitating evacuation under general anaesthetic. This tends to be more common where the cervix is closed and the gestation sac is intact (missed miscarriage). The advantages are that a general anaesthetic is avoided, as are the potential complications of evacuation.

Conservative management

This is the favoured option for incomplete miscarriages when the uterus is small or when, on scan, there is minimal evidence of retained products. It is acceptable management in women with missed miscarriages who do not wish to undergo either of the former options.

Whichever method is chosen, products should be sent for histological examination, as a small number will prove to be evidence of gestational trophoblastic disease.

 Medical and expectant management are an effective alternative to surgical treatment in confirmed miscarriage.

Recurrent miscarriage

Recurrent miscarriage should be investigated by examining the karyotype of both parents and, if possible, any fetal products. Maternal blood should be examined for lupus anticoagulant and anticardiolipin antibodies on at least two occasions 6 weeks apart. An ultrasound scan should be arranged to assess ovarian morphology for polycystic ovarian syndrome and the uterine cavity. Women with persistent lupus anticoagulant and anticardiolipin antibodies can be treated with low-dose aspirin and heparin during subsequent pregnancies. Those with karyotypic abnormalities should be referred to a clinical geneticist. Cervical cerclage carried out at 14–16 weeks in cases of cervical incompetence reduces the incidence of preterm delivery but has not been shown to improve fetal survival.

 Genetic abnormalities are the commonest cause of isolated miscarriage but a relatively uncommon cause of recurrent pregnancy loss.

Psychological aspects of miscarriage

In western Europe most women now confirm their pregnancies considerably earlier than was usual in previous generations. A spontaneous miscarriage is often regarded medically as not serious, and is rarely investigated when it occurs for the first time. Follow-up is often left in primary care and few women receive gynaecological attention or an explanation of their loss. Although there is no evidence to associate miscarriage with an overall increased risk of psychiatric morbidity, almost half of all women are considerably distressed at 6 weeks following miscarriage, and often feel angry, alone and guilty. Women who have had a previous miscarriage and no live child, women who have had a previous termination of pregnancy and those with a previous psychiatric history are most at risk of becoming depressed in the months following miscarriage. Women who have had many miscarriages are particularly vulnerable, and should probably receive gynaecological support and counselling.

Women who lose pregnancies in the second and third trimesters face the same risks of postpartum 'mood disorder' as a delivered population, and their grief reactions are usually more severe. They will, therefore, be considerably distressed, with the features of a typical grief reaction for up to 6 months following the loss of their pregnancy. Their psychological recovery may be assisted by granting their pregnancy the dignity afforded to a full-term infant with a burial, naming, etc. However, rigid 'grieving procedures' should be avoided even for full-term stillborn infants. Women and their partners should be allowed the flexibility to manage their baby's death in the way that they find most suitable.

ECTOPIC PREGNANCY

The term 'ectopic pregnancy' refers to any pregnancy occurring outside the uterine cavity.

The most common site of extrauterine implantation is the Fallopian tube, but it may occur in the ovary as an ovarian pregnancy, in the abdominal cavity as an abdominal pregnancy or in the cervical canal as a cervical pregnancy (Fig. 20.6).

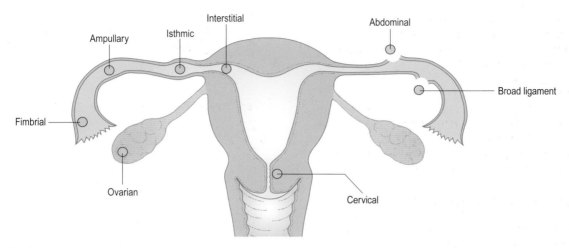

Fig. 20.6 Sites of implantation of ectopic pregnancies.

Tubal pregnancy occurs in 1/100 pregnancies in the UK, although this incidence varies substantially in different populations. Tubal pregnancy may occur in the ampulla, the isthmus or the interstitial portion of the tube and the outcome will depend on the site of implantation.

Predisposing factors

The majority of cases of ectopic pregnancy have no identifiable predisposing factor but a previous history of ectopic pregnancy, sterilization, pelvic inflammatory disease and subfertility all increase the likelihood of an ectopic pregnancy (Table 20.1). The increased risk for an intrauterine device (IUD) applies only to pregnancies that occur despite the presence of the IUD. Because of their effectiveness as contraceptives, ectopic rates per year in IUD users are lower than in women not using contraception.

Clinical presentation

Acute presentation

The classic pattern of symptoms includes amenorrhoea, lower abdominal pain and uterine bleeding. The abdominal pain usually precedes the onset of vaginal bleeding, and may start on one side of the lower abdomen, but rapidly becomes generalized as blood loss extends into the peritoneal cavity. Subdiaphragmatic irritation by blood produces referred shoulder tip pain and syncopal episodes may occur.

The period of amenorrhoea is usually 6–8 weeks, but may be longer if implantation occurs in the interstitial

Table 20.1 Risk factors for ectopic pregnancy	
	Relative risk
Previous history of pelvic inflammatory disease	4
Previous tubal surgery	4.5
Failed sterilization	9
Intrauterine contraceptive device in situ	10
Previous ectopic pregnancy	10–15

Case study
Subacute presentation

A 22-year-old woman, para 0, was admitted with vaginal bleeding after 8 weeks of amenorrhoea. She had had a positive home pregnancy kit test, and described passing some tissue per vaginam. Ultrasound scan showed an empty uterus, although serum beta-hCG was still positive. A presumptive diagnosis of incomplete miscarriage was made, and evacuation of the uterus was carried out uneventfully. She was discharged the following day but was readmitted that night with lower abdominal pain; a ruptured ampullary ectopic was found at laparotomy. Some days later, histology of the original curettage was reported as 'decidua with Arias–Stella type reaction, no chorionic villi seen'.

Case study
Acute presentation

An 18-year-old woman, para 0, was brought into casualty collapsed with lower abdominal pain. On admission she was shocked with a blood pressure of 80/40, a pulse of 120 beats/minute and a tender, rigid abdomen. Vaginal examination revealed a slight red loss, a bulky uterus and marked cervical excitation, with a tender mass in the right fornix. At laparotomy, 800 ml of fresh blood was removed from the peritoneal cavity and a ruptured right tubal ectopic pregnancy was found. Subsequently, a history of recurrent pelvic infections and irregular periods was elicited.

portion of the tube or in abdominal pregnancy. Clinical examination reveals a shocked woman with hypotension, tachycardia and signs of peritonism including abdominal distension, guarding and rebound tenderness. Pelvic examination is usually unimportant because of the acute pain and discomfort, and should be undertaken with caution. This type of acute presentation occurs in no more than 25% of cases.

Subacute presentation

After a short period of amenorrhoea, the patient experiences recurrent attacks of vaginal bleeding and abdominal pain. Any woman who develops lower abdominal pain following an interval of amenorrhoea should be considered as a possible ectopic pregnancy. In the subacute phase, it may be possible to feel a mass in one fornix.

Pathology

Implantation may occur in a variety of sites, and the outcome of the pregnancy will depend on the site of implantation. Abdominal pregnancy may result from direct implantation of the conceptus in the abdominal cavity or on the ovary, in which case it is known as

primary abdominal pregnancy, or it may result from extrusion of a tubal pregnancy with secondary implantation in the peritoneal cavity, which is known as secondary abdominal pregnancy. Implantation of the conceptus in the tube results in hormonal changes that mimic normal pregnancy. The uterus enlarges and the endometrium undergoes decidual change. Implantation within the fimbrial end or ampulla of the tube allows greater expansion before rupture occurs, whereas implantation in the interstitial portion or the isthmic part of the tube presents with early signs of haemorrhage or pain (Fig. 20.7).

Trophoblastic cells invade the wall of the tube and erode into blood vessels. This process will continue until the pregnancy bursts into the abdominal cavity or into the broad ligament, or the embryo dies, thus resulting in a tubal mole. Under these circumstances, absorption or tubal miscarriage may occur. Expulsion of the embryo into the peritoneal cavity or partial miscarriage may also occur, with continuing episodes of bleeding from the tube.

Diagnosis

Ectopic pregnancy should always be suspected where early pregnancy is complicated by pain and bleeding.

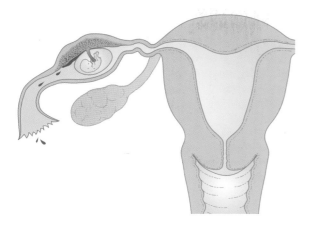

Fig. 20.7 Penetration of the tubal wall by trophoblastic tissue.

While the diagnosis of acute ectopic pregnancy rarely presents a problem, diagnosis in the subacute phase may be much more difficult. The condition may be mistaken for a threatened or incomplete miscarriage. It may also be confused with acute salpingitis or appendicitis with pelvic peritonitis. It may sometimes be confused with rupture or haemorrhage of an ovarian cyst.

If sufficient blood loss has occurred into the peritoneal cavity, the haemoglobin level will be low and the white cell count is usually normal or slightly raised. Serum beta-hCG measurement will exclude ectopic pregnancy if negative, with a specificity of greater than 99%, and urinary hCG with modern kits that can be used on the ward or in the Accident and Emergency Department will detect 97% of pregnancies. In the presence of a viable intrauterine pregnancy, the serum hCG will double over a 48-hour period in 85% of cases (compared to 15% of ectopic pregnancies). Serial measurements of serum hCG levels in conjunction with ultrasound diagnosis can distinguish early intrauterine pregnancy from miscarriage or ectopics in up to 85% of cases but laparoscopy is usually used to confirm the diagnosis. Ultrasound scan of the pelvis may demonstrate tubal pregnancy in 2% of cases or suggest it by other features such as free fluid in the peritoneal cavity, but is mainly of help in excluding intrauterine pregnancy. Intrauterine pregnancy can usually be identified by transabdominal scan at 6 weeks gestation and somewhat sooner by transvaginal scan at 5–6 weeks gestation. Occasionally, there may be no clinical signs of an ectopic pregnancy but if curettings submitted for histopathology show evidence of decidual reaction and the Arias–Stella phenomenon then it is advisable to consider laparoscopy.

Management

In patients who are haemodynamically compromised blood should be taken for urgent cross-matching and transfusion. Laparotomy should be performed as soon as possible, with removal of the damaged tube.

Surgical management

Once the diagnosis is confirmed, the options for treatment are:

- **Salpingectomy:** If the tube is badly damaged, or the contralateral tube appears healthy, the correct treatment is removal of the affected tube. If implantation has occurred in the interstitial portion of the tube, then it may be necessary to resect part of the uterine horn in addition to removing the tube.
- **Salpingotomy:** Where the ectopic pregnancy is contained within the tube, it may be possible to conserve the tube by removing the pregnancy and reconstituting the tube. This is particularly important where the contralateral tube has been lost. The disadvantage is the persistence of trophoblastic tissue, requiring further surgery or medical treatment in up to 6% of cases.

Subsequent intrauterine pregnancy rates are similar after both types of treatment, although the risk of recurrent ectopic pregnancy is greater after salpingotomy. Both can be carried out as an open procedure or laparoscopically. The laparoscopic approach is associated with quicker recovery time, shorter stay in hospital and less adhesion formation and is the method of choice if the patient is stable.

Medical management

Medical treatment of an ectopic pregnancy involves the administration of methotrexate, either systemically or by injection into the ectopic pregnancy by laparoscopic visualization or by ultrasound guidance. Medical treatment is not suitable for all cases of ectopic pregnancy. It is most effective where the ectopic is less than 2 cm in size and the hCG level is less than 1500 IU/l. Systemic side effects occur in 20% of cases and abdominal pain in 40%. Tubal rupture requiring surgery occurs in 5–10% of cases.

After an ectopic pregnancy treated by any method, 85–90% of subsequent pregnancies will be intrauterine but only 60% of women will manage to conceive spontaneously, reflecting global tubal disease.

Management of other forms of extrauterine pregnancy

Abdominal pregnancy

Abdominal pregnancy presents a life-threatening hazard to the mother. The placenta implants outside the uterus and across the bowel and pelvic peritoneum. Any attempt to remove it will result in massive haemorrhage, which is extremely difficult to control. The fetus should be removed by laparotomy and the placenta left in situ to reabsorb or extrude spontaneously.

Cervical pregnancy

Cervical pregnancy often presents as the cervical stage of a spontaneous miscarriage. Occasionally, it is possible to remove the conceptus by curettage but haemorrhage can be severe, and in 50% of cases it is necessary to proceed to hysterectomy to obtain adequate haemostasis.

TROPHOBLASTIC DISEASE

Abnormality of early trophoblast may arise as a developmental anomaly of placental tissue and results in the formation of a mass of oedematous and avascular villi. There is usually no fetus but the condition can be found in the presence of a fetus. The placenta is replaced by a mass of grape-like vesicles known as a *hydatidiform mole* (Fig. 20.8).

Invasion of the myometrium without systemic spread occurs in about 16% of cases of benign mole and is known as *invasive mole* or *chorioadenoma destruens*. Frankly malignant change occurs in 2.5%, and is known as *choriocarcinoma*.

Incidence

The overall prevalence of this condition is about 1.5/1000 pregnancies in the UK but is much higher in

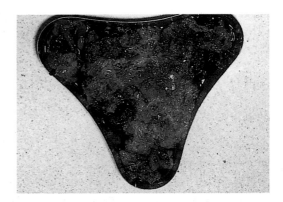

Fig. 20.8 Vesicles of a hydatidiform mole.

parts of Asia. It is relatively more common at the extremes of reproductive age.

Pathology

Molar pregnancy is thought to arise from fertilization by two sperm and can be diploid with no female genetic material (*complete mole*) or may exhibit triploidy (*partial mole*). Benign mole remains confined to the uterine cavity and decidua. The histopathology exhibits a villous pattern, which is also found in the invasive mole. However, invasive molar tissue penetrates the myometrium deeply and may result in serious haemorrhage. Choriocarcinoma comprises plexiform columns of trophoblastic cells without villous patterns. Widespread blood-borne metastases are a feature of this disease, which, until recent years, carried a very high mortality rate. Metastases may occur locally in the vagina but most commonly appear in the lungs. Theca lutein cysts occur in about one-third of all cases as a result of high circulating levels of hCG. These regress spontaneously with removal of the molar tissue. Around 50% of cases of choriocarcinoma are not associated with molar pregnancy.

Clinical presentation

Molar pregnancy most commonly presents as bleeding in the first half of pregnancy, and spontaneous miscarriage often occurs at about 20 weeks gestation. Occasionally, the passage of a grape-like villus heralds the presence of a mole. The uterus is large for dates in about half of cases but this is not a reliable sign as it may sometimes be small for dates. Severe hyperemesis, pre-eclampsia and unexplained anaemia are all factors suggestive of this disorder. The diagnosis can be confirmed by ultrasound scan and by the presence of very high levels of hCG in the blood or urine.

Management

Once the diagnosis is established, the pregnancy is terminated by suction curettage. Adequate replacement of blood loss is essential. Although there is an increased risk of blood loss there is a theoretical concern over the routine use of oxytocic agents because of the potential to disseminate trophoblastic tissue through the venous system. If possible these should be commenced once the evacuation has been completed. Occasionally repeat evacuation may be requires if there is persistent bleeding or a raised serum hCG but routine second evacuation is not helpful. All cases of molar pregnancy in the UK should be registered with one of the trophoblastic disease screening centres, which will arrange follow up. Serial estimations of hCG are performed for a period of 6 months or 2 years, initially every 2 weeks. If hCG levels reach normal within 6 weeks of evacuation of the mole, follow-up will be for 6 months, otherwise follow-up will be for 2 years but in the second year samples are collected at intervals of 3 months.

If the histological evidence shows malignant change, chemotherapy with methotrexate and actinomycin D is employed and produces good results. In the UK, management of these cases is concentrated in specialized centres.

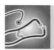

Case study
Trophoblastic disease

A 27-year-old primigravid woman attended the clinic with a history of 12 weeks of amenorrhoea, complaining of bright vaginal blood loss and lower abdominal discomfort. Abdominal examination revealed that the uterine fundus was 16 weeks in size. There was fresh blood in the vagina and the cervical os was closed. There was a high titre of hCG in the urine and an ultrasound scan showed a ground-glass appearance in the uterine cavity with no evidence of fetal parts. Suction evacuation of molar tissue was performed the following day, and recovery was uneventful.

> **!** It must be remembered that choriocarcinoma sometimes can occur following a miscarriage or a normal-term intrauterine pregnancy.

Pregnancy is contraindicated until 6 months after the serum hCG levels fall to normal. Oestrogen-containing oral contraceptives and hormone replacement therapy can be used as soon as hCG levels are normal. The risk recurrence in subsequent pregnancies is 1/74 and serum hCG levels should be checked 6 weeks after any subsequent pregnancy.

ESSENTIAL INFORMATION

Miscarriage

- Pregnancy loss before 24 weeks
- Complicates 15–20% of pregnancies
- Commonly associated with chromosome abnormalities
- Does not always require surgical treatment

Recurrent miscarriage

- Defined as three consecutive pregnancy losses
- Investigations should include screening for antiphospholipid antibodies, chromosome abnormalities and polycystic ovarian syndrome
- Chances of successful subsequent pregnancy are more than 60% without any treatment
- Women with antiphospholipid antibodies should be offered treatment with low-dose aspirin and heparin

Ectopic pregnancy

- 1% of pregnancies are ectopic
- Most important cause of maternal death in early pregnancy
- Atypical presentations are common
- Commonest site for ectopic pregnancy is the ampullary region of the Fallopian tube
- Can be accurately diagnosed by a combination of ultrasound and hCG measurement
- Laparoscopic treatment is associated with lower morbidity

Trophoblastic disease

- Affects 1/650 pregnancies in the UK
- Partial moles are triploid, complete moles diploid
- Treated initially by surgical evacuation of the uterus
- 50% of choriocarcinomas occur without a history of molar pregnancy
- Requires follow-up with serial hCG measurement

21 Contraception and termination of pregnancy

The ability to control fertility by reliable artificial methods has transformed both social and epidemiological aspects of human reproduction. Family size is determined by a number of factors, including social and religious customs, economic aspirations, knowledge of contraception and the availability of reliable methods to regulate fertility.

Artificial methods of contraception act by the following pathways:

- Inhibition of ovulation
- Prevention of implantation of the fertilized ovum
- Barrier methods of contraception, whereby the spermatozoa are physically prevented from gaining access to the cervix.

The effectiveness of any method of contraception is measured by the number of unwanted pregnancies that occur during 100 women years of exposure, i.e. during 1 year in 100 women who are normally fertile and are having regular coitus. This is known as the 'Pearl index' (Table 21.1).

BARRIER METHODS OF CONTRACEPTION

These techniques involve a physical barrier that prevents spermatozoa from reaching the female upper genital tract. Barrier methods also offer protection against sexually transmitted infection. The relative risk of pelvic inflammatory disease is 0.6 for women using these methods. Women who use another method of contraception to prevent pregnancy may use a condom as well to reduce the risk of infection.

Male condoms

The basic condom consists of a thin, stretchable latex film, which is moulded into a sheath, lubricated and packed in a foil wrapper. The sheath has a teat end to collect the ejaculate. The disadvantages of sheaths are that they need to be applied before intercourse and that they reduce the level of sensation for the male partner. The advantages are that they are readily available, that

Table 21.1
Comparative failure rates – pregnancy rates (/100 women) during the first year of use

Method	Typical use	Perfect use
Diaphragm	8–10	6
Male condom	15	2–3
Progestogen-only pill	10	1.2
Combined oral contraceptive pill	2.7	0.27
IUD (Cu T 380A)	0.8	0.6
Female sterilization	0.5*	0.5*
Depo-Provera	0.3	0.3
Male sterilization	0.05*	0.05*
Mirena	0.1	0.1
None	85	85

* 5-year failure rate.

they are without side effects for the female partner and that they provide a degree of protection against infection. They have an efficiency of 97–98% with careful use, although typical failure rates can be as high as 15 pregnancies per 100 women years. Common reasons for failure are leakage of sperm when the penis is withdrawn, putting the condom on after genital contact, use of lubricants that cause the latex to break and mechanical damage. Condoms should be unrolled completely on to the penis before genital contact occurs and held when the penis is withdrawn to avoid leakage.

Female condoms

Female condoms are less widely used than the male equivalent but have a similar failure rate and give similar protection against infection. They are made of polyurethane and are suitable for a single episode of intercourse only.

Diaphragms and cervical caps

The female equivalent of the sheath is the diaphragm. The modern diaphragm consists of a thin latex rubber dome attached to a circular metal spring. These diaphragms vary in size from 45 mm to 100 mm in diameter. The size of the diaphragm required is ascertained by examination of the woman. The size and position of the uterus are determined by vaginal examination and the distance from the posterior vaginal fornix to the pubic symphysis is noted. The appropriate measuring ring is inserted. This usually varies between 70 mm and 80 mm and, when correctly in position, the anterior edge of the ring or diaphragm should lie behind the pubic symphysis and the lower posterior edge should lie comfortably in the posterior fornix (Fig. 21.1).

The woman should be advised to insert the diaphragm either in the dorsal position or in the kneeling position while bending forwards. The diaphragm can be removed by simply hooking an index finger under the rim from below and pulling it out. The diaphragm should be smeared on both sides with a contraceptive cream, and it is usually advised that it should be inserted dome down. However, some women prefer to insert the diaphragm with the dome upwards.

The diaphragm must be inserted prior to intercourse and should not be removed until at least 6 hours later. The main advantage of this technique is that it is free of side effects to the woman, apart from an occasional reaction to the contraceptive cream. The main disadvantages are that the diaphragm must be inserted before intercourse and typical failure rates are between 8 and 10 pregnancies per 100 women years.

There are a variety of vault and cervical caps, which are of much smaller diameter than the diaphragm. These are suitable for women with a long cervix or with some degree of prolapse, but otherwise have no particular advantage over the diaphragm.

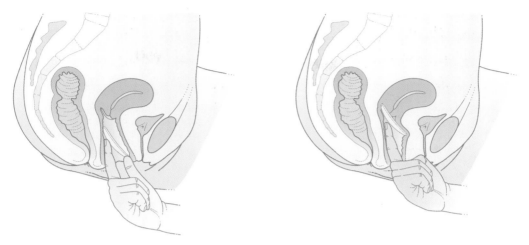

Fig. 21.1 Insertion of a vaginal diaphragm to cover the cervix and anterior vaginal wall.

Spermicides and sponges

Spermicides are only effective, in general, if used in conjunction with a mechanical barrier. Pessaries or suppositories have a water-soluble or wax base and contain a spermicide. They must be inserted approximately 15 minutes before intercourse. Common spermicides are nonoxynol-9 and benzalkonium. Creams consist of an emulsified fat base and tend not to spread. Care in insertion is essential so that the cervix is covered.

Jellies or pastes have a water-soluble base that spreads rapidly at body temperature. They therefore have an advantage over creams, as they spread throughout the vagina.

Foam tablets and foam aerosols contain bicarbonate of soda so that carbon dioxide is released on contact with water. The foam spreads the spermicide throughout the vagina. Pregnancy rates vary with different agents, but average around 9–10 per 100 women years.

Sponges consist of polyurethane foam impregnated with nonoxynol-9. The failure rate is between 10% and 25%, and their use in isolation is not recommended. They are inserted at least 15 minutes before intercourse and can be left in for a maximum of 12 hours.

INTRAUTERINE CONTRACEPTIVE DEVICES

Intrauterine contraception is used by 6–8% of women in the UK. A wide variety of intrauterine devices (IUDs) have been designed for insertion into the uterine cavity (Fig. 21.2). These devices have the advantage that, once inserted, they are retained without the need to take alternative contraceptive precautions. It seems likely that they act mainly by preventing fertilization. This is a result of a reduction in the viability of ova and the number of viable sperm reaching the tube.

The first device to be widely used was the Graefenberg ring, which was made of a silver–copper alloy. Introduced in the 1930s, it ran into considerable difficulties with haemorrhage, infection, miscarriages and uterine perforation. Later inert plastic devices such as the Lippes loop were associated with a significant increase in menstrual blood flow in many users. The development of copper IUDs has been associated with improved contraceptive efficacy and a lessening of excess menstrual blood loss.

Types of device

The devices are either inert or pharmacologically active.

Inert devices

Lippes loops, Saf-T-coils and Margulis spirals are plastic or plastic-coated devices. They have a thread attached that protrudes through the cervix and allows the woman to check that the device is still in place. Inert devices tend to be relatively large. They are not now available but may still be found in situ in some older users.

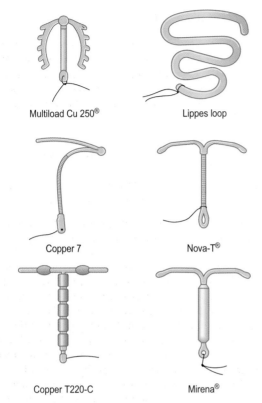

Multiload Cu 250®   Lippes loop

Copper 7   Nova-T®

Copper T220-C   Mirena®

Fig. 21.2 Some intrauterine contraceptive devices; on the right the levonorgestrel intrauterine system.

Pharmacologically active devices

The addition of copper to a contraceptive device produces a direct effect on the endometrium by interfering with endometrial oestrogen-binding sites and depressing uptake of thymidine into DNA. It also impairs glycogen storage in the endometrium. Examples of such devices are the Copper-T or Copper-7 (first generation), the Multiload Copper-250 (second generation) and the Copper-T 380 (third generation).

Devices containing progestogen

The levonorgestrel-releasing intrauterine system or Mirena® contains 52 mg of levonorgestrel (Fig. 21.2); this provides protection against pregnancy for 5 years with a failure rate of 0.3–1.1%, comparable to third-generation copper devices.

The levonorgestrel-containing device also suppresses the normal build up of the endometrium so that, unlike most IUDs, it causes a reduction in menstrual blood loss. However, there is a high incidence of irregular scanty bleeding in the first 3 months after insertion of the device. Unlike previous progestogen-containing devices it does not appear to be associated with a higher risk of ectopic pregnancy. The superior efficacy of third-generation copper IUDs and the levonorgestrel-releasing system means that these are now considered the devices of choice.

Life span of devices

The Cu T 380 is licensed for 8 years in the UK (13 in the USA). Other copper devices and the Mirena® are licensed for 5 years. However, IUDs do not need to be replaced in women over 40. They should be left in place until 2 years after the menopause if this occurs under 50 and 1 year otherwise.

Insertion of devices

The optimal time for insertion of the device is in the first half of the menstrual cycle. With postpartum women, the optimal time is 4–6 weeks after delivery. Insertion at the time of therapeutic abortion is safe and can be performed when motivation is strong. It is unwise to insert IUDs following miscarriage because of the risk of infection. Devices may be inserted within a few days of delivery but there is a high expulsion rate. Ideally, the woman should be placed in the lithotomy position. A cervical smear should be taken, and a swab taken for culture if there is any sign of infection. The uterus is examined bimanually and its size, shape and position are ascertained. The cervix is swabbed with an antiseptic solution and a vulsellum can be applied to the anterior lip of the cervix, although this is not essential and may cause discomfort.

The passage of a uterine sound will indicate the depth and direction of the uterine cavity and the dimensions of the cavity may be assessed by devices known as cavimeters, which measure its length and breadth. Many IUDs are available in different sizes, and cavimeters help to choose the appropriate IUD.

Insertion devices vary in construction but generally consist of a stoppered plastic tube containing a plunger to extrude the device, which may be linear or folded. The device is inserted in the plane of the lumen of the uterus and care is taken not to push it through the uterine fundus.

Attempts at insertion of a device where the cervical canal is tight may result in vagal syncope. Acute pain following insertion may indicate perforation of the uterus.

The woman should be instructed to check the loop strings regularly and to notify her doctor immediately if the strings are not palpable.

Complications

The complications of IUDs are summarized in Figure 21.3.

Pregnancy rates

Pregnancy rates vary according to the type of device used, from 2–6/100 women years for non-medicated IUDs and 0.5–2/100 for early generation copper devices to less than 0.3/100 women years for third-generation copper and levonorgestrel IUDs. If pregnancy does occur with an IUD in situ and its strings are easily grasped, it is sensible to remove it to reduce the incidence of a septic miscarriage, there being a high incidence of miscarriage in such pregnancies. If it is not accessible, it should be left and removed at the time of delivery. The risk of failure of the IUD diminishes with each year after insertion.

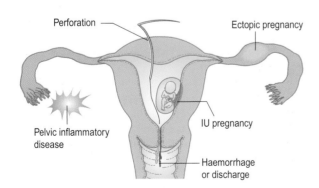

Fig. 21.3 Complications of IUDs.

Perforation of the uterus

About 0.1–1% of devices perforate the uterus. In many cases, partial perforation occurs at the time of insertion and later migration completes the perforation. If the woman notices that the tail of the device is missing, then it must be assumed that one of the following has occurred:

- The device has been expelled
- The device has turned in the uterine cavity and drawn up the strings
- The device has perforated the uterus and lies either partly or completely in the peritoneal cavity.

If there is no evidence of pregnancy, an ultrasound examination of the uterus should be performed. If the device is located within the uterine cavity (Fig. 21.4), then it is removed and, unless part of the loop or strings is visible, it will generally be necessary to remove the device with formal dilatation of the cervix under general or local anaesthesia. If the device is not found in the uterus, a radiograph of the abdomen will reveal the site in the peritoneal cavity (Fig. 21.4) It is advisable to remove all extrauterine devices by either laparoscopy or laparotomy. Inert devices can probably be left with impunity, but copper devices promote considerable peritoneal irritation and should certainly be removed.

Pelvic inflammatory disease

Pre-existing pelvic inflammatory disease is a contra-indication to this method of contraception. There is a small increase in the risk of acute pelvic inflammatory disease in IUD users but this is largely confined to the first 3 weeks after insertion. If pelvic inflammatory disease does occur, antibiotic therapy is commenced and, if the response is poor, the device should be removed. If the infection is severe, it is preferable to complete 24 hours of antibiotic therapy before removing the device.

Abnormal uterine bleeding

Increased menstrual loss occurs in most women with an IUD but can be tolerated by the majority. However, in 15% of such women it is sufficiently severe to necessitate removal of the device. It can be controlled by drugs such as tranexamic acid or mefenamic acid. Intermenstrual bleeding may also occur but if the loss is

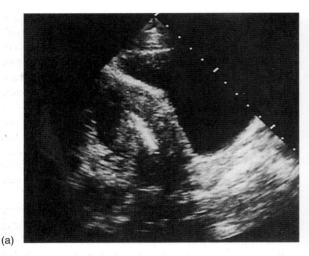

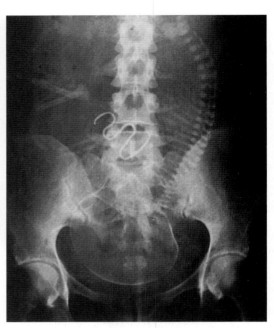

Fig. 21.4 (a) Ultrasound diagnosis of a plastic IUD. (b) Radiography of the abdomen showing an IUCD and a full-term pregnancy.

slight it does not constitute a reason for removal. Amenorrhoea occurs in up to 20% of women using the Mirena® and average menstrual blood loss is reduced by 75%.

Pelvic pain

Pain occurs either in a chronic low-grade form or as severe dysmenorrhoea. The incidence is widely variable, with up to 50% of women suffering some pain. However, the pain may be acceptable if it is not severe, and this is a decision that has to be made by the patient in relation to the convenience of the method.

Vaginal discharge

Vaginal discharge may be due to infection but most women with an IUD develop a slight watery or mucoid discharge.

Ectopic pregnancy

Compared with women having unprotected intercourse, the incidence of pregnancy is lower in women with an IUD in situ (1.2/1000 women years). However, should pregnancy occur, there is a higher risk (10%) of the pregnancy being extrauterine. It is therefore essential to think of this diagnosis in any woman presenting with abdominal pain and irregular vaginal bleeding who has an IUD in situ.

> **!** Ectopic pregnancy should be excluded in any woman who conceives with an IUD in situ.

HORMONAL CONTRACEPTION

Oral contraception is given as a combination of oestrogen or progestogen, as a combined pill, or as progesterone only.

Combined pill

The combined pill contains 20–50 µg of ethinylestradiol (ethinyloestradiol) and 150–4000 µg of progestogen. The progestogens used are derived from 17-hydroxyprogesterone or 19-norsteroids (Table 21.2). The pill is taken for 21 days, followed by a 7-day pill-free interval during which there is a withdrawal bleed. Every-day (ED) preparations include seven placebo pills that are taken instead of a pill-free week. The concentration of

Table 21.2
Progestogen content of contraceptive pills

Combined
Norethisterone (Norimin®, Ovysmin®)
Norgestrel (Eugynon®)
Levonorgestrel (Eugynon 30®, Microgynon®)
Desogestrel (Mercilon®)
Gestodene (Femodene®)

Progestogen only
Norethisterone (Norriday®)
Levonorgestrel (Neogest®)

the hormones may be the same throughout the 21 days (monophasic preparations) or vary across the cycle (biphasic and triphasic preparations) in order to reduce breakthrough bleeding.

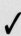 If a pill is missed for more than 12 hours (or absorption is uncertain because of vomiting or antibiotics) alternative methods of contraception should be used for the next 7 days. If this would include the pill-free week, the woman should be advised to start the next pill packet without the normal break.

Progestogen-only pill

Progestogen-only pills contain either norethisterone or levonorgestrel and are taken continuously on the basis of one tablet daily. Because of the low dose, they should be taken at the same time every day.

Mode of action

Combined and triphasic pills act by suppressing gonadotrophin secretion and, in particular, the luteinizing hormone peak. The endometrium becomes unsuitable for nidation and the cervical mucus becomes hostile. Progesterone-only pills alter the endometrial maturation and affect cervical mucus. Ovulation is suppressed in only 40% of women.

Contraindications

There are various contraindications to the pill, some being more absolute than others.

The absolute contraindications include pregnancy, pulmonary embolism, deep vein thrombosis, sickle-cell disease, porphyria, liver disease and jaundice – particularly where it is associated with a previous pregnancy or carcinoma of the breast. It is necessary to maintain a high level of vigilance in women with varicose veins, diabetes, hypertension, renal disease and chronic heart failure but none of these conditions constitutes an absolute contraindication and, in some cases, the adverse effects of a pregnancy may substantially outweigh any hazard from the pill. Women who smoke and those over the age of 35 years have a significantly increased risk of thromboembolic disease.

The occurrence of migraine for the first time, severe headaches or visual disturbances, or transient neurological changes are indications for immediate cessation of the pill. There are a series of minor side effects that may sometimes be used to advantage or may be offset by using a pill with a different combination of steroids (Table 21.3).

Other therapeutic uses

Therapeutic uses other than contraception include the treatment of menorrhagia, premenstrual syndrome, endometriosis and dysmenorrhoea.

Major side effects

The risk of venous thrombosis is increased from 5/100 000 to 15/100 000 women per year and is further increased in smokers and women with a previous history of venous thrombosis. This compares to a risk in pregnancy and the puerperium of 60/100 000 women. Several studies have suggested that so called 'third-generation' combined pills containing desogestrel or gestodene are associated with a twofold greater risk of venous thrombosis than those containing other progestogens, although the risk of venous thrombosis in these 'second-generation' pills was lower in these studies than had previously been reported.

There is an increase in arterial disease, with a 1.6–5.4-fold increase in stroke and 3–5-fold increase in myocardial infarction (although there is no significant increase in women under 25 or in non-smokers). However, both these conditions are rare in women under 35 so the overall risk remains low, with deaths from venous thrombosis attributable to the combined pill of no more than 1–2/million women years.

Table 21.3
Minor side effects of combined oral contraception

Oestrogenic effects	Progestogenic effects
Fluid retention and oedema	Premenstrual depression
Premenstrual tension and irritability	Dry vagina
Increase in weight	Acne, greasy hair
Nausea and vomiting	Increased appetite with weight gain
Headache	Breast discomfort
Mucorrhoea, cervical erosion	Cramps of the legs and abdomen
Menorrhagia	Decreased libido
Excessive tiredness	
Vein complaints	
Breakthrough bleeding	

There is a small increase in the relative risk of breast (relative risk 1.24) and cervical cancer (relative risk 1.5–2) in pill users. This risk is highest in current users and declines with time after stopping the pill.

There is an increase in gallstone formation and cholecystitis and an increase in glucose intolerance.

The progestogen-only pill has a higher failure rate and is more likely to be associated with irregular bleeding. If it fails there is a higher risk of ectopic pregnancy.

Beneficial effects

In addition to the prevention of unwanted pregnancy, the use of the combined pill is associated with a 30% reduction in blood loss at menstruation, a lower incidence of ectopic pregnancy (0.4/1000) and some protection against pelvic inflammatory disease and benign ovarian cysts. Pill users also have a reduced risk of both endometrial and ovarian cancer of up to 50%, depending on the length of use.

Counselling

It is important to obtain a complete general history and examination before prescribing the pill, and also to perform annual check-ups and cervical cytology. There are a large number of compounds commercially available, and some pills marketed by different companies contain the same compounds at the same concentrations.

Interaction between drugs and contraceptive steroids

Many drugs affect the contraceptive efficacy of the pill, and therefore additional precautions should be taken (Table 21.4). Vomiting and diarrhoea also result in loss of the pill and hence the return of fertility – particularly with the low-dose pills now widely in use. Progestogen-only pills must be taken every day if they are to be effective.

Failure rates

The failure rate of combined pills is 0.27–2.7/100 women years. The failure rate for progestogen-only preparations is higher and varies between 0.9 and 4.3/100 women years.

The pill and surgery

The pill increases the risk of deep vein thrombosis and should therefore be stopped at least 6 weeks before major surgery. It should not be stopped before minor procedures – particularly before laparoscopic sterilization procedures. The risk of an unwanted pregnancy occurring before admission is substantially greater than the risk of thromboembolism.

The pill and lactation

Combined preparations tend to inhibit lactation and are therefore best avoided. The pill of choice at this time

Table 21.4
Interaction of various drugs with oral contraceptives

Interacting drug	Effects of interaction
Analgesics	Possible increased sensitivity to pethidine
Anticoagulants	Possible reduction of effect of anticoagulant – increased dosage of anticoagulant may be necessary
Anticonvulsants	Possible decrease in contraceptive reliability
Tricyclic antidepressants	Reduced antidepressant response; increase in antidepressant toxicity
Antihistamines	Possible decrease in contraceptive reliability
Antibiotics	Possible decrease in contraceptive reliability Possibility of breakthrough bleeding (this is most likely with rifampicin)
Hypoglycaemic agents	Control of diabetes may be reduced
Antiasthmatics	Asthmatic condition may be exacerbated by concomitant oral contraceptive
Systemic corticosteroids	Increased dosage of steroids may be necessary

is the progestogen-only pill as it has minimal effect on lactation and may indeed promote it.

Injectable compounds

There are currently two main types. Depo-Provera® contains 150 mg of medroxyprogesterone acetate and is given as a 3-monthly intramuscular injection. Implanon® is a single Silastic rod containing etono-gestrel that is inserted subdermally in the upper arm and is effective for up to 3 years. An earlier type of implant, the levonorgestrel-releasing Norplant® Silastic rod, has been discontinued but some women may still have this in place. They work by making the cervical mucus hostile, the endometrium hypotrophic and by suppressing ovulation.

Failure rates are low, at 0.2/100 women years in the first year rising to 3.9/100 over 5 years. Failures mostly relate to women already pregnant at the time of implantation so it is essential that depot injections are given at the time of termination or within the first 5 days of menstruation.

Parenteral progestogen-only contraceptives are long-acting but easily reversible, effective, avoid first-pass effect liver metabolism, require minimal compliance and avoid the side effects associated with oestrogens. However, they may cause irregular bleeding or amenorrhoea, which can be a source of anxiety because of the possibility of pregnancy. Removal of the implants may be difficult and should only be carried out by a doctor trained in the procedure. Some women will experience systemic progestogenic effects such as mood changes and weight gain or symptoms of oestrogenic deficiency.

EMERGENCY CONTRACEPTION

After unprotected intercourse, missed combined pill or burst condom, a single 750 mg levonorgestrel tablet is taken within 72 hours of intercourse, followed by a second dose exactly 12 hours later. The levonorgestrel-only method has fewer side effects than the previously used combined method and is available to women over 16 from pharmacists. Side effects include nausea, vomiting (an additional pill should be taken if vomiting occurs within 2–3 hours of the first dose) and bleeding. The woman should be advised that:

- Her next period might be early or late
- She needs to use barrier contraception until then and should continue taking the oral contraceptive
- She needs to return if she has any abdominal pain or if the next period is absent or abnormal.

If the next period is more than 5 days overdue, pregnancy should be excluded. Emergency contraception prevents 85% of expected pregnancies. Efficacy decreases with time from intercourse.

NON-MEDICAL METHODS OF CONTRACEPTION

The most fertile phase of the menstrual cycle occurs at the time of ovulation. In a 28-day cycle, this occurs between day 12 and day 14 of the cycle. It is associated with changes in cervical mucus that a woman can learn to recognize by self-examination and hormone changes that can be measured by home urine testing kits. Avoidance of the fertile period can be an extremely effective method in well-motivated couples.

Natural methods of family planning include the following.

- The *rhythm method* – avoiding intercourse mid-cycle and for 3–4 days either side of mid-cycle. The efficacy of this method depends on being able to predict the time of ovulation.
- *Coitus interruptus (withdrawal)* – a traditional and still widely used method of contraception that relies on withdrawal of the penis before ejaculation. It is not a particularly reliable method of contraception.
- *Lactational amenorrhoea method.* Breastfeeding has historically been the most important means of family 'spacing'. Ovulation resumes on average 4–6 months later in women who continue to breastfeed. During the first 6 months after birth this is an effective method of contraception in mothers who are fully breastfeeding and amenorrhoeic, with failure rates as low as 2/100 women.

STERILIZATION

Contraceptive techniques have the major advantage that they are easily reversible and provide a high level of protection against pregnancy. They have the disadvantage that they require a conscious act on behalf of the individual before intercourse. When family size is complete or there is a specific medical contraindication to continuing fertility, sterilization becomes the contraceptive method of choice. Around 30% of couples use sterilization for contraception and this increases to 50% in those aged over 40.

Counselling

It is essential to counsel both partners about the nature of the procedures and their implications and to discuss whether it is better for the male or female partner to be sterilized. In many cases, only one partner will be seeking sterilization, in which case only one point of view needs to be considered. It is important to ensure that there is a full discussion of the alternatives.

Counselling should include reference to the intended method, its risks and failure rates (1/200 for female sterilization, 1/2000 for male sterilization). Women should be warned of the increased risk of ectopic pregnancy in the event of failure.

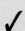
The reported failure rate for third-generation/levonorgestrel IUDs is comparable to that of sterilization but male sterilization has a significantly lower failure rate.

With the improvements brought about by micro-surgery, it is no longer acceptable to say that sterilization is irreversible and the patient should be counselled according to the technique to be used. The partner to be sterilized will be a matter of choice and motivation. If one partner has a reduced life expectancy from chronic illness, then that partner should be sterilized.

Women should be advised to continue to use other contraception until the period following sterilization and men until they have had two consecutive semen analyses showing azoospermia 2–4 weeks apart at least 8 weeks after the procedure.

Timing of sterilization

The operation can be performed at any time in the menstrual cycle. A pregnancy test should be performed preoperatively if a woman has a late or missed period or thinks she may be pregnant.

Techniques

Female sterilization

The majority of procedures involve interruption of the Fallopian tubes but may vary from the application of clips on the tubes to total hysterectomy. In general terms, the more radical the procedure the less likely there is to be a failure. However, very low failure rates can now be achieved using methods with high reversibility prospects and these should be the methods of choice.

Laparoscopic sterilization

The use of the laparoscope for sterilization procedures has substantially reduced the duration of hospital stay. This is the method of choice in the UK but an open approach through a mini-laparotomy may be more

adequate provision is made for this after the termination. The procedure can be combined with sterilization. This has the advantage of preventing further terminations for the woman who is certain that she has completed her family. There is little evidence that this is associated with an increase in the rate of complications or later contraceptive failure. However, because of the increase in the 'regret rate' for the sterilization, an interval procedure is generally recommended. IUD insertion can be carried out at the same time as termination and is not associated with an increased risk of perforation or failure. If the oral contraceptive is being used, this can be started on the same or following day.

CRIMINAL ABORTION

Miscarriage induced by a variety of techniques makes up a substantial percentage of miscarriage in some countries. Where the indications for legal miscarriage are liberal, criminal abortion is infrequent but in many countries it contributes to a high percentage of apparently spontaneous miscarriages. The World Health Organization estimates that 250 000 women per year in the world die as a result of abortions, most of which are illegal. Mortality from abortion in the UK has fallen from a rate of 37/million maternities to 1.4/million since 1967. There have been no deaths from illegal abortion in the UK since 1982.

ESSENTIAL INFORMATION

Intrauterine devices

- Prevent implantation
- Inert or pharmacologically active
- Best for older multiparous women
- Can be inserted at time of delivery
- Replace after 3–5 years
- Failure rate 2/100 women years
- Complications: perforation, pelvic inflammatory disease, abnormal bleeding, ectopic pregnancy

Combined oral contraceptive pill

- Suppress gonadotrophins
- Oestradiol and progestogen
- Pregnancy, thromboembolism and liver disease contraindicate
- 1.3/100 000 mortality
- Failure rate 0.5/100 women years

Sterilization

- 1/2000 failure rate (female)
- Increased risk of ectopic pregnancy if procedure fails
- Permanence
- Risks of surgery
- Alternatives

Termination of pregnancy

- Methods
  - surgical
  - medical
- Complications
  - bleeding
  - infection
  - infertility
  - retained tissue
  - regret

22 Genital tract infections

The female genital tract provides direct access to the peritoneal cavity. Infection may extend to any level of the tract and, once it reaches the Fallopian tubes, is usually bilateral.

The genital tract has a rich anastomosis of blood and lymphatic vessels that serve to resist infection, particularly during pregnancy.

There are other natural barriers to infection:

- The physical apposition of the pudendal cleft and the vaginal walls
- Vaginal acidity – the low pH of the vagina in the sexually mature female provides a hostile environment for most bacteria; this resistance is weakened in the prepubertal and postmenopausal female
- Cervical mucus, which acts as a barrier in preventing the ascent of infection
- The regular monthly shedding of the endometrium.

LOWER GENITAL TRACT INFECTIONS

The commonest infections of the genital tract are those that affect the vulva and vagina. Infections that affect the vagina also produce acute and chronic cervicitis.

Symptoms

Swelling and reddening of the vulval skin is accompanied by soreness, pruritus and dyspareunia. When the infection is predominantly one of vaginitis, the symptoms include vaginal discharge, pruritus, dyspareunia and often dysuria. Cervicitis is associated with purulent vaginal discharge, sacral backache, lower abdominal pain, dyspareunia and dysuria. The proximity of the cervix to the bladder often results in coexistent trigonitis and urethritis, particularly in the case of gonococcal infections.

Chronic cervicitis is present in about 50–60% of all parous women. In many cases, the symptoms are minimal. There may be a slight mucopurulent discharge, which is not sufficient to trouble the woman and may simply present as an incidental finding that does not justify active treatment. In the more severe forms of the condition, there is profuse vaginal discharge, chronic sacral backache, dyspareunia and occasionally post-coital bleeding. Bacteriological culture of the discharge is usually sterile. The condition may cause subfertility because of hostility of the cervical mucus to sperm invasion.

Signs

These will depend on the cause. The appearance of the vulval skin is reddened, sometimes with ulceration and excoriation. In the sexually mature female, the vaginal walls may become ulcerated, with plaques of white monilial discharge adherent to the skin or, in protozoal infections, the discharge may be copious with a greenish-white, frothy appearance.

Bartholin's glands are sited between the posterior part of the labia minora and the vaginal walls, and these two glands secrete mucus as a lubricant during coitus. Infection of the duct and gland results in closure of the duct and formation of a Bartholin's cyst or abscess. The condition is often recurrent and causes pain and swelling of the vulva. Bartholinitis is readily recognized by the site and nature of the swelling.

In cervicitis the cervix appears reddened and may be ulcerated, as with herpetic infections, and there is a mucopurulent discharge as the endocervix is invariably involved. The diagnosis is established by examination and taking cervical swabs for culture.

Common organisms

Vaginal candidiasis

Candida albicans is a yeast pathogen that occurs naturally on the skin and in the bowel. Infection may be asymptomatic or associated with an increased or changed vaginal discharge associated with soreness and itching in the vulva area. There is no evidence of male to female sexual transmission. White curd-like collections attached to the vaginal epithelium may be seen on speculum examination, although these are not present in all cases.

Candidal infections are particularly common during pregnancy, in women taking the contraceptive pill and in underlying conditions involving immuno-suppression (e.g. HIV infection, diabetes or long-term steroids). In each instance, vaginal acidity is increased above normal and bacterial growth in the vagina is inhibited in such a way as to allow free growth of yeast pathogens, which thrive well in a low-pH environment. *Candida* hyphae and spores can also be seen in a wet preparation and can be cultured.

Trichomoniasis

Trichomonas vaginalis is a flagellated single-celled proto-zoal organism that may infect the cervix, urethra and vagina. In the male the organism is carried in the urethra or prostate and infection is sexually transmitted. The organisms are often seen on the Papanicolaou smear even in the absence of symptoms. The commonest presentation is with abnormal vaginal bleeding but other symptoms include vaginal soreness and pruritus. The vaginal pH is usually raised above 4.5. A fresh wet preparation in saline of vaginal discharge will show motile trichomonads (Fig. 22.1). The characteristic flagellate motion is easily recognized and the organism can be cultured.

Genital herpes

The condition is caused by herpes simplex virus (HSV) type 2 and, less commonly, type 1. It is a sexually transmitted disease. Primary HSV infection is usually a systemic infection with fever, myalgia and occasionally meningism. The local symptoms include vaginal discharge, vulval pain, dysuria and inguinal lymph-adenopathy. The discomfort may be severe enough to cause urinary retention. Vulval lesions include skin vesicles and multiple shallow skin ulcers (Fig. 22.2). The infection is also associated with cervical dysplasia.

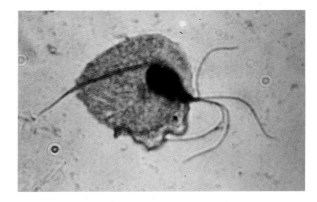

Fig. 22.1 *Trichomonas vaginalis.*

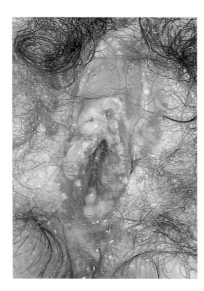

Fig. 22.2 Herpetic vulvitis. Lesions can also occur in the cervix and in the perivulvar region.

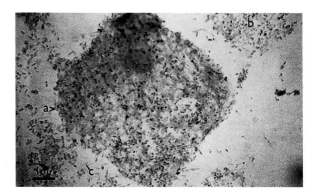

Fig. 22.3 Clue cells in bacterial vaginosis. These are epithelial squamous cells with multiple bacteria adherent to their surface.

Partners may be asymptomatic and the incubation period is 2–14 days.

The diagnosis is made by sending fluid from vesicles for viral culture or antigen detection. After the initial infection the virus remains latent in the sacral ganglia. Recurrences may be triggered by stress, menstruation or intercourse, but are normally of shorter duration and less severe than the primary episode. Serum antibodies are raised in well-established lesions.

Bacterial vaginosis

This is due to an overgrowth of a number of anaerobic organisms including *Gardnerella* spp. It is not sexually transmitted. It may be asymptomatic or cause a smelly vaginal discharge and vulval irritation. It is associated with an increased risk of pelvic inflammatory disease, urinary tract infection and puerperal infection. Diagnosis is made by finding three of the following:

- An increase in vaginal pH of more than 4.5
- A typical thin homogenous vaginal discharge
- A fishy odour produced when 10% potassium hydroxide is added to the discharge
- Clue cells on Gram-stained slide of vaginal fluid (Fig. 22.3).

Gonococcal and chlamydial vulvovaginitis

These are associated with extensive pelvic infection (see below) but may also be asymptomatic or indicated merely by vaginal discharge and dysuria.

Syphilis

The initial lesion appears 10–90 days after contact with the spirochaete *Treponema pallidum*. The primary lesion or chancre is an indurated, firm papule, which may become ulcerated and has a raised firm edge. This lesion most commonly occurs on the vulva but may also occur in the vagina or cervix. The primary lesion may be accompanied by inguinal lymphadenopathy. The chancre heals spontaneously within 2–6 weeks.

Some 6 weeks after the disappearance of the chancre, the manifestations of secondary syphilis appear. A rash develops which is maculopapular and is often associated with alopecia. Papules occur, particularly in the anogenital area and in the mouth, and give the typical appearance known as condylomata lata.

Swabs taken from either the primary or secondary lesions are examined microscopically under dark-ground illumination, and the spirochaetes can be seen. The serological tests have been described in a previous chapter.

The disease then progresses from the secondary phase to a tertiary phase. It may mimic almost any disease process and affect every system in the body, but the common long-term lesions are cardiovascular and neurological.

Genital warts (condylomata acuminata)

Vulval and cervical warts (Fig. 22.4) are caused by a human papilloma virus (HPV). The condition is commonly, although by no means invariably, transmitted by sexual contact. The incubation period is up to 6 months. The incidence has risen significantly over the last 15 years, particularly in women aged 16–25.

The warts have an appearance similar to those seen on the skin in other sites, and in the moist environment of the vulval skin are often prolific – particularly during pregnancy. There is frequently associated pruritus and vaginal discharge. The lesions may spread to the perianal region, and in some cases become confluent and subject to secondary infections. Diagnosis is usually made by clinical examination

> ! Vaginal discharge in a child may also be associated with the presence of a foreign body, and this possibility should always be excluded.

Treatment of lower genital tract infections

When the diagnosis has been established by examination and the bacteriological tests, the appropriate treatment can be instituted. The treatment for chlamydia and gonorrhoea is discussed below under infections of the upper genital tract. Whenever a diagnosis of sexually transmitted infection is made, it is essential to screen patients (and their partners) for other infections.

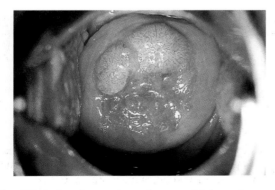

Fig. 22.4 Papilloma virus infection of the cervix: condylomata acuminata.

Vulval and vaginal monilial infections can be treated by topical or oral preparations. These include a single dose of clotrimazole given as a pessary, or fluconazole taken orally. Recurrent infections can be treated by oral administration of ketoconazole and fluconazole. The patient's partner should be treated at the same time, and any predisposing factors such as poor hygiene or diabetes should be corrected.

Trichomonas infections and bacterial vaginosis are treated with metronidazole 400 mg taken twice a day for 5 days, which must be taken by both sexual partners if recurrence of the infection is to be avoided. Metronidazole may be administered as a single dose of 2 g, but high-dose therapy should be avoided in pregnancy. Topical treatment with metronidazole gel or clindamycin cream is also effective for bacterial vaginosis.

Non-specific vaginal infections are common, and are treated with vaginal creams, including hydrargaphen, povidone–iodine, di-iodohydroxyquinoline or sulphonamide creams.

Syphilis is treated in the first instance with penicillin and, if this fails, for example in the case of coinfection, with penicillin-resistant strains of the gonococcus, doxycycline hydrochloride or acrosoxacin can be used.

Infections of the vagina associated with menopausal atrophic changes are treated by the appropriate hormone replacement therapy using an oral or vaginal oestrogen preparation, or lactic acid pessaries where oestrogens are contraindicated. The same therapy may be used, with the local application of oestrogen creams, in juvenile vulvovaginitis.

Infections of Bartholin's gland are treated with the antibiotic appropriate to the organism. If abscess formation has occurred, the abscess should be 'marsupialized' by excising an ellipse of skin and sewing the skin edges to wall off the abscess cavity (Fig. 22.5). This reduces the likelihood of recurrence of the abscess.

Vulval warts are treated with either physical or chemical diathermy using podophyllin applied directly to the surface of the warts. Any concurrent vaginal discharge should also receive the appropriate therapy.

Herpetic infections are notoriously resistant to treatment and highly prone to recurrence. The best available treatment is aciclovir (acyclovir) administered in tablet form 200 mg five times daily for 5 days or locally as a 5% cream.

Acute cervicitis usually occurs in association with generalized infection of the genital tract and is diagnosed and treated according to the microbiology. Medical treatment is rarely effective in chronic cervicitis because

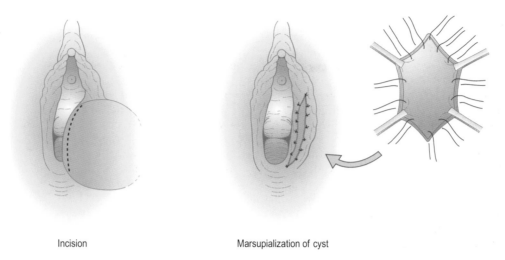

Incision   Marsupialization of cyst

Fig. 22.5 Marsupialization of a Bartholin's cyst or abscess. The incision is made over the medial aspect of the cyst (left) and the lining is sutured to the skin (right).

it is difficult to identify an organism and antibiotics do not penetrate the chronic microabscesses of the cervical glands. If the cervical swab is negative, the next most effective management is diathermy of the endocervix under general anaesthesia. Following diathermy, an antibacterial cream should be placed in the vagina and the woman should be advised that the discharge may increase in amount for 2–3 weeks but will then diminish. She should also be advised to avoid intercourse for 3 weeks as coitus may cause secondary haemorrhage.

INFECTIONS OF THE UPPER GENITAL TRACT

Acute infection of the endometrium, myometrium, Fallopian tubes and ovaries are usually the result of ascending infections from the lower genital tract causing pelvic inflammatory disease (PID).

However, infection may be secondary to appendicitis or other bowel infections, which sometimes give rise to a pelvic abscess. Perforation of the appendix with pelvic sepsis remains a common cause of tubal obstruction and subfertility. Pelvic sepsis may also occur during the puerperium and after termination. Retained placental tissue and blood provide an excellent culture medium for organisms from the bowel, including *Escherichia coli*, *Clostridium welchii* or *C. perfringens*, *Staphylococcus aureus* and *Streptococcus faecalis*.

Pelvic inflammatory disease affects approximately 1.7% of women between 15 and 35 years of age per year in the developed world. Up to 20% of women with PID will have a further episode within 2 years. The disease is most common between the ages of 15 and 24 years, and particular risk factors include multiple sexual partners and procedures involving transcervical instrumentation. PID is an important cause of infertility. After a first episode 8% of women will have evidence of tubal infertility; subsequent episodes approximately double this figure. Women with a past history of PID are 10 times more likely to have an ectopic pregnancy when they conceive.

> ✓ 40% of women who have had three or more episodes of PID have tubal damage.

Symptoms and signs

The symptoms of acute salpingitis include :

- Acute bilateral lower abdominal pain: Salpingitis is almost invariably bilateral; where the symptoms are unilateral, an alternative diagnosis should be considered
- Deep dyspareunia

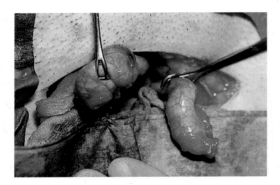

Fig. 22.6 Acute salpingitis: the tubes are swollen and engorged.

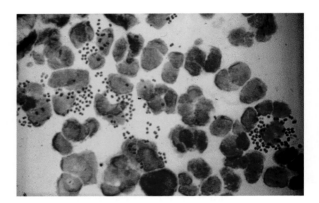

Fig. 22.7 *Neisseria gonorrhoeae.*

- Abnormal menstrual bleeding
- Purulent vaginal discharge.

The signs include:

- Signs of systemic illness with pyrexia and tachycardia
- Signs of peritonitis with guarding or rebound tenderness
- On pelvic examination, acute pain on cervical excitation and thickening in the vaginal fornices, which may be associated with the presence of cystic tubal swellings due to pyosalpinges or pus-filled tubes; fullness in the pouch of Douglas suggests the presence of a pelvic abscess (Fig. 22.6)
- An acute perihepatitis occurs in 10–25% of women with chlamydial PID, which may cause right upper quadrant abdominal pain, deranged liver function tests and multiple filmy adhesions between the liver surface and parietal peritoneum, and is known as the *Fitz-Hugh–Curtis syndrome*
- A pyrexia of 38°C or more, sometimes associated with rigors.

Common organisms

Pelvic inflammatory disease is thought to be the result of polymicrobial infection with primary infection by *Chlamydia trachomatis* or *Neisseria gonorrhoeae* (or both) allowing opportunistic infection with other aerobic bacteria and anaerobes.

Chlamydia

Chlamydia trachomatis is an obligate intracellular Gram-negative bacterium. It is the commonest bacterial sexually transmitted infection in Europe and North America and is thought to be the causative agent in at least 60% of cases of PID in those areas. Prevalence rates vary from 11% to 30% in women attending genito-urinary medicine clinics, with the peak incidence in the UK in women aged 20–24. The main sites of infection are the columnar epithelium of the endocervix, urethra and rectum but many women remain asymptomatic. Ascent of infection to the upper genital tract occurs in about 20% of women with cervical infection.

Gonorrhoea

Neisseria gonorrhoea is a Gram-negative intracellular diplococcus (Fig. 22.7). Infection is commonly asymptomatic or associated with vaginal discharge. In cases of PID it spreads across the surface of the cervix and endometrium and causes tubal infection within 1–3 days of contact. It is the principle cause for 14% of cases of PID and occurs in combination with *Chlamydia* in a further 8%.

Differential diagnosis

It is often difficult to establish the diagnosis of acute pelvic infection with any degree of certainty. The predictive value of clinical signs and symptoms when compared to laparoscopic diagnosis is 65–90%. The differential diagnosis includes the following.

- **Tubal ectopic pregnancy:** Initially pain is unilateral in most cases. There may be syncopal episodes and signs of diaphragmatic irritation with shoulder tip pain. The white cell count is normal or slightly raised

but the haemoglobin level is low, whereas in acute salpingitis the white cell count is raised and the haemoglobin concentration is normal.
- **Acute appendicitis.** The most important difference in the history lies in the unilateral nature of the condition. Pelvic examination does not usually reveal as much pain and tenderness but it must be remembered that the two conditions sometimes coexist, particularly where the infected appendix lies adjacent to the right fallopian tube.
- **Acute urinary tract infections.** These may produce similar symptoms but rarely produce signs of peritonism and are commonly associated with urinary symptoms.
- **Torsion or rupture of an ovarian cyst.**

Investigations

When the diagnosis of acute salpingitis is suspected, the woman should be admitted to hospital. After completion of the history and general examination, swabs should be taken from the vaginal fornices and cervical canal and sent to the laboratory for culture and antibiotic sensitivity. A midstream specimen of urine should also be sent for culture. An additional endocervical swab should be taken for detection of *Chlamydia* by enzyme-linked immunoassay (ELISA) or, preferably, polymerase chain reaction (PCR). Urethral swabs may identify chlamydial infection not detected by endocervical swabs. PCR assays of urine samples have a similar of better sensitivity (90%) compared to genital tract swabs and offer a potential means for screening for chlamydial infection in asymptomatic women.

Examination of the blood for differential white cell count, haemoglobin estimation and C-reactive protein may help to establish the diagnosis. Blood culture is indicated if there is a significant pyrexia. The diagnosis of mild to moderate degrees of PID on the basis of history and examination findings is unreliable and, where the diagnosis is in doubt, laparoscopy is indicated.

 Negative swabs do not exclude the possibility of pelvic inflammatory disease.

Management

When the patient is unwell and exhibits peritonitis, high-grade fever, vomiting or a pelvic inflammatory

mass, she should be admitted to hospital and managed as follows.

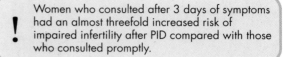 Women who consulted after 3 days of symptoms had an almost threefold increased risk of impaired infertility after PID compared with those who consulted promptly.

- Fluid replacement by intravenous therapy – vomiting and pain often result in dehydration.
- When PID is clinically suspected, antibiotic therapy should be commenced pending the results of microbiological tests. Antibiotic therapy prescribed for clinically diagnosed PID should be effective against *C. trachomatis*, *N. gonorrhoeae* and the anaerobes characterizing bacterial vaginosis. If the woman is acutely unwell, treatment should be started with an antibiotic such as cefuroxime and metronidazole given intravenously with oral doxycycline until the acute phase of the infection begins to resolve. Treatment with oral metronidazole and doxycycline should then be continued for 7 and 14 days respectively.
- Pain relief with non-steroidal anti-inflammatory drugs.
- If the uterus contains an intrauterine device, it should be removed as soon as antibiotic therapy has been commenced.
- Bed rest – immobilization is essential until the pain subsides.
- Abstain from intercourse.

Patients who are systemically well can be treated as outpatient, with a single dose of azithromycin and a 7-day course of doxycycline, reviewed after 48 hours.

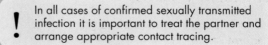 In all cases of confirmed sexually transmitted infection it is important to treat the partner and arrange appropriate contact tracing.

Indications for surgical intervention

In most cases, conservative management results in complete remission. Laparotomy is indicated where the condition does not resolve with conservative management and where there is a pelvic mass.

In most cases, the mass will be due to a pyosalpinx or tubo-ovarian abscess. This can either be drained or a salpingectomy can be performed.

CHRONIC PELVIC INFECTION

Acute pelvic infections may progress to a chronic state with dilatation and obstruction of the tubes forming bilateral hydrosalpinges with multiple pelvic adhesions (Fig. 22.8).

Symptoms and signs

Symptoms are varied but include:

- Chronic pelvic pain
- Chronic purulent vaginal discharge
- Epimenorrhagia and dysmenorrhoea
- Deep-seated dyspareunia.

Chronic salpingitis is also associated with infection in the connective tissue of the pelvis known as *parametritis*.

On examination, there is a purulent discharge from the cervix. The uterus is often fixed in retroversion, and there is thickening in the fornices and pain on bimanual examination.

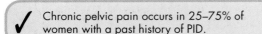

✓ Chronic pelvic pain occurs in 25–75% of women with a past history of PID.

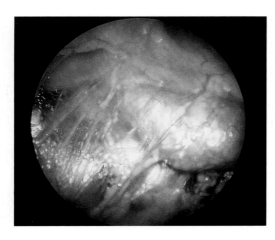

Fig. 22.8 Chronic pelvic inflammatory disease: a sheet of fine adhesions covering the tubes and ovary, which is buried beneath the tube.

Management

Conservative management of this condition is rarely effective and the problem is only eventually resolved by clearance of the pelvic organs. Women with a history of PID are 8 times more likely to have a hysterectomy than the general population.

HUMAN IMMUNODEFICIENCY VIRUS

Human immunodeficiency virus (HIV)-1 and HIV-2 are RNA retroviruses characterized by their tropism for the human CD4+ (helper) T lymphocyte. The proportion of cells infected is initially low and there is a prolonged latent phase between infection and clinical signs. Transmission occurs by sex, infected blood products, shared needles, breastfeeding and at the time of delivery. Risk groups include intravenous drug abusers and their partners, the partners of bisexual men, haemophiliacs, prostitutes and immigrants from high-risk areas. Although HIV infection is more common in men in the developed world, anonymous testing shows that 0.3% of pregnant women in London are infected and it is now the most common cause of death in African American females aged 24–35 years in the USA. Vertical transmission rates can be reduced from 40% to less than 5% by antenatal treatment with antiretroviral drugs, delivery by elective caesarean section and avoidance of breastfeeding.

The main clinical states can be identified as:

- A 'flu-like' illness 3–6 months after infection, associated with seroconversion
- Asymptomatic impaired immunity
- Persistent generalized lymphadenopathy
- Acquired immunodeficiency syndrome (AIDS)-related complex with pathognomonic infections or tumours.

Common opportunistic infections include *Candida*, HSV, HPV, *Mycobacterium* spp., *Cryptosporidium* spp., *Pneumocystis carinii* and cytomegalovirus. Non-infective manifestations include weight loss, diarrhoea, fever, dementia, Kaposi's sarcoma and an increased risk of cervical cancer.

The diagnosis is made by detecting antibodies to the virus, although these may take up to 3 months to appear.

ESSENTIAL INFORMATION

Vulvovaginitis

- Commonest infection of genital tract
- Presents as pruritus, dyspareunia or discharge
- Common causes are *Trichomonas*, bacterial vaginosis and *Candida*
- Predisposing factors include pregnancy, diabetes, contraceptive pill
- Can be diagnosed by examination of fresh wet preparation of vaginal discharge

Herpes genitalis

- Caused by herpes simplex virus
- Presents with pain, bleeding and vesicles or shallow ulcers on the vagina/vulva
- Associated with cervical dysplasia
- Tends to be recurrent but with decreasing severity
- Can be transmitted to the neonate during vaginal delivery if active

Infections of the cervix

- Acute (associated with generalized infection) or chronic
- Discharge, dyspareunia, low abdominal pain or backache, urinary symptoms and postcoital bleeding
- Can cause subfertility
- Difficult to isolate an organism when chronic
- Treatment includes appropriate antibiotics and cautery

Upper genital tract infection

- Usually from ascending lower genital tract infection
- Can follow abortion or normal delivery
- Commonly due to *C. trachomatis* or *N. gonorrhoeae* when sexually transmitted
- Presents as pain, fever, discharge and irregular periods
- Bilateral pain on cervical excitation and raised white cell count
- Differential diagnosis includes ectopic pregnancy, urinary tract infection and appendicitis
- Management includes fluid replacement, antibiotics, analgesia and rest
- Surgery is indicated to confirm diagnosis if in doubt, for drainage of pelvic mass and to clear pelvis in unresponsive chronic disease
- Major cause of infertility worldwide, resulting in tubal obstruction in 40% of cases after three or more attacks

HIV infection

- Retrovirus infection of T-helper cells and central nervous system
- Transmitted by sex, blood transfusion or to offspring
- Diagnosis by serology, differential lymphocyte count or opportunistic infection
- Can be asymptomatic, cause generalized malaise and lymphadenopathy or AIDS
- Rates of vertical transmission can be reduced by drug treatment, elective caesarean section and avoiding breastfeeding
- Incidence in heterosexuals increasing

menopause; in its most extreme form the fibroid is converted into a stony mass.

- **Infection and abscess formation** are rare complications that are particularly likely to affect submucous fibroids following septic abortion or occasionally following a tumour, particularly if radiotherapy is used.
- **Necrobiosis** – impairment of blood supply is particularly likely to occur in pedunculated subserous fibroids but there are special forms of necrosis such as red degeneration, which is seen in pregnancy. The cut surface of the tumour has a dull reddish hue and the appearance is associated with aseptic degeneration and local haemolysis.
- **Sarcomatous change** – the incidence of malignant change in fibroids has been variably reported to be between 0.13% and 1%.

Symptoms and signs

Some 50% of women with fibroids are asymptomatic and the condition may be discovered during routine pelvic examination – either at the time of cervical cytology or in the management of a pregnancy.

Where symptoms do occur, they are often related to the site of the fibroids. The common presenting symptoms are as follows.

- **Menstrual disorders:** Submucous and intramural fibroids commonly cause menorrhagia. They do not influence the length of the menstrual cycle. Submucous fibroids may cause irregular vaginal bleeding, particularly if the surface of the fibroid becomes necrotic or ulcerated, or if endometrial carcinoma is also present.
- **Pain:** Colicky uterine pain may occur with pedunculated fibroids as the uterus attempts to expel them. Pain may also occur during pregnancy if red degeneration occurs or if torsion of a subserous fibroid results in necrosis of the tumour. The pain will be persistent until necrosis is complete.
- **Pressure symptoms:** A large mass of fibroids may become apparent because of palpable enlargement of the abdomen or because of pressure on the bladder or rectum.
- **Complications of pregnancy.** Recurrent miscarriage is more common in women with submucous fibroids. Fibroids tend to enlarge in pregnancy and are more likely to undergo red degeneration. A large fibroid in the pelvis may obstruct labour or make

caesarean section more difficult. There is no evidence that they increase the risk of intrauterine growth restriction or premature labour.

- **Infertility.** Fibroids are found in 3% of women with infertility, and up to 30% of women with uterine fibroids will have difficulty in conceiving. Submucous and intramural fibroids are more likely to impair infertility than subserous ones. The mechanism may be mediated by both mechanical and hormonal effects.

The diagnosis can usually be confirmed by ultrasound scans of the pelvis. However, a solid ovarian tumour may be mistaken for a subserous fibroid and a fibroid undergoing cystic degeneration may mimic an ovarian cyst.

Management

Most fibroids are asymptomatic and do not require treatment. Occasionally it may be necessary to remove a large asymptomatic fibroid because of the difficulty of excluding the diagnosis of ovarian tumour or sarcoma.

Medical treatment

Progestogens and non-steroidal anti-inflammatory drugs have no effect on the size of fibroids but may be of value in controlling menstrual loss. A reduction of up to 50% in size can be achieved using gonadotrophin-releasing hormone (GnRH) analogues. However, the long-term use of these drugs is limited by their effect on bone density and the fibroids return to their original size when treatment is stopped. They may be of value in reducing the size and vascularity of fibroids prior to myomectomy. Danazol and the antiprogesterone mifepristone have also been shown to reduce the size of fibroids but are not as effective as GnRH analogues.

Uterine artery embolization

This involves the catheterization of the uterine arteries via the femoral artery and the injection of polyvinyl particles to reduce the blood supply to the uterus. The fibroid shrinks because of ischaemia. The advantages of this technique is that avoids the risks of major surgery and allows the preservation of fertility. The side effects include pain from uterine ischaemia and the risk of sepsis in the degenerating fibroid. At present its use is recommended only in selected centres.

Surgical treatment

Where the preservation of reproductive function is not important, the surgical treatment of choice is hysterectomy. Indeed, fibroids account for about a third of all hysterectomies in the UK. In younger women, or where the preservation of reproductive function is important, the removal of the fibroids by surgical excision or myomectomy is indicated. This procedure involves incision of the pseudocapsule of the fibroid, enucleation of the bulk of the tumour and closure of the cavity by interrupted absorbable sutures. Myomectomy is associated with greater morbidity than hysterectomy because of the occurrence of haematoma formation in the cavity of the excised fibroid and also because of infection. It is also impossible to be certain that all fibroids are removed without causing excessive uterine damage; there is always a possibility that residual seedling fibroids may regrow.

 Recurrence of fibroids occurs in up to 40% of cases after myomectomy.

Endoscopic resection of some submucous or subserous fibroids can be performed using the hysteroscope or laparoscope respectively. This is associated with a lower morbidity and a recurrence rate comparable to the open procedure. If the fibroid is more than 3 cm in diameter, GnRH analogues should be given for 3 months prior to surgery to reduce the size of the fibroid.

Adenomyosis

Adenomyosis is a condition characterized by the invasion of endometrial glands and stroma into the myometrium. It is difficult to diagnose until the uterus is subjected to histological examination and therefore the diagnosis is often overlooked.

Symptoms and signs

This condition, unlike endometriosis, occurs in parous women and usually arises in the fourth decade. It is associated with menorrhagia and dysmenorrhoea of increasing severity. On clinical examination, the uterus is symmetrically enlarged and tender. The condition is rare after the menopause.

Pathology

The macroscopic appearances of the uterus are those of diffuse enlargement. Adenomyosis and myomas often coexist, although the uterus is rarely enlarged to the size seen in the presence of myomas. The posterior wall of the uterus is usually thicker than the anterior wall. The cut surface of the uterus presents a characteristic, whorl-like trabeculated appearance but occasionally circumscribed nodules with dark haemorrhagic spots can be seen in the myometrium.

The microscopic diagnosis is based on the finding of islands of endometrial tissue buried deep within the myometrium. The aberrant endometrium does not respond to progesterone and the appearances are always those of proliferative endometrium. It is very rare for malignant change to occur in these lesions.

The only certain way of diagnosing adenomyosis preoperatively is by the use of magnetic resonance imaging (MRI). The nature of MRI of endometrial tissue can be seen within the myometrium, and provides a high degree of accuracy in diagnosing adenomyosis (Fig. 23.7).

Treatment

Hysterectomy is generally curative. The ovaries should be conserved, depending on the age of the patient. Medical therapy as for endometriosis is effective in some cases and symptomatic relief of dysmenorrhoea can be obtained with prostaglandin synthetase inhibitors.

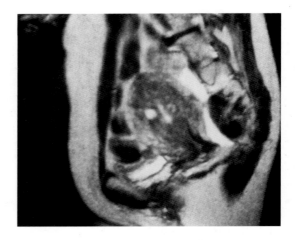

Fig. 23.7 Sagittal view using MRI of a uterus enlarged by adenomyosis.

MALIGNANT DISEASE OF THE UTERUS

Endometrial carcinoma

Adenocarcinoma of the endometrium is a common gynaecological tumour with an annual incidence of 13/100 000 women in the UK. It is the commonest gynaecological cancer in the USA. It presents after the menopause in three-quarters of all cases. Cancer of the body of the uterus is the predominant genital tract malignancy in women over the age of 50 years. The peak age of incidence occurs at the age of 61 years, and less than 8% of cases occur in women under the age of 45.

There are specific risk factors associated with an increased incidence of corpus carcinoma.

- **Obesity:** The ovarian stroma continues to produce androgens after the menopause, which are converted to the oestrogen estrone in adipose tissue. As there is no corresponding increase in progesterone to oppose the effects of excess oestrogen on the endometrium, this results in endometrial hyperplasia and malignancy in obese patients. This is a strong risk factor; approximately half of the women who develop endometrial carcinoma are grossly overweight.
- **Parity:** The incidence of corpus carcinoma is twice as high in nulliparous women.
- **Late menopause:** The incidence is significantly increased in women who have a menopause after the age of 50 years. Early menarche may also be a risk factor.
- **Diabetes mellitus:** Abnormalities of glucose tolerance are associated with a twofold increase in the incidence of endometrial carcinoma and there is also an increased incidence of hypertensive disease, although this is probably a secondary association.
- **Exogenous oestrogens:** Unopposed oestrogen action, particularly as used for hormone replacement therapy in the menopause, is associated with an increased incidence of endometrial carcinoma. The addition of a progestogen for 7 days of each month can reduce this risk, and the combined oral contraceptive pill reduces the incidence of the disease. Although used for its anti-oestrogenic effects in breast cancer, tamoxifen acts as an oestrogen agonist in the endometrium, see below
- **Endogenous oestrogens:** Oestrogen-producing ovarian tumours and polycystic ovarian tumours are both associated with an increase in the risk of endometrial cancer.
- **Family history:** A small proportion of women with endometrial cancer have a family history of cancers of the breast, ovary and gut (Lynch II syndrome).
- **Breast cancer:** Women with a history of breast cancer are twice as likely to develop endometrial cancer. In addition the drug tamoxifen, which is commonly used in the treatment of breast cancer, has an has oestrogenic effect on the endometrium causing hyperplasia and probably further increasing the risk of endometrial cancer in these patients.
- **Endometrial hyperplasia:** Prolonged stimulation of the endometrium with unopposed oestrogen may lead to hyperplasia of the endometrium with periods of amenorrhoea followed by heavy or irregular bleeding. If this is associated with cellular atypia, there is a 23% risk of an eventual progression to endometrial carcinoma.

Symptoms

The commonest symptom is postmenopausal bleeding. However, in the premenopausal woman, endometrial carcinoma is associated with irregular vaginal bleeding and menorrhagia. A serous bloodstained and offensive discharge may also accompany the history of abnormal bleeding.

Pathology

Adenocarcinoma of the endometrium may occur in a diffuse form and cover the whole surface of the endometrium, or it may be circumscribed in the form of a localized polypoid growth. The microscopic appearances include changes in the architecture with the development of closely packed polyhedral cells with dark-staining nuclei and considerable numbers of mitoses. In many tumours, the cells may retain their normal characteristics. The stromal cells almost always show marked reactive inflammatory infiltration with round cells and leukocytes. The virulence of the tumour is related to the degree of histological dedifferentiation.

Endometrial cancer grows locally for a long period of time and expands the uterus (Fig. 23.8). The tumour spreads by direct invasion into the myometrium and then transcervically, transtubally and by spillage of

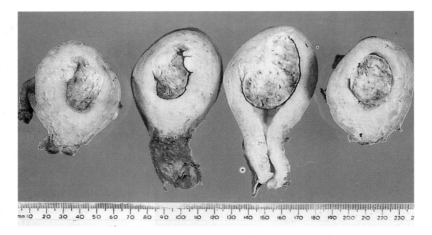

Fig. 23.8 Endometrial adenocarcinoma. Multiple sections showing a large endometrial carcinoma invading the substance of the myometrium.

carcinomatous material. Lymphatic spread occurs in 25% of cases with disease clinically confined to the uterus, is the primary method of extrauterine extension and involves the external and internal iliac nodes and the aortic nodes. In lesions involving the fundus of the uterus, spread may occur along the lymphatics of the round ligament and metastasise to the superficial or deep inguinal nodes.

Some 75% of cases are of the endometrioid type. Clear-cell serous and mixed patterns are found less commonly, serous papillary lesions having a poor prognosis irrespective of stage or differentiation.

Diagnosis

The diagnosis of the tumour is established by endometrial biopsy. This should be accompanied by hysteroscopy to identify focal abnormalities that might be missed by blind curettage. This can be carried out as an outpatient procedure or under general anaesthesia. Where endometrial thickness is less than 5 mm, as assessed by ultrasound, a significant endometrial lesion is unlikely. Invasion of carcinoma into the rectum or bladder can be recognized by cystoscopy and proctoscopy. The most accurate method of determining the depth of invasion of an endometrial carcinoma is by MRI, when the tumour can be clearly seen to breach the non-resonant subendometrial layer.

Treatment

The mainstay of treatment is total abdominal hysterectomy and bilateral salpingo-oophorectomy. Patients at high risk of extrauterine disease should undergo full pelvic lymphadenectomy (as determined by preoperative MRI or computed tomography (CT) scan). The value of routine lymphadenectomy for all patients with endometrial cancer remains controversial.

Adjuvant radiotherapy is given to patients with proven or, in the absence of lymph node sampling, those at high risk of, extrauterine spread. Although this has not been shown to improve long-term survival in these patients, it does reduce the risk of vaginal and pelvic recurrence. Patients with advanced disease (stages III and IV; Table 23.1) are treated by debulking the tumour followed by radiotherapy. About 25% of tumours will respond to hormonal therapy using high-dose progestogens but the duration of response may be limited. Cytotoxic drugs such as carboplatin and doxorubicin are used in the treatment of recurrent disease but response rates are low (20%).

Prognosis

Prognostic factors include age, node involvement, depth of myometrial invasion, degree of differentiation, positive cytology and tumour type. In cases of super-

Table 23.1
The FIGO classification of endometrial carcinoma

The FIGO classification of endometrial carcinoma takes into account the distribution of the tumour and the depth of penetration of the myometrium and histological grading.

Stage I Carcinoma confined to the corpus:
      Stage IA: Superficial
      Stage IB: Penetrating less than half the depth of the myometrium
      Stage IC: Penetrating into the outer half of the myometrium but not breaching the serosal surface.

Stage II The carcinoma involves the cervix but does not extend outside the uterus:
      Stage IIA: Involving glands only
      Stage IIB: Involving the cervical stroma.

Stage III The tumour has extended outside the uterus but not the pelvis:
      Stage IIIA: Spread to uterine serosa and/or adnexa and/or positive peritoneal cytology
      Stage IIIB: Vaginal metastases
      Stage IIIC: Pelvic and/or para-aortic lymph nodes involved.

Stage IV The tumour extends beyond the pelvis:
      Stage IVA: Spread to bladder and rectum
      Stage IVB: Spread to distant organs or inguinal nodes.

The tumours are further grouped according to the degree of differentiation:
G1:   Highly differentiated
G2:   Differentiated with solid areas
G3:   Solid or undifferentiated adenocarcinoma.

ficial invasion the 5-year survival for patients with stage I disease is greater than 80% compared with 66% for patients where the outer half of the myometrium is involved. Serous papillary and clear cell carcinomas have a poorer prognosis, with 5-year survival rates of 50% and 35% respectively.

Malignant mesenchymal tumours of the uterus

Non-epithelial cancers account for only 3% of uterine malignancies. In general they arise from either myometrial smooth muscle (leiomyosarcomas) or stroma of the endometrium (stromal sarcomas). Mixed müllerian duct or carcinosarcomas contain malignant elements from both the endometrial epithelium and stroma.

Stromal sarcomas

These tumours, arising from the stroma of the endometrium, account for 15% of uterine sarcomas. They tend to present in a younger age group (45–50 years) than other uterine tumours with vaginal discharge and bleeding. Endometrioid stromal sarcoma is found in association with adenomyosis and endometriosis. It can

be classified as low- or high-grade, depending on the number of mitotic figures and similarity to the non-glandular elements of the endometrium. Malignant mixed mesodermal sarcomas contain elements of both smooth muscle and stroma.

Mixed müllerian tumours (carcinosarcomas)

These tumours (Fig. 23.9) consist of both epithelial and mesenchymal elements. The epithelial elements are usually endometrioid but can be squamous or a mixture. The stromal elements are either heterologous (chondroblastoma, osteosarcoma, fibrosarcoma) or homologous (leiomyosarcoma, presarcoma). The mean age at presentation is 65. An enlarged, irregular uterus with tumour protruding through the cervical os is a common finding at examination. Extrauterine spread occurs early and only 25% of patients have disease limited to the endometrium at the time of diagnosis.

 A significant number of patients with mixed müllerian tumours will give a history of previous pelvic irradiation.

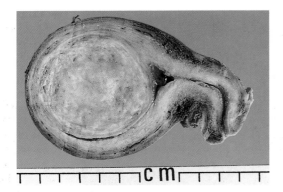

Fig. 23.9 Large mixed müllerian tumour.

Leiomyosarcoma

These smooth muscle tumours arise in the myometrium of the uterus and account for only 1.3% of uterine malignancies. They are uncommon (0.7/100 000), with a peak incidence at the age of 52, about 10 years later than the peak incidence for fibroids. Between 5 and 10% arise in existing fibroids, although the risk of malignant change occurring in a fibroid is small (0.3–0.8%). Leiomyosarcomas are classified according to the degree of differentiation. They may present with pain, post-menopausal bleeding or a rapidly growing 'fibroid' but are often asymptomatic and diagnosed following hysterectomy for fibroids. Treatment is by hysterectomy and bilateral salpingo-oophorectomy. Adjuvant radiotherapy and chemotherapy reduces the risk of local recurrence but does not improve long-term survival.

 Rapid growth of a 'fibroid', especially when associated with pain and irregular bleeding, may indicate malignant change.

Treatment

This is by hysterectomy, with removal of as much macroscopic disease as possible, followed by radiotherapy. Prognosis for low-grade stromal sarcomas is similar to that for endometrioid tumours, but poor for others, with a 20–40% 5-year survival.

TUMOURS OF THE FALLOPIAN TUBES

Primary Fallopian tube cancers are extremely rare, accounting for 0.16–1% of all gynaecological malig-

Case study
Leiomyosarcoma in a young woman

A 26-year-old woman presented for investigation of subfertility and was found to have a 3 cm diameter fibroid arising from the posterior surface of her uterus. This was not considered to be the cause of her difficulties in conceiving, and shortly after laparoscopy she conceived. The pregnancy was uneventful except that she developed episodes of abdominal pain and the fibroid showed rapid growth and enlarged to fill the pouch of Douglas. Because of the obstruction caused by the fibroid, which had enlarged to a diameter of 10 cm, it was necessary to deliver the child by caesarean section. In the 6 weeks after delivery, the patient continued to complain of pain and, unexpectedly, the fibroid did not regress. Ten weeks after delivery, a myomectomy was performed, with a difficult removal of an adherent, necrotic fibroid in the pouch of Douglas. Histology showed numerous mitotic figures with a highly malignant leiomyosarcoma and, despite a further laparotomy, radiotherapy and chemotherapy, the woman died from widespread metastatic disease 8 weeks later. This was a very rare event but demonstrates the rapid blood-borne metastatic disease associated with this type of sarcoma, which has an exceedingly poor prognosis.

nancies. The mean age at diagnosis is 52 years, with a range of 18–80 years. The symptoms include abnormal vaginal bleeding and a canary-yellow discharge. Tubal cancers are predominantly adenocarcinomas, which are histologically similar to epithelial ovarian tumours and are best treated by radiotherapy. In fact, most of these tumours are first diagnosed at the time of laparotomy and are therefore surgically excised with subsequent treatment with chemotherapy.

LESIONS OF THE OVARY

Ovarian enlargement is commonly asymptomatic, and the silent nature of malignant ovarian tumours is the major reason for the advanced stage of presentation.

Ovarian tumours may be cystic or solid, functional, benign or malignant. There are common factors in the presentation and complications of ovarian tumours and it is often difficult to establish the nature of a tumour without direct examination.

Symptoms

Tumours of the ovary that are less than 10cm in diameter rarely produce symptoms. The common presenting symptoms include:

- Abdominal enlargement – in the presence of malignant change, this may also be associated with ascites
- Symptoms from pressure on surrounding structures such as the bladder and rectum
- Symptoms relating to complications of the tumour (Fig. 23.10): These include:
  - **Torsion:** Acute torsion of the ovarian pedicle results in necrosis of the tumour; there is acute pain and vomiting followed by remission of the pain when the tumour has become necrotic
  - **Rupture:** The contents of the cyst spill into the peritoneal cavity and result in generalized abdominal pain
  - **Haemorrhage** into the tumour is an unusual complication but may result in abdominal pain and shock if the blood loss is severe
  - **Hormone-secreting tumours** may present with disturbances in the menstrual cycle. In androgen-secreting tumours the patient may present with signs of virilization. Although a greater proportion of the sex-cord stromal type of tumour (see

below) are hormonally active, the commonest type of secreting tumour found in clinical practice is the epithelial type.

Signs

On examination, the abdomen may be visibly enlarged. Percussion over the swelling will demonstrate central dullness and resonance in the flanks. These signs may be obscured by gross ascites. Small tumours can be detected on pelvic examination and will be found by palpation in one or both fornices. However, as the tumour enlarges, it assumes a more central position and, in the case of dermoid cysts, is often anterior to the uterus. Most ovarian tumours are not tender to palpation; if they are painful the presence of infection or torsion should be suspected. Benign ovarian tumours are palpable separately from the uterine body and are usually freely mobile.

BENIGN OVARIAN TUMOURS
Functional cysts of the ovary

These cysts occur only during menstrual life and rarely exceed more than 6 cm in diameter.

Follicular cysts

Follicular cysts (Fig. 23.11) are the commonest functional cysts in the ovary and may be multiple and bilateral. The cysts rarely exceed 4 cm in diameter, the walls consisting of layers of granulosa cells and the

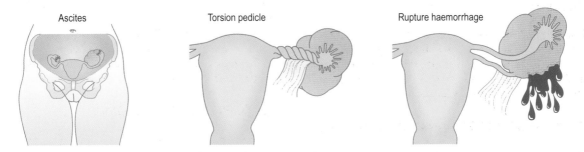

Fig. 23.10 Common complications of ovarian tumours that precipitate a request for medical advice.

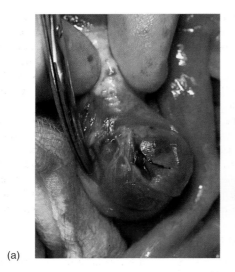

(a)

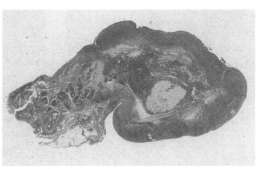

(b)

Fig. 23.11 (a) Small follicular cyst near mid-cycle. (b) Histological features.

contents of clear fluid, which is rich in sex steroids. These cysts commonly occur during treatment with clomiphene or human menopausal gonadotrophin (Fig. 23.12). They may produce prolonged unopposed oestrogen effects on the endometrium, resulting in cystic glandular hyperplasia of the endometrium.

Management

These cysts regress spontaneously but if they have not involuted after 60 days the diagnosis should be revised. The size and growth of the cysts can be monitored by ultrasound scans.

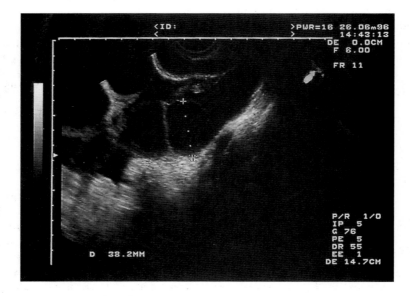

Fig. 23.12 Pelvic ultrasound showing ovarian hyperstimulation with multiple follicles.

The prolonged and heavy menstrual loss caused by unopposed oestrogen action can be offset by the administration of a progestogen for 1 week followed by 'medical curettage', or through surgical intervention by cervical dilatation and uterine curettage.

Lutein cysts

There are two types of luteinized ovarian cyst.

- **Granulosa lutein cysts**, functional cysts of the corpus luteum, may be 4–6 cm in diameter and occur in the second half of the menstrual cycle. Persistent production of progesterone may result in amenorrhoea or delayed onset of menstruation. These cysts often give rise to pain and therefore present a problem in terms of differential diagnosis, as the history and examination findings mimic tubal ectopic pregnancy. Occasionally, haemorrhage occurs into the cyst, which may rupture and lead to a haemoperitoneum. The cysts usually regress spontaneously and require surgical intervention only when they give rise to symptoms of intra-abdominal haemorrhage.
- **Theca lutein cysts** commonly arise in association with high levels of chorionic gonadotrophin and are therefore seen in cases of hydatidiform mole. The cysts may be bilateral and can, on occasion, give rise to haemorrhage if they rupture. Once the cysts have been formed, they can be detected by ultrasound. They usually undergo spontaneous involution but surgical intervention may be necessary if there is significant haemorrhage from the ovaries.

Benign neoplastic cysts

These tumours may be cystic or solid and arise from specific cell lines in the ovary. The full World Health Organization classification of ovarian tumours illustrates the complexity of tumours arising from the ovary; only the commoner ones will be discussed in this section.

Epithelial tumours

Serous cystadenomas

These cysts, in conjunction with mucinous cystadenomas, form the commonest group of cystic ovarian tumours. The cysts may be unilocular, lined by a layer of cuboidal epithelium, or multilocular with papillary growths extending from both internal and external surfaces of the tumour. It is often difficult to differentiate between benign and malignant appearances. The wall of the tumour sometimes contains calcified granules known as *psammoma bodies*. The growths may be bilateral and may be large enough to fill the peritoneal cavity.

The tumours often replace all normal ovarian tissue; if this is the case, the whole ovary should be removed. If the tumour is small, it may be possible to perform a local resection and to conserve ovarian tissue. If both ovaries are extensively involved or there is reason to believe that the tumours are malignant, it is better to perform bilateral oophorectomy and hysterectomy.

Mucinous cystadenomas

These tumours are multilocular and often reach enormous dimensions, with tumours weighing in excess of 100 kg recorded in the literature. The fluid content consists of mucin, and the epithelium lining the cysts presents a characteristic appearance of a secretory epithelium of tall columnar cells with a pseudostratified appearance. This appearance is similar to the epithelium lining the endocervix. The demarcation between epithelial cells and stroma is sharply defined. There is little tendency to form papillae. These tumours are less likely to become malignant than the serous variety.

The only treatment is to remove the tumour surgically.

Care should be taken to avoid rupture of the cysts because mucinous epithelium may implant in the peritoneal cavity, giving rise to a condition known as pseudomyxoma peritonei. Huge amounts of gelatinous material may accumulate in the peritoneal cavity.

Brenner cell tumours

Brenner cell tumours are commonly solid and occur in women after the age of 50 years. They are only rarely malignant. The histological features of these tumours include nests of epithelial cells surrounded by fibromatous connective tissue groundwork.

The cut surface of the tumour is similar to that of an ovarian fibroma apart from a rather yellowish tinge. The tumours are occasionally bilateral and can be safely treated by local excision.

Sex cord stromal tumours

Hormone-secreting tumours of the ovary are a small but important group.

Granulosa cell tumours

Arising from ovarian granulosa cells, these tumours (Fig. 23.13) produce oestrogens and constitute some 3% of all solid ovarian tumours. Approximately 25% exhibit the characteristics of malignancy. As granulosa cell tumours can present at any age, the symptoms depend on the age of occurrence. Tumours arising before puberty produce precocious sexual development and, in women of the reproductive age, prolonged oestrogen stimulation results in cystic glandular hyperplasia and irregular and prolonged vaginal bleeding. Around 50% of cases occur after the menopause and present with postmenopausal bleeding. If the tumour is histologically benign, the surgery should be limited to oophorectomy. If there is evidence of malignancy, pelvic clearance is indicated.

Thecomas or theca cell tumours arise from the spindle-shaped thecal cells but are often mixed with granulosa cells and are oestrogen secreting. The presence of a thecoma in one ovary is commonly associated with diffuse thecomatosis in the contralateral ovary.

Arrhenoblastomas or androblastomas

These are tumours of Sertoli–Leydig cells. They are rare androgen-secreting tumours that occur most frequently in the decade between 20 and 30 years of age. The clinical manifestations include the onset of amenor-rhoea, loss of breast tissue, increasing facial and body hirsutism, deepening of the voice and enlargement of the clitoris. The diagnosis is established by the exclusion of virilizing adrenal tumours and the identification of a tumour in one ovary. The condition is treated by excision of the affected ovary. Approximately 25% of these tumours are malignant.

Germ cell tumours

Tumours of germ cell origin may replicate stages resembling the early embryo.

Mature cystic teratoma (dermoid cyst)

Benign cystic teratomas account for 12–15% of true ovarian neoplasms. They contain a large number of embryonic elements such as skin, hair, adipose and muscle tissue, bone, teeth and cartilage (Fig. 23.14). Some of the components can be recognized on radiography.

These tumours are often chance findings as they are commonly asymptomatic unless they undergo torsion or rupture, when the release of sebaceous material causes an acute chemical peritonitis. Dermoid cysts tend to be anterior to the uterus. They are bilateral in 12% of cases, and, although usually benign, become malignant in approximately 2%. Some specialized elements in these tumours become predominant. The growth of thyroid tissue (struma ovarii) may induce a state of hyperthyroidism.

These cysts should be excised from the ovary with conservation of ovarian tissue. They are frequently bilateral and it is important to examine both ovaries before proceeding to surgical excision.

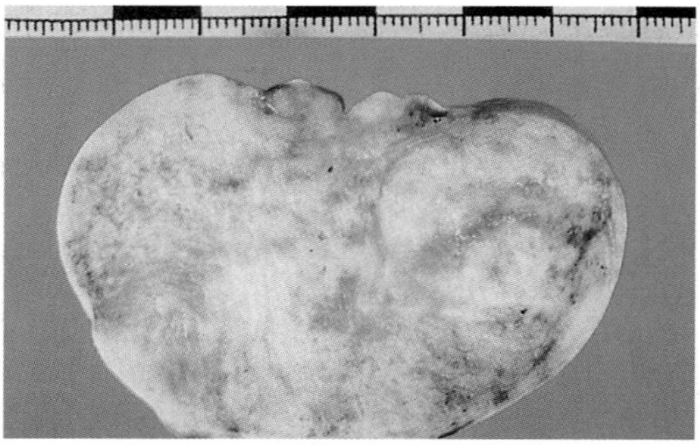

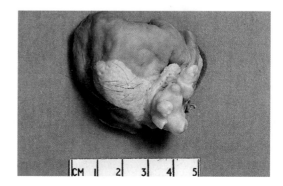

Fig. 23.13 Granulosa cell /theca cell tumour. This shows haemorrhagic areas in the solid white surface of the cut tumour.

Fig. 23.14 Dermoid cyst (benign cystic teratoma) containing teeth and hair.

Dermoid cysts are the commonest solid ovarian neoplasm found in young women.

Fibromas

These solid tumours of the ovary are rare. They may be associated with the presence of ascites or hydrothorax – a condition known as Meigs' syndrome.

Tumour-like conditions

This group includes endometriotic cysts, pregnancy luteomas and germinal cell cysts. The treatment depends on the nature of the tumour and normally involves simple excision of the cysts.

Endometriotic cysts

Endometriomas contain chocolate-coloured fluid representing the accumulation of altered blood, and have a thick fibrous capsule (Fig. 23.15). The lining may consist of endometrial cells but in old cysts these may disappear. Management is discussed below.

MALIGNANT OVARIAN TUMOURS

Ovarian cancer is the fourth commonest cause of death from malignant disease in women in the UK. It follows breast, large intestine and lung cancer in frequency and accounts for approximately 5% of all cancer deaths in women. There are approximately 17 new cases of ovarian cancer per year for every 100 000 women in England and Wales. The incidence increases with age from fewer than 5/100 000 in women under 35 to 40/100 000 in women over 45.

The 5-year survival figure is approximately 35–40%. The poor survival rate is attributable to late diagnosis and the resistant nature of many of these tumours.

Aetiology

Although the cause of epithelial ovarian cancer remains unknown, there are now several well-defined factors associated with the disease.

Genetic

About 1% of cases of ovarian cancer occur in women whose families show an autosomal dominant pattern of inheritance of breast and ovarian cancer. Female members of these families have a 40% lifetime risk of developing the disease. Many of these women have been shown to have defects in the *BRCA1* gene locus on chromosome 17, although the exact nature of the defect varies among different families. Women with only a single affected relative also have a two- to threefold increased relative risk of getting ovarian cancer.

Parity and fertility

Multiparous women are at 40% less risk than nulliparous women of developing ovarian cancer, whereas women who have had unsuccessful treatment for infertility seem to be at increased risk. The use of the contraceptive pill may produce up to a 60% reduction in the incidence of the disease in long-term pill users.

Pathology
Primary ovarian carcinoma

The distribution of histological types of ovarian cancers is as follows.

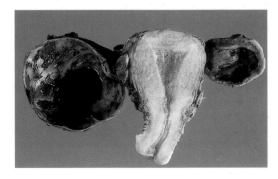

Fig. 23.15 Bilateral endometriomas removed at hysterectomy.

Epithelial type

Tumours of this type, such as serous and mucinous cystadenocarcinomas, make up 85% of cases; 0–15% of these cases are of borderline malignancy. All can be papillary, solid or exophytic. They are described by their gross morphological features, the proportion of stromal tissue they contain and their degree of differentiation.

- **Serous cystadenocarcinoma** is the most common histological type of ovarian carcinoma (40%) and is usually unilocular. They may be bilateral. These tumours are more likely to contain solid areas than their benign counterparts.
- **Mucinous cystadenocarcinomas:** These multicystic tumours (Fig. 23.16) are characterized by mucin-filled cysts lined by columnar glandular cells, and may be associated with tumours of the appendix and gall bladder. The cysts are commonly multilocular.
- **Endometrioid cystadenocarcinomas** resemble endometrial adenocarcinomas and are associated with uterine carcinomas in 20% of cases.
- **Clear-cell cystadenocarcinoma** is the most common ovarian malignancy found in association with ovarian endometriosis. The unilocular thin-walled cysts are lined by epithelium with a typical hobnail appearance and clear cytoplasm.
- **Brenner or transitional cell cystadenocarcinoma** is often found in association with mucinous tumours

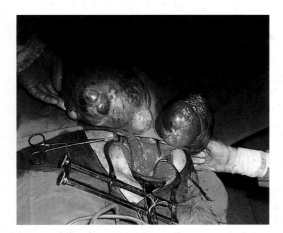

Fig. 23.16 Bilateral multicystic malignant ovarian tumours.

but has a better prognosis than similar tumours arising from the bladder.

Tumours of low malignant or borderline potential account for 10–15% of primary epithelial carcinomas and occur in any of the histological types already mentioned but are most commonly associated with mucinous tumours. There are cytological changes of malignancy including cellular atypia with increased mitosis and multilayering but without invasion. They may present as stage III disease but have a significantly better prognosis than invasive disease, with a 5-year survival of more than 95% for stage I lesions. There is a 10–15% incidence of late recurrence.

Sex cord stromal tumours

These tumours are relatively rare as they make up only 6% of primary ovarian cancers.

- **Granulosa cell tumours:** These solid, unilateral, haemorrhagic tumours are the most common oestrogen-secreting lesions, although some epithelial tumours also secrete oestrogens. They are characterized histologically by the presence of *Call–Exner bodies*.
- **Sertoli–Leydig cell tumours:** Approximately 25% of these are malignant, and, as with benign tumours, they may present with signs and symptoms of androgen excess.

Germ cell tumours

- **Dysgerminomas:** These solid tumours may be small or large enough to fill the abdominal cavity. The cut surface of the tumour has a greyish-pink colour and the microscopic appearance is characteristic. The tumour consists of large polygonal cells arranged in alveoli or nests separated by septa of fibrous tissue. The 5-year survival rate is only 27%.
- **Teratomas:** The malignant or immature form of teratoma is most commonly solid, unilateral and heterogenous with multiple tissue elements. These tumours may produce human chorionic gonadotrophin, alpha-fetoprotein or thyroxine.
- **Endodermal sinus or yolk sac tumours.** Although these tumours make up only 10–15% of germ cell tumours, they are the most common germ cell tumour in children. They are solid, encapsulated tumours containing microcysts lined by flat mesothelial cells.

Secondary ovarian carcinomas

The ovaries are a common site for secondary deposits (metastases) from primary sources in the breast, genital tract, gastrointestinal system and haematopoietic system.

Krukenberg's tumours are metastatic deposits from the gastrointestinal system. They are solid growths that are almost always bilateral and retain the shape of the ovary. The cut surface is variegated in appearance and, although predominantly solid, it often contains areas of cystic degeneration.

The stroma is often richly cellular and may appear to be myomatous. The epithelial elements occur as clusters of well-marked acini with cells exhibiting mucoid change. These cells are often known as signet cells. Secondary ovarian tumours may be much larger than the primary lesion, and tumour deposits in the liver, in particular, suggest primary malignancies in the bowel.

The mechanism by which tumour deposits occur in the ovary is not clear, but there are four possible methods that are likely:

- Direct implantation of cancer cells on the surface of the ovary after transcoelomic spread from the primary site
- Lymphatic metastasis
- Blood-borne spread
- Extension of tumour by direct spread from contiguous structures.

The same principles apply to the spread of primary ovarian tumours.

Staging of ovarian carcinoma

Staging of ovarian carcinoma (Table 23.2) is important in determining both prognosis and the method of management. Ideally, it should be staged at the time of laparotomy with inspection and biopsy of the peritoneum and diaphragm, cytological examination of any peritoneal fluid and selective sampling of the pelvic and para-aortic lymph nodes.

 Up to 20% of apparently stage I and II lesions will have nodal involvement.

Diagnosis

Ovarian carcinoma commonly remains asymptomatic until late in the course of the disease and is detected as a

---

Table 23.2
FIGO classification of ovarian carcinoma

Stage I	Growth limited to the ovaries:	
	Stage IA:	Growth limited to one ovary, no ascites and no tumour present on the external surface; capsule intact
	Stage IB:	Growth limited to both ovaries, no ascites and no tumour present on the external surface; capsule intact
	Stage IC:	Stage 1A or 1B where there is tumour on the surface of either ovary; or with ruptured capsules or with ascites containing malignant cells or positive peritoneal washings
Stage II	Growth involving one or both ovaries with pelvic extension:	
	Stage IIA:	Extension and/or metastases to the uterus and tubes
	Stage IIB:	Extension to other pelvic tissues
	Stage IIC:	Stage IIA and IIB with tumour on the surface of either ovary or positive peritoneal washings or malignant ascites
Stage III	Growth involving one or both ovaries with peritoneal implants outside the pelvis or positive retroperitoneal or inguinal lymph nodes:	
	Stage IIIA:	Microscopic seeding of abdominal peritoneal surfaces
	Stage IIIB:	Macroscopic disease outside the pelvis less than 2 cm in diameter
	Stage IIIC:	Abdominal implants greater than 2 cm and/or positive nodes
Stage IV	Growth involving one or both ovaries with distant metastases including parenchymal (but not superficial) liver metastases and pleural effusions containing malignant cells	

mass on pelvic examination. Where symptoms do occur, these are due to distension, torsion or bleeding (causing pain), pressure effects on adjacent structures and hormone effects (postmenopausal bleeding, virilization). The clinical findings are of a solid or cystic mass arising from the pelvis. The uterus is felt separately. There may be associated ascites. An ultrasound scan will usually exclude other causes of pelvic mass such as fibroids and show features of malignant change such as solid areas within the cyst or free fluid. A chest X-ray should be done to look for pleural effusions. CT or MRI scans (Fig. 23.17) may give an indication of

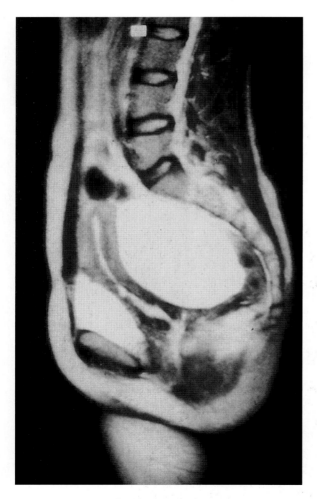

Fig. 23.17 MRI of a large ovarian cyst. The tumour can be seen distending the uterus and elongating the endometrium.

spread but will not usually alter management. Ovarian carcinoma is associated with increased serum levels of a number of oncofetal proteins, of which CA125 is the most important. However, 15% of ovarian carcinomas will have normal levels.

Management

Treatment is based on surgical excision or debulking and chemotherapy. Surgery involves abdominal hysterectomy, bilateral salpingo-oophorectomy, omentectomy and careful inspection and sampling of peritoneal surfaces and retroperitoneal lymph nodes. The aim is to remove all macroscopic disease or, failing this, to leave no tumour deposits of greater than 2 cm in diameter. Subsequent prognosis is proportional to the amount of disease remaining after primary surgery, and such optimal debulking should be possible in up to 75% of tumours in experienced hands. Surgery is followed by chemotherapy.

Chemotherapy

Traditionally this has been used as adjuvant therapy in all but well or moderately differentiated stage 1A tumours. However, the results of a recently completed Medical Research Council study suggest that, even in early-stage disease, there may be a survival advantage in giving such treatment.

The platinum-based drugs cisplatin and carboplatin are currently the mainstay of treatment. These are given parenterally at 3–4 weekly intervals for up to 6 courses. The main side effects are marrow suppression, neurotoxicity and renal toxicity (less with carboplatin). The overall response rate is 60–80%, and this is further improved if combined therapy with alkylating agents such as cyclophosphamide is used. The use of another drug, paclitaxel, in the treatment of primary disease remains controversial.

Although chemotherapy prolongs median survival and the disease-free interval, it has had little impact on 5-year survival.

Radiotherapy

This can be given as external beam or by intraperitoneal instillation of phosphorus-32 but is less widely used.

Borderline tumours

These can be treated by unilateral oophorectomy in young women wishing to preserve their reproductive capacity, although careful, long-term follow-up is required.

Germ cell tumours

These are more common in young women, and chemotherapy may be curative without hysterectomy. These patients should, therefore, be referred to specialist gynaecological oncology centres for treatment.

Follow-up and treatment of recurrence

This is carried out by measurement of tumour markers, clinical examination and imaging. Further surgery after chemotherapy (interval debulking) or for recurrence does not appear to improve survival but may be of palliative value. The response to further chemotherapy depends on the interval between original treatment and recurrence. Where this is short, response is poor, although some platinum-resistant tumours will respond to paclitaxel. In the absence of effective second-line treatment, the routine use of second-look staging operations has no value.

Prognosis

The overall 5-year survival is now 35–40%. This figure has improved somewhat over recent decades but the prognosis remains poor compared to the other main gynaecological cancers. The 5-year survival figures depend on the stage and on whether the tumour has or has not been completely removed (Table 23.3).

The impact of eruption of the tumour through the capsule is seen in the difference in survival in the various grades of stage I lesion (Table 23.4).

Screening for ovarian cancer

Because the prognosis for early-stage disease is better than that for advanced disease it has been suggested that, if the disease could be diagnosed earlier in asymptomatic women, overall survival might be improved. The two main methods that have been proposed for use in screening are ultrasound and CA125 measurement.

Ultrasound examination. As many cysts in premenopausal women are functional (follicular or corpus luteum) more than one measurement may be required. Suspicious features are increasing size, internal septa, solid areas within the cyst and increased blood flow (Doppler). False-positive results may be due to benign ovarian tumours (which might need to be removed in

Table 23.3
Survival, stage and tumour removal (5-year survival, %)

Stage	Incomplete tumour excision	Complete tumour excision
I	–	62
II	15	50
III	8	30
IV	5	–

Table 23.4
Survival rates for stage I tumours

Stage	5-year survival (%)
Stage IA low potential malignancy	95
Stage IA carcinomas	69
Stage IB low potential malignancy	92
Stage IB carcinomas	43
Stage IC carcinomas	40

Case study
Malignant ovarian tumour

A 39-year-old woman with two children attended a gynaecological clinic accompanied by her general practitioner. She had no gynaecological symptoms but requested abdominal hysterectomy and removal of her ovaries on the basis of her family history. She was one of seven sisters, and she produced copies of the death certificates of three of her sisters, all of whom had died from ovarian cancer. The request was agreed, and pelvic clearance was performed. The histology of her ovaries was normal. This procedure was performed in the mid-1970s, and while this woman was in hospital recovering from her surgery, news came through to the ward that a fourth sister had been admitted to hospital with advanced ovarian cancer, from which she subsequently died. The two remaining sisters were located and offered pelvic clearance. One had a small Brenner cell tumour and subsequently died from bowel carcinoma. The remaining sister, along with the original sister, have both survived.

any case), endometriosis and inflammatory masses. Screening needs to be done centrally and requires some operator expertise.

CA125 is a glycoprotein shed by 85% of epithelial tumours. Cut-off levels of between 30IU/l and 65 IU/l have been used for screening. CA125 lacks sufficient specificity if used alone but can be used as a primary screen to identify candidates for ultrasound. It has the advantage that it does not require specialist expertise or equipment at the point of collection. False positives occur in other malignancies (liver, pancreas), endometriosis, pelvic inflammatory disease and early pregnancy. Sensitivity can be improved by looking at serial measurements in women with borderline values. Up to 50% of stage 1 tumours will have a value of less than 35 IU/l.

Ultrasound, either used alone or in combination with CA125, now appears to have sufficient sensitivity and specificity for screening but most studies to date have not compared long-term death rates in screened and unscreened populations. Several large multicentre studies

randomizing women into screened and unscreened controls are in progress but at the moment the value of screening the general population remains unproven. Women with hereditary disease should be offered testing where possible to see if they are carriers of an abnormal *BRCA* gene. Carriers may be offered annual screening with ultrasound and CA125 and prophylactic oophorectomy when their family is complete. Even in this groups the effect of such an approach on increased survival is unproven.

ENDOMETRIOSIS

This terms describes the presence of extrauterine implants of endometrial-like tissue consisting of glands and stroma, often surrounded by an inflammatory response. These implants have receptors for oestrogen and progesterone and the capacity to respond to stimulation by these hormones. Endometriosis affects up to 15% of fertile women and 40–50% of women presenting with infertility.

Pathology

Aberrant endometrial deposits occur in many different sites (Fig. 23.18). Endometriosis commonly occurs in the ovaries (Fig. 23.19), the uterosacral ligaments and the rectovaginal septum. It may also occur in the pelvic peritoneum covering the uterus, tubes, rectum, sigmoid colon and bladder. Remote ectopic deposits of endometrium may be found in the umbilicus, laparotomy

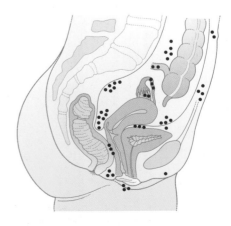

Fig. 23.18 Common sites of endometriotic deposits.

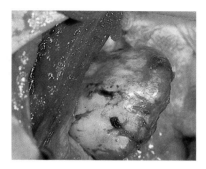

Fig. 23.19 Endometriotic patches on the surface of the ovary.

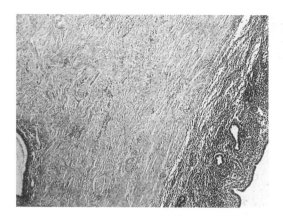

Fig. 23.21 High-powered magnification showing active epithelial lining of the cavity of an endometriotic deposit in scar tissue.

scars (Fig. 23.20), hernial scars, the appendix, vagina, vulva, cervix, lymph nodes and, on rare occasions, the pleural cavity.

Ovarian endometriosis occurs in the form of small superficial deposits on the surface of the ovary or as larger cysts known as endometriomas (Fig. 23.15) which may grow up to 10 cm in size. These cysts have a thick, whitish capsular layer and contain altered blood, which has a chocolate-like appearance. For this reason, they are known as chocolate cysts. Endometriomas are often densely adherent both to the ovarian tissue and to other surrounding structures.

These cysts are likely to rupture and, in 8% of cases, patients with endometriosis present with symptoms of acute peritoneal irritation.

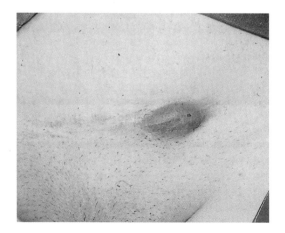

Fig. 23.20 Endometriosis in a caesarean section scar. The dark tender mass at the left of the wound becomes tender and enlarged during menstruation.

The microscopic features of the lesions may be of endometrium (Fig. 23.21) that cannot be distinguished from the normal tissue lining the uterine cavity, but there is wide variation and, in many long-standing cases, desquamation and repeated menstrual bleeding may result in the loss of all characteristic features of endometrium. Underneath the lining of the cyst, there is often a broad zone containing phagocytic cells with haemosiderin. There is also a broad zone of hyalinized fibrous tissue. One of the characteristics of endometriotic lesions is the intense fibrotic reaction that surrounds them, and this may also contain muscle fibres. The intensity of this reaction often leads to great difficulty in dissection at the time of any operative procedure. The pathogenesis of endometriosis remains obscure. Sampson (1921) originally suggested that the condition was associated with retrograde spill of endometrial cells during menstruation and that some of these cells would implant under appropriate conditions in the peritoneal cavity and on the ovaries. This hypothesis does not account for endometriotic deposits outside the peritoneal cavity. An alternative theory suggests that endometrial lesions may arise from metaplastic changes in epithelium surfaces throughout the body.

Symptoms and signs

Although the diagnosis of endometriosis is most commonly made in the third decade of life, the first symptoms usually occur at an earlier age. It is more common in women of low parity. A substantial number of women are asymptomatic and present only with a history of subfertility. The mechanism of the association between subfertility and endometriosis is unknown, and cannot be explained in most instances by distension or obstruction of the tubes. An alternative explanation is that endometriosis is commonly associated with the LUF (luteinized unruptured follicles) syndrome.

The commonest symptom is crescendic dysmenorrhoea. Pelvic pain and swelling commence in the week preceding menstruation and dysmenorrhoea persists until the completion of the period. If an endometrioma ruptures, generalized abdominal pain and peritonism may occur.

If the uterus becomes fixed or there is any adnexal mass adherent in the pouch of Douglas, deep-seated dyspareunia results. Menstrual disorders are not a common feature of endometriosis but if the ovaries are extensively involved the cycle may shorten and under these circumstances menorrhagia may also occur.

The symptoms produced by lesions outside the peritoneal cavity depend on the site of the lesion. Involvement of bowel may result in rectal bleeding or, if the lesion has caused scarring and fibrosis, in bowel obstruction. Lesions of the bladder may cause haematuria. Cutaneous lesions at the umbilicus, in skin wounds and at the vulva will bleed externally on a cyclical basis. Occasionally, lesions in the thorax cause recurrent haemothorax or haemoptysis.

Diagnosis

In a small number of cases, the lesion is visible on the surface but in most patients nothing abnormal is visible or palpable on pelvic examination. In well-established disease, the uterus is often fixed in retroversion. There is thickening in the uterosacral ligaments and, if the ovaries are involved, there may be fixed cystic swellings palpable in the pelvis.

The diagnosis can be established only by direct inspection by laparoscopy or at the time of laparotomy. Cysts can be identified by ultrasound or by magnetic resonance imaging. Endometriosis is associated with an elevated serum CA125 level.

 It is important to remember that endometriosis is found in asymptomatic women and in those with pain it may not correlate with, or be the cause of, their symptoms.

Management

Medical therapy

Endometriosis is a difficult condition to treat, and therapy is determined by the presenting symptoms and the nature of the endometriotic lesion. It is often necessary to combine both medical and surgical treatment if the best results are to be obtained.

 Recurrence is common after all forms of treatment with symptoms returning in a third of women with mild disease and three-quarters of those with severe disease within 5 years.

Endometriotic deposits respond in the same way as normal endometrium. Thus, pregnancy usually induces marked regression of the lesions. However, as the condition is commonly associated with infertility, this is rarely a practical solution to the problem and medical treatment does not improve fertility rates in patients presenting with infertility. Medical therapy depends on the concept of inducing a pseudopregnancy and is most effective in the treatment of small lesions. These effects can be achieved by administration of various drugs.

- The combined oral contraceptive pill is effective in reducing non-menstrual pain and dyspareunia, although less effective for dysmenorrhoea unless given continuously. Its major advantage is that it can be used indefinitely but the reduction in the amount of disease may be less than other treatments.
- Progestogens act through pituitary suppression of gonadotrophins, resulting in anovulation and a mildly hypo-oestrogenic state. The effectiveness is similar to that of other treatments, with 70–80% of patients reporting symptomatic improvement. Up to 75% of patients will be amenorrhoeic. Other side effects include weight gain, acne, bloating, depression and breakthrough bleeding. Dydrogesterone 10 mg three times daily is usually sufficient to inhibit menstruation and to produce regression of small lesions. A similar effect can be achieved with oral medroxyprogesterone acetate 10 mg three times a day over 9 months. Levonorgestrel, as part of the Mirena® intrauterine system, has been used in the treatment of endometriosis.

An alternative approach to therapy is to induce a pseudomenopause. The decision on which drugs to use depends principally upon their side-effect profiles, because they relieve pain associated with endometriosis equally well.

Danazol is a weak impeded androgen that causes marked gonadotrophin inhibition with minimal overt sex hormone stimulation. This produces suppression of all endogenous stimuli to the endometrium and allows regression to occur in endometriotic deposits. Given in adequate dosage, the drug induces complete suppression of menstruation, but cessation of therapy results in the resumption of menstruation within 6 weeks. The required dosage is between 200 and 600 mg daily for 6–9 months. The drug may produce side effects that are not tolerable and may necessitate cessation of therapy. These include weight gain, oedema, fatigue, depression, increased hair growth, acne and reduced breast size. Up to 90% of patients report significant improvement in symptoms after 6 months of treatment.

Gestrinone, which is a synthetic trienic 19-norsteroid, may be used as an alternative therapy. The drug acts by inhibiting ovarian steroidogenesis and is taken twice weekly. It has similar side effects to danazol but in a smaller proportion of patients.

Gonadotrophin-releasing hormone analogues (GnRHa) are synthetic peptides that bind competitively to pituitary GnRH receptors, causing downregulation in the release of follicle-stimulating hormone and luteinizing hormone. These compounds can be administered as monthly depot injections or implants (leuprorelin, goserelin) or as a twice-daily nasal spray (nafarelin, buserelin). Menopausal side effects such as flushes, vaginal dryness and breast atrophy are common, but androgenic side effects are minimal. Long-term use is limited to 6 months because of a reversible loss of bone density. These side effects can be ameliorated by the concurrent administration of 'add-back' hormone replacement therapy without any apparent reduction in effectiveness.

None of these treatments are compatible with pregnancy during the period of treatment, with the possible exception of progestogens given during the luteal phase. Symptomatic treatment of pain with non-steroidal anti-inflammatory drugs may be an effective 'non-hormonal' alternative.

Surgical treatment

Skin lesions can be cured by excision. Diathermy or laser ablation of small lesions is associated with improvement in symptoms and fertility rates in women with mild to moderate degrees of disease. A laparoscopic approach is associated with lower morbidity and subsequent problems with adhesions but requires a high degree of expertise in patients with severe disease. Postoperative medical treatment may prolong the length of time patients remain pain-free.

Where large endometriomatous deposits occur, as with ovarian endometriomas, medical therapy is rarely effective and it is necessary to resect these lesions. Every attempt should be made to conserve ovarian tissue in these circumstances. In a limited number of situations where conservation of reproductive potential is important, pain relief can be achieved by presacral neurectomy. This procedure involves surgical transection of the presacral plexus with excision of tissue between the right ureter and superior haemorrhoidal vessels.

If all these procedures fail or there is no desire for conservation of reproductive function, then pelvic clearance is indicated with total hysterectomy and bilateral salpingo-oophorectomy. Even after such surgery, peritoneal deposits of disease may remain and approximately 10% of patients will experience a recurrence of the symptoms after hysterectomy, even with removal of both ovaries.

ESSENTIAL INFORMATION

Congenital abnormalities of the uterus

- Due to failure of müllerian ducts to fuse or develop
- Usually asymptomatic unless menstrual flow obstructed
- May cause recurrent abortion, malpresentation or retained placenta
- May be associated with abnormalities of the renal tract

Benign uterine tumours

- Commonest are endometrial polyps and fibroids
- 20% of women over 30 years old have fibroids
- Symptoms depend on size and site and include menstrual disorders, pressure symptoms and complications of pregnancy
- May undergo secondary change including necrosis or malignant change (0.13–1%)
- Management depends on size and need to preserve reproductive function

Endometrial carcinoma

- Disease of postmenopausal women
- Risk factors include obesity, nulliparity, late menopause, glucose intolerance and unopposed oestrogens
- Commonly presents as postmenopausal bleeding
- Spreads by direct invasion but tends to remain localized within the uterus initially
- Well-differentiated early stage disease can be treated by hysterectomy alone; more advanced lesions require radiotherapy ± progestational agents
- Has 90% 5-year survival if diagnosed early

Functional ovarian cysts

- Usually less than 6 cm in size
- May arise from follicles, corpus luteum or as a result of exogenous gonadotrophins

- Can produce sex steroids and affect menstruation
- Can be monitored by ultrasound
- Usually regress spontaneously
- Require surgical intervention if the source of significant intraperitoneal bleeding

Benign ovarian neoplasia

- May be solid, cystic or mixed
- Commonly present as asymptomatic abdominal mass but occasionally with hormone effects or pain
- Mostly serous or mucinous epithelial tumours but germ cell tumours more common in younger patients
- Differential diagnosis includes endometriosis, functional cysts and malignant tumours

Malignant ovarian tumours

- Fourth commonest cause of cancer deaths in women
- Affect 1/75 women by the age of 75 years
- Cause unknown – ?'super-ovulation'
- 75% cases present with advanced disease
- Most cases are epithelial in type
- Prognosis depends on stage at diagnosis and extent of residual disease after initial surgery
- 5-year survival 35–40%
- Incidence increases with age
- Shows an autosomal dominant pattern of inheritance in 1% of cases

Endometriosis and adenomyosis

- 'Ectopic' endometrium
- Commonest sites are ovaries, uterosacral ligaments and pelvic peritoneum
- May arise from metaplastic change or implantation
- Presents as subfertility and/or crescendic dysmenorrhoea
- Management is to induce pseudopregnancy or pseudomenopause, or surgical excision

24 Lesions of the lower genital tract

BENIGN LESIONS OF THE VULVA

There have been numerous changes in the classification of vulvar disease, and the previous terminology of 'vulval dystrophies' has been discarded. The classification now recommended is summarized in Table 24.1.

This classification is based on histological appearances. Where there is histological evidence of cellular atypia, the lesion should be classified as vulvar intraepithelial neoplasia. Other dermatoses include psoriasis, lichen planus, lichen simplex chronicus, *Candida* infection and condyloma acuminatum. Mixed epithelial conditions may occur, and it is recommended that both descriptions should be used under these circumstances.

Non-neoplastic epithelial disorders

Lichen sclerosus (lichen sclerosus et atrophicus)

This most commonly affects postmenopausal women. It is characterized by pale, thin vulval skin with loss of

---

Table 24.1
Classification of disorders of vulval skin

Non-neoplastic epithelial disorders of skin and mucosa:
    Lichen sclerosus (lichen sclerosus et atrophicus)
    Squamous cell hyperplasia (formerly hyperplastic dystrophy)
    Other dermatoses

Vulvar intra-epithelial neoplasia (VIN):
    Squamous VIN
        VIN I: Mild dysplasia (formally mild atypia)
        VIN II: Moderate dysplasia (formally moderate atypia)
        VIN III: Severe dysplasia (formally severe atypia).
    Non-squamous VIN
        Paget's disease

The epithelial disorders are associated in about 5% of cases with malignant change, the development of which is always preceded by atypical changes.

Treatment

It is important to inspect the vulva with good light and magnification, and biopsy the skin to establish an accurate diagnosis (Fig. 24.2). Common infections, such as with *Trichomonas* and *Candida*, should be excluded, and a full history of onset, previous treatments, other skin complaints and illnesses such as diabetes should be taken. General advice on hygiene and potential irritants, clothing and barrier creams should be given. Treatment is medical, with long-term follow-up for early detection of malignant change. The mainstay of treatment is topical steroids, using short courses of high-potency

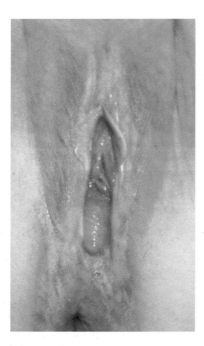

Fig. 24.1 Lichen sclerosus. The histological findings are of thinning of the epithelium, subepidermal hyalinization and the presence of a deep band of inflammatory cells.

the labia minora, often accompanied by narrowing of the introitus and fissuring of the skin. The condition also affects the perineum and perianal skin (Fig. 24.1). Vulval pruritus and soreness are the usual presenting symptoms and superficial dyspareunia is common.

Other dermatoses

Vulval skin can be affected by a wide range of conditions that affect other skin surfaces; these include allergic dermatitis, psoriasis, intertrigo and lichen planus.

Aetiology

The cause of non-neoplastic epithelial disorders is unknown. Lichen sclerosus is associated with a high incidence (21%) of autoimmune disorders, including pernicious anaemia, hypothyroidism and hyperthyroidism.

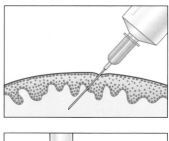
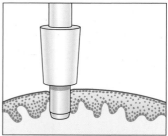
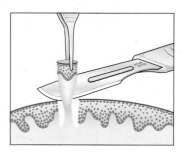

Fig. 24.2 Diagnosis of vulval skin lesions using Keye's punch biopsy under local anaesthetic.

creams such as clobetasol propionate applied twice a day for 6 weeks followed by a moderately potent steroid such as betamethasone for a further 6 weeks. Where maintenance therapy is needed to control symptoms this should be with low-potency creams such as 0.1% hydrocortisone to avoid steroid thinning of the skin. Surgery is indicated for excision of suspicious lesions or to restore normal function where the anatomy has been distorted.

If all conservative therapy fails, it may be necessary to remove the affected skin by simple vulvectomy or excision biopsy or LASER ablation of visible lesions. However, the conditions have a tendency to reoccur.

Benign tumours of the vulva

Benign cysts of the vulva include sebaceous cysts, epithelial inclusion cysts and wolffian duct cysts (Fig. 24.3), which arise from the labia minora and the per-urethral region, and Bartholin's cysts, which have been described elsewhere. A rare cyst may arise from a peritoneal extension along the round ligament, forming a hydrocele in the labium major. Benign solid tumours include fibromas, lipomas and hidradenomas. True squamous papillomas appear as warty growths and rarely become malignant. All these lesions are treated by simple biopsy excision.

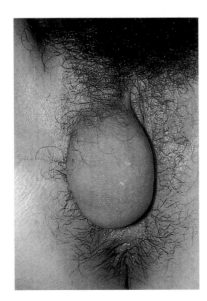

Fig. 24.3 Benign vulval cyst arising from remnant of the wolffian duct.

VULVAL AND VAGINAL TRAUMA

Injuries to the vulva and vagina may result in severe haemorrhage and haematoma formation. Vulval bruising may be particularly severe because of the rich venous plexus in the labia, and commonly results from falling astride. Lacerations of the vagina are often associated with coitus. Vulval haematomas often subside with conservative management but sometimes need drainage. It is important to suture vaginal lacerations and to be certain that the injury does not penetrate into the peritoneal cavity.

NEOPLASTIC LESIONS OF THE VULVA
Vulval intraepithelial neoplasia

Vulval intraepithelial neoplasia (VIN) is a condition characterized by disorientation and loss of epithelial architecture extending through the full thickness of the epithelium but not penetrating the basement membrane. The grading (Table 24.1) is based on the extent to which normal epithelium is replaced by abnormal dysplastic cells. There is an association with similar changes to the cervix (CIN) and in the perianal region (PAIN), although the link with human papilloma virus (HPV) infection is not as clear as it is in the cervix. Around 40% of cases occur in women under the age of 41 years. It was originally known as Bowen's disease.

Vulval intraepithelial neoplasia may be asymptomatic. Where symptoms do occur these include vulval soreness, pruritus and the feeling of a 'lump'. The clinical manifestations range from erythematous or ulcerated areas to slightly raised areas on the vulva.

A further variant that arises from the apocrine glands is known as *Paget's disease*. The appearance of the lesions is variable, but they are popular and raised, may be white, grey, dull red or various shades of brown, and may be localized or widespread. These conditions are rare, with an incidence of 0.53/100 000, and commonly occur in women over the age of 50 years.

> **!** Paget's disease is associated with underlying adenocarcinoma or primary malignancy elsewhere in 20% of cases.

Management

The only satisfactory treatment of this condition is local excision. Recurrence occurs in up to 50% of cases within 4 years. It is important to establish the diagnosis by biopsy and to search for any other sites of intra-epithelial neoplasia, which are commonly found in association with the vulval lesion, particularly the cervix and vagina. Up to 20% of patients will have occult squamous carcinoma in areas excised for suspected VIN and the risk of subsequent progression to invasive disease is 5%, so that long-term follow-up with excision biopsy of suspicious lesions is essential.

Carcinoma of the vulva

Carcinoma of the vulva accounts for 4% of female malignancies. 90% of the lesions are squamous cell carcinomas, 5% are adenocarcinomas, 1% are basal carcinomas and 0.5% are malignant melanomas. Carcinoma of the vulva most commonly occurs in the sixth and seventh decades. Predisposing conditions include VIN and lichen sclerosus, and there is an association with chronic vulvitis, diabetes, hypertension and obesity.

Symptoms

The patient with vulval carcinoma experiences pruritus and notices a raised lesion on the vulva, which may ulcerate and bleed (Fig. 24.4). Malignant melanomas are usually single, hyperpigmented and ulcerated. The tumour most frequently develops on the labia majora (50% of cases) but may also grow on the prepuce of the clitoris, the labia minora, Bartholin's glands and in the vestibule of the vagina.

Natural history

The disease tends to progress from an area of VIN through carcinoma-in-situ to invasion. Spread occurs both locally and through the lymphatic system. The lymph nodes involved are the superficial and deep inguinal nodes and the femoral nodes (Fig. 24.5). Pelvic lymph nodes, except in primary lesions involving the clitoris, have usually only secondary involvement. In particular, the external iliac and obturator nodes are

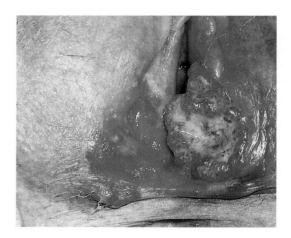

Fig. 24.4 Ulcerative squamous cell carcinoma of the vulva.

involved. Vascular spread is late and rare. The disease usually progresses slowly and the terminal stages are accompanied by extensive ulceration, infection, haemorrhage and remote metastatic disease. In some 30% of cases, lymph nodes are involved on both sides. Stages are defined by the International Federation of Obstetrics and Gynaecology (FIGO) on the basis of surgical rather than clinical findings (Table 24.2).

Therapy

Stage IA disease can be treated by wide local excision. Stage 1B lesions that are at least 2 cm lateral to the midline are treated by wide local excision and unilateral groin node dissection. All other stages are treated by wide radical local excisions or radical vulvectomy and bilateral groin node dissection. This procedure involves extensive removal of the vulval and bilateral inguinal nodes and pelvic lymphadenectomy (Fig. 24.6). Postoperative radiotherapy has a role to play in patients where the tumour extends close to the excision margin or there is involvement of the groin nodes. Preoperative radiotherapy may be used in cases of extensive disease to reduce the tumour volume. Complications of radical vulvectomy include wound breakdown and lymphoedema (30%), secondary bleeding, thromboembolism and psychological morbidity. Response to chemotherapy (bleomycin) is generally poor. Patients are followed up at intervals of 3–6 months for 5 years.

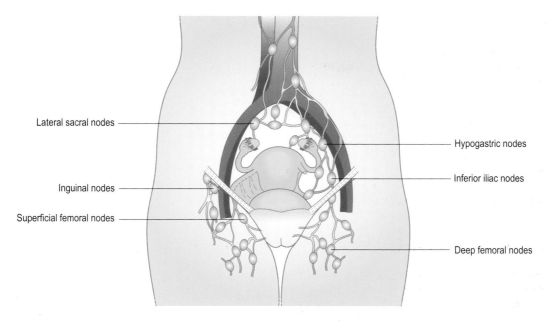

Fig. 24.5 Lymphatic drainage of the vulva.

Table 24.2
FIGO Staging of vulval cancer

Stage I   Tumour confined to the vulva – 2 cm or less in diameter. Nodes are not involved.
    A. Lesions less than 1 mm depth invasion
    B. Other lesions less than 2 cm in diameter
Stage II   Tumour confined to the vulva – more than 2 cm in diameter. Nodes are not involved.
Stage III   Tumour of any size with:
    Adjacent spread to the lower urethra and/or the vagina, the perineum and the anus, and/or
    unilateral lymph node involvement.
Stage IV   Tumour of any size with bilateral groin lymph node involvement:
    A. Infiltrating the bladder mucosa or the rectal mucosa, or both, including the upper part of the
    urethral mucosa
    B. Fixed to the bone or other distant metastases. Fixed or ulcerated nodes in either one or both
    groins.

Prognosis

Prognosis is determined by the size of the primary lesion and lymph node involvement. The overall survival rate in operable cases without lymph node involvement is 90% and is up to 98% where the primary lesion is less than 2 cm in size. This falls to 50–60% with node involvement and is less than 30% in patients with bilateral lymph node involvement. Malignant melanoma and adenocarcinoma have a poor prognosis, with a 5-year survival of 5%.

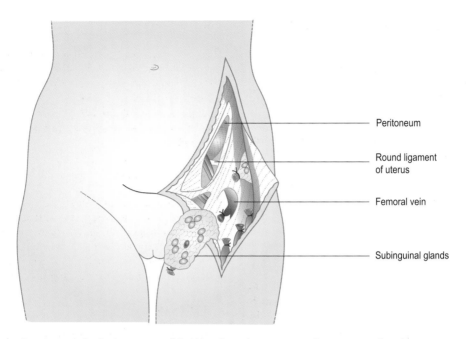

Fig. 24.6 Block dissection of the lymph nodes in surgical treatment of malignant disease of the vulva.

Peritoneum

Round ligament of uterus

Femoral vein

Subinguinal glands

BENIGN TUMOURS OF THE VAGINA

Vaginal cysts

Congenital

Cysts arise in the vagina from embryological remnants; the commonest varieties are those arising from Gartner's duct (wolffian duct remnants). These are not rare and occur in the anterolateral wall of the vagina. They are usually asymptomatic and are found on routine examination.

Histologically, the cysts are lined by cuboidal epithelium but sometimes a flattened layer of stratified squamous epithelium is seen.

The cysts are treated by simple surgical excision and rarely give rise to any difficulties.

Vaginal inclusion cysts

Inclusion cysts arise from inclusion of small particles or islands of vaginal epithelium under the surface. The cysts commonly arise in episiotomy scars and contain yellowish thick fluid. They are treated by simple surgical excision.

Endometriosis

Endometriotic lesions may appear anywhere in the vagina, but occur most commonly in the posterior fornix. The lesions may appear as dark brown spots or reddened ulcerated lesions. The diagnosis is established by excision biopsy. If the lesions are multiple, then medical therapy should be instituted as for lesions in other sites.

Solid benign tumours

These lesions are rare but may represent any of the tissues that are found in the vagina. Thus, polypoid tumours may include fibromyomas, myomas, fibromas, papillomas and adenomyomas. These tumours are treated by simple surgical excision.

Neoplastic lesions of the vaginal epithelium

Vaginal intraepithelial neoplasia

Vaginal intraepithelial neoplasia (VAIN) is usually multicentric and tends to be multifocal and associated with similar lesions of the cervix. The condition is asymptomatic and tends to be discovered because of a positive smear test or during colposcopy for abnormal cytology, often after hysterectomy. There is a risk of progression to invasive carcinoma but the disease remains superficial until then and can be treated by surgical excision, laser ablation or cryosurgery.

Vaginal adenosis

This is the presence of columnar epithelium in the vaginal epithelium and has been found in adult females whose mothers received treatment with diethylstilboestrol during pregnancy. The condition commonly reverts to normal squamous epithelium but in about 4% of cases the lesion progresses to vaginal adenocarcinoma. It is therefore important to follow these women carefully with serial cytology.

MALIGNANT VAGINAL TUMOURS

Primary malignancies of the vagina are very rare. The lesions include squamous cell carcinomas and sarcomas and, rarely, chorioepitheliomas.

Carcinoma of the vagina

Invasive carcinoma of the vagina may be a squamous carcinoma or, occasionally, an adenocarcinoma. Primary lesions arise in the sixth and seventh decades, but are rare in the UK. In recent years, there has been an increase in adenocarcinomas in young women, which has been associated with the administration of diethylstilboestrol during the pregnancies of their mothers. These tumours are of the clear-cell or mesonephric variety.

Secondary deposits from cervical carcinoma and endometrial carcinoma are relatively common in the upper third of the vagina and can sometimes occur in the lower vagina through lymphatic spread.

Symptoms

The symptoms include irregular vaginal bleeding and offensive vaginal discharge when the tumour becomes necrotic and infection supervenes. Infection may also cause pain, and local spread into the rectum, bladder or urethra may result in fistula formation. The tumour may appear as an exophytic lesion or as an ulcerated, indurated mass.

Method of spread

Tumour spread, as previously stated, occurs by direct infiltration or by lymphatic extension. Lesions involving the upper half of the vagina follow a pattern of spread similar to that of carcinoma of the cervix. Tumours of the lower half of the vagina follow a similar pattern of spread to that of carcinoma of the vulva.

Treatment

The diagnosis is established by biopsy of the tumour, and careful evaluation of tumour extension and staging is made before commencing treatment (Table 24.3).

The primary method of treatment is by radiotherapy – both by external beam therapy and by interstitial gamma-ray sources.

Surgical treatment includes radical vaginectomy and anterior or posterior exenteration, but this is rarely used as the primary therapy.

Prognosis

Results of treatment depend on the initial staging and on the method of therapy. Stages I and II have a 5-year survival of around 60% but this figure falls to 30–40%

Table 24.3
Clinical staging of vaginal carcinoma

Stage 0:	Intraepithelial carcinoma
Stage I:	Limited to the vaginal walls
Stage II:	Involves the subvaginal tissue but has not extended to the pelvic wall
Stage III:	The tumour has extended to the lateral pelvic wall
Stage IV:	The lesion has extended to involve adjacent organs (IVA) or has spread to distant organs (IVB)

for stages III and IV. Adenocarcinoma of the vagina, which often occurs in young females, also responds well to irradiation.

Sarcoma botryoides

This is a rare tumour of mixed mesodermal origin that occurs in girls aged 2–3 years. The tumour grows rapidly and may appear at the introitus as a grape-like mass. Combined treatment with radiotherapy and surgery seems to offer the best prospect for cure and may allow conservation of the bladder and rectum, although it is not possible to conserve reproductive function.

LESIONS OF THE CERVIX

Examination of the cervix

Routine examination of the cervix involves direct inspection with a good light and exposure with a bivalve or Sims speculum. The size, shape and consistency of the cervix should be noted and the nature of any discharge recorded. The external cervical os is circular in shape, and in parous women the os is a transverse slit (Fig. 24.7). The nature of the epithelium should be observed, as it will vary according to the hormonal status of the woman. The normal ectocervix is covered with stratified squamous epithelium and the endocervical canal by columnar epithelium. The junction between these two epithelia is known as the *squamo-columnar junction (SCJ)*, and it may be situated at any point across the cervix. The area adjacent to the SCJ is the *transformation zone* and it is in this area that most abnormal changes occur.

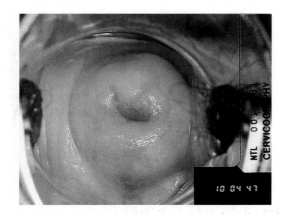

Fig. 24.7 Normal multiparous cervix.

The term *cervical ectopy* or *cervical ectropion* (sometimes incorrectly described as a cervical erosion) is used where the endocervical epithelium appears to advance on to the ectocervix and gives a bright red, velvety appearance. In fact, this reflects no more than the dynamic behaviour of the transformation zone and the SCJ. During pregnancy and adolescence, and in some women on oral contraception, the endocervical epithelium advances outwards, whereas at the menopause, shrinkage occurs with diminution of the exposed area of the transformation zone. In most cases, cervical ectropion is asymptomatic but it is sometimes associated with leukorrhoea and postcoital bleeding.

Management

These conditions are benign and should be treated only when they produce symptoms. Treatment of symptomatic cervical ectopy is by diathermy or cryosurgery. Squamous epithelium grows over the region previously covered by columnar epithelium. For 2 weeks after treatment, the discharge may worsen, with separation of the cauterized epithelium, but within a month the symptoms will either recede or disappear.

Benign neoplasms of the cervix

Cervical polyps

Benign polyps arise from the endocervix and are pedunculated, with a covering of endocervical epithelium and a central fibrous tissue core. The polyps present as bright red, vascular growths that may be identified on routine examination; the presenting symptoms may include irregular vaginal blood loss or postcoital bleeding.

Less frequently, the polyps arise from the squamous epithelium, when the appearance will resemble the surface of the vaginal epithelium.

Small polyps can be avulsed in the outpatient clinic by grasping them with polyp forceps and rotating through 360°. Larger polyps may need ligation of the pedicle and excision of the polyp under general anaesthesia.

Cervical fibroids

Cervical leiomyomas are similar to fibroids in other sites of the uterus. They are commonly pedunculated but may be sessile and grow to a size that will fill the vagina and distort the pelvic organs.

Symptoms are similar to those caused by other cervical polyps and, in addition, the attempted extrusion of fibroid polyps may cause colicky uterine pain, particularly at the time of menstruation.

Treatment is by surgical excision. Many of these lesions have a thick pedicle that must be transfixed and ligated before excision of the polyp. Malignant change in the form of sarcomatous degeneration is extremely rare and is no more frequent than sarcomatous change arising in the myometrium.

Screening for cervical cancer

It has been recognized for 60 years that cervical cytology could be used to identify women with cervical cancer. The aim of modern screening programmes is mainly the detection of the non-invasive precursor of the disease, cervical intra-epithelial neoplasia (CIN) in the asymptomatic population in order to reduce mortality and morbidity. The NHS national cervical screening programme was introduced in England and Wales in 1988 and by 1991 80% of all women between the ages of 20 and 65 were being tested on a 5-yearly basis. Since then mortality from cervical cancer has fallen by 7% a year. Currently all women aged between 20 and 65 are invited for screening every 3–5 years. It has been estimated that cervical screening reduces the risk of dying of cervical cancer by 75%.

Technique (see also History taking and examination in gynaecology)

It is essential to obtain a good view of the cervix. The speculum should be introduced with a minimum of artificial lubricant. Cells are taken from around the cervix from the whole of the transformation zone by taking a smear with a 360° sweep using an Ayres or Aylesbury spatula. Although preinvasive lesions arising from the endocervical epithelium (cervical glandular intraepithelial neoplasia, CGIN) can be identified by cervical cytology, the method is primarily for screening for squamous lesions and cannot reliably exclude endocervical disease.

Cytology

Apart from assessing the cells for signs of malignant change, a smear from the upper third of the vagina can also be used for assessment of hormone status.

The preparation is stained using the Papanicolaou technique. With this method, the nuclei stain blue, the superficial cell cytoplasm pink and the intermediate parabasal cell cytoplasm stains blue/green (Fig. 24.8). The squamous epithelium of the vagina and cervix is composed of four layers as follows (Fig. 24.9).

- **Basal cells:** These lie on the basement membrane and are not usually exfoliated

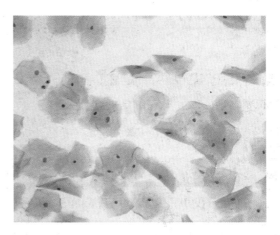

Fig. 24.8 Normal cervical smear showing superficial (pink) and intermediate (blue/green) exfoliated cervical cells (low-power magnification).

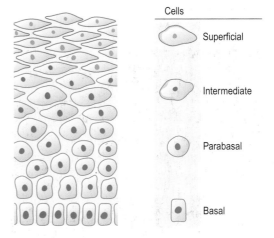

Fig. 24.9 Cell layers in the stratified squamous epithelium of the cervix and vagina.

- **Parabasal cells:** These cells are oval in shape and have a centrally placed nucleus with a cytoplasm that is basophilic
- **Intermediate squamous cells:** These cells are polygonal in shape and have a basophilic cytoplasm, except in the presence of infection when it becomes eosinophilic; the cells lie singly or in clumps with either a flattened or a folded appearance
- **Superficial or mature squamous cells:** Polygonal cells with a pyknotic nucleus and a cytoplasm that is eosinophilic.

Endocervical cells, which are tall and cylindrical, may be seen as well as endometrial cells. Hormone status is assessed by counting the number of squamous cells with a pyknotic nucleus in relation to the rest of the squamous cell population; this is known as the karyopyknotic index (KPI). The KPI is high (50–60%) in the proliferative phase of the cycle and low (0–10%) in the secretory phase.

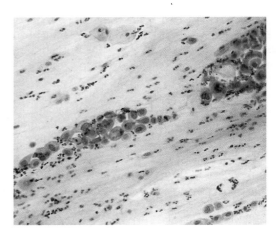

Fig. 24.10 Moderate dyskaryosis. The cells are smaller and the nuclear–cytoplasmic ratio higher when compared to normal cells.

Classification of cervical cytology

The terminology used in the UK for reporting cervical smears was introduced by The British Society for Clinical Cytology in 1986 (Table 24.4). Approximately 10% of smears will be reported as unsuitable for analysis if the cervical cells are obscured by inflammatory or red blood cells.

The term *dyskaryosis* is used to describe those cells that lie between normal squamous and frankly malignant cells and exhibit degrees of nuclear change consistent with malignancy (Fig. 24.10). Cells showing abnormalities that fall short of dyskaryosis are described as borderline. Atypical glandular cells may represent premalignant disease of the endocervix or endometrium.

Malignant cells show nuclear enlargement at the expense of cytoplasmic mass (Fig. 24.11). The nuclei may assume a lobulated outline. There is increased intensity of staining of the nucleus and an increase in the number of mitotic figures.

The Bethesda system of classification used in the United States (Table 24.4) differs by combining moderate and severe dyskaryosis as high-grade squamous intraepithelial lesions (SIL) and using the term atypical squamous cells of undetermined significance (ASCUS) instead of borderline.

The correlation between cytology and histological changes in the cervix is poor, with 30–40% of women with mild dyskaryosis having CIN II or greater. The

Table 24.4 Classification of cervical smears	
UK system	**US Bethesda system**
Negative	Within normal limits
Borderline nuclear abnormalities	ASCUS
? Glandular neoplasia	
Wart virus change	Low-grade SIL
Mild dyskaryosis	
Moderate dyskaryosis	High-grade SIL
Severe dyskaryosis	
Invasive cancer	Invasive cancer

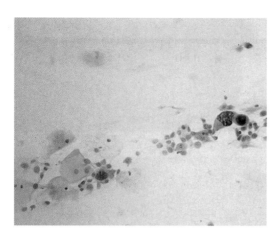

Fig. 24.11 Carcinoma cells. Note the large nuclei and abnormal distribution of chromatin.

overall false-negative rate varies from 2% to 26%. CIN will be detected in 2–3% of the screened population.

Colposcopy

The presence of dyskaryosis or malignant cells on cytology is an indication for examination by colposcopy. A borderline smear will be repeated after 6 months and if borderline changes persist colposcopy is also advised. In some centres, colposcopy for mild dyskaryosis is also deferred until after two successive smears 6 months apart are abnormal. Persistently 'inadequate' smears also require colposcopic examination to exclude any coincidental abnormality.

Colposcopy is inspection of the cervix using a binocular microscope with a light source (colposcope). It is usually an outpatient procedure performed using a speculum to expose the cervix. Squamous neoplasia most often occurs in the areas adjacent to the junction of the columnar (velvety red) and squamous (smooth pink) epithelium or SCJ. If this can not be seen in its entirety, CIN can not be excluded by colposcopic examination and a cone biopsy will be required.

Pathophysiology

The junction of the squamous epithelium that lines the ectocervix and the columnar glandular epithelium of the endocervix, the SCJ, moves in relation to the anatomical external cervical os. Changes in oestrogen such as occur during puberty, pregnancy or while on the pill move the SCJ outwards, exposing columnar epithelium to the lower pH of the vagina. This reacts by undergoing transformation back to squamous epithelium by a process of squamous metaplasia. The area that lies between the current SCJ and that reached as it moves outwards across the ectocervix is the transformation zone and it is here that most preinvasive lesions occur.

It follows then that an adequate colposcopic examination requires that all the SCJ is visualized in order that the entire transformation zone can be inspected.

Neoplastic cells have an increased amount of nuclear material in relation to cytoplasm and less surface glycogen than normal squamous epithelium. They are associated with a degree of hypertrophy of the underlying vasculature. These features are exploited in colposcopic examination. When exposed to 5% acetic acid the nuclear protein will be coagulated, giving the neoplastic cells a characteristic white appearance (Fig. 24.12), but they will not react with Schiller's iodine, unlike the normal squamous epithelium, which will stain dark brown (Fig. 24.13). The increased capillary vascularity may be visible through the epithelium as red dots or punctation or a 'crazy paving' mosaic pattern.

Colposcopic appearances

Cervical intraepithelial neoplasia appears as a white area with a well-defined edge following application of 5% acetic acid solution (Fig. 24.12). Small blood vessels beneath the epithelium may be seen as dots (punctation) or a crazy paving pattern (mosaicism). CIN can also be identified by the use of Schiller's iodine solution which stains normal cervical epithelium dark brown

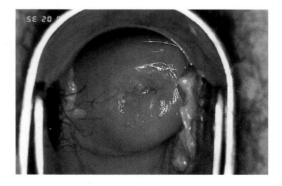

Fig. 24.12 Colposcopy of CIN 1. The acetowhite appearance of the anterior lip of the cervix indicates the presence of CIN.

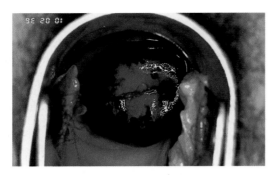

Fig. 24.13 Colposcopic appearances of CIN2. The abnormal epithelium fails to stain with iodine.

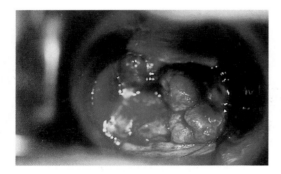

Fig. 24.14 Colposcopic appearance of invasive carcinoma of the cervix.

(Fig. 24.13). The diagnosis is confirmed by biopsies taken from the most abnormal-looking areas. Early invasive disease (cancer of the cervix) is characterized by a raised or ulcerated area with abnormal vessels, friable tissue and coarse punctation with marked mosaicism. It feels hard on palpation and often bleeds on contact. In more advanced disease the cervix becomes fixed or replaced by a friable warty looking mass (Fig. 24.14).

Human papilloma virus

Certain types of HPV are found in association with neoplastic changes in the cervix. Types 6 and 11 are associated with low-grade CIN and condylomata, whereas serotypes 16, 18, 45 and 56 are associated with all grades of CIN and carcinoma of the cervix. These viruses are identified by their DNA sequences.

Factors that point towards an aetiological role for the virus in carcinoma of the cervix include:

- Continued expression of the DNA in transforming epithelium
- Gene products which transform epithelial cells
- The particular types of HPV associated with carcinoma of the cervix will transform cells in vitro
- Women with the type 16 HPV have a 10-fold increased risk of developing CIN.

The immune response to this virus group appears to be relatively ineffective, and anti-HPV titres do not reflect the ability to resist further infection.

Human papilloma virus DNA is present in 95% of squamous cell cervical cancers and 60% of adenocarcinomas but it must be remembered that 10–30% of normal subjects will also be found to have HPV DNA present in cervical epithelium.

The role of testing for high-risk HPV serotypes in cervical screening remains unclear. The sensitivity of these tests for cervical neoplasia is much higher than that for conventional cytology but not all women with high-risk HPV will develop clinical disease. It is possible that HPV status may help to determine whether women with low-grade disease should be treated or the frequency that cytological screening needs to be carried out in the general population.

In theory the incidence of cervical cancer could be reduced by immunization against HPV and progress has been made towards producing type-specific vaccines. Phase I and II trials are currently under way but it is likely to be some time before their effectiveness will be known.

Cervical intraepithelial neoplasia

This is a histological diagnosis, usually made from colposcopically directed biopsy, of changes in the squamous epithelium characterized by varying degrees of loss of differentiation and stratification and nuclear atypia (Fig. 24.15). It may extend up to 5 mm below the surface of the cervix by involvement of crypt epithelium in the transformation zone, but does not extend below the basement membrane. The aetiology is the same as that of invasive disease but with a peak incidence 10 years earlier. In the UK CIN is graded as mild (CIN 1), moderate (CIN 2) or severe (CIN3) depending on the proportion of the epithelium replaced by abnormal cells. In the USA CIN 2 and CIN 3 are grouped together as high-grade CIN and CIN 1 is classified as low-grade.

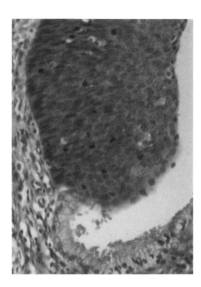

Fig. 24.15 Histological appearance of CIN 3.

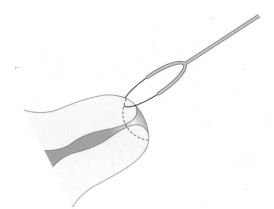

Fig. 24.16 Large loop excision of the cervix.

In 25% of cases, CIN 1 will progress to higher-grade lesions over 2 years, 30–40% of CIN 3 to carcinoma over 20 years. Around 40% of low-grade lesions (CIN 1) will regress to normal within 6 months without treatment.

Cervical glandular intraepithelial neoplasia is the equivalent change occurring in the columnar epithelium and is associated with the development of adenocarcinoma of the cervix. Two thirds of cases coexist with CIN. Cervical cytology can not be used to reliably detect adenocarcinoma of the cervix or CGIN and screening has had no impact its incidence.

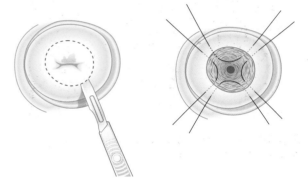

Fig. 24.17 Cone biopsy of the cervix (left); four mattress sutures are usually adequate to control bleeding from the cervical stump (right).

Treatment

Low-grade CIN can be managed by cytological and colposcopic surveillance at 6 monthly intervals as progress to invasive disease does not occur within 6 months or it can be treated as for higher-grade lesions (see below).

Higher-grade lesions (CIN2 and 3 and dyskaryotic glandular cells) are an indication for immediate treatment either by excision or destruction of the affected area (usually the whole of the transformation zone).

Destructive therapies include LASER ablation and coagulation diathermy. Excision can be carried out using scalpel, LASER or using a diathermy loop wire (large loop excision of the transformation zone, LLETZ; (Fig. 24.16). LASER and LLETZ can be carried out under local anaesthetic. Ectocervical lesions can be adequately treated by removing tissue to a depth of 8 mm but where the SCJ cannot be seen or a lesion of the glandular epithelium is suspected a deeper 'cone' biopsy is required to ensure that all of the endocervix is sampled (Fig. 24.17). Patients are advised to abstain from intercourse and not to use tampons for 4 weeks after treatment to reduce the risk of infection. Hysterectomy is rarely indicated for treatment of CIN but may be used if indicated for another reason such as heavy periods.

Complications of cone biopsy

The commonest complication is haemorrhage. This may be primary, i.e. within 12 hours of operation, or secondary, usually between the fifth and 12th post-operative day. Haemorrhage may be profuse but can be controlled by compression with vaginal packing or by resuturing the cervix. Secondary haemorrhage is commonly associated with infection and the management therefore includes blood transfusion and antibiotic therapy.

Later complications include cervical stenosis with dysmenorrhoea and haematometra. Cone biopsy may also cause cervical incompetence and subsequent midtrimester miscarriage.

Follow-up

Approximately 5% of women will have persistent or recurrent disease following treatment. Cervical cytology and/or colposcopy are used to carry out follow-up. Two examinations are carried out in the first 12 months after treatment followed by annual smears for 4 years before returning to the normal 3-yearly screening programme.

Cervical cancer

Cervical cancer is the second commonest female cancer worldwide. In many countries this is the most common cause of death from cancer in women. In the UK the annual incidence in 1997 was 9.3/100 000 women with 2740 new cases and 1222 deaths. Cervical cancer has a direct relationship to sexual activity. Associated risk factors are early age of first intercourse, number of partners, smoking and infection with human papillomavirus.

In contrast to other gynaecological cancers, cervical cancer affects young women, with a peak incidence at 45.

Pathology

There are two types of invasive carcinoma of the cervix. Approximately 70–80% of lesions are squamous cell carcinoma and 20–30% adenocarcinomas. Histologically the degree of invasion may be (Table 24.5):

- **Early stromal** where invasion is less than 3 mm below basement membrane
- **Microinvasive** where invasion is less than 5 mm below basement membrane
- **Invasive** where invasion is more than 5 mm below the basement membrane.

The spread of tumour

Cervical carcinoma spreads by direct local invasion and via the lymphatics and blood vessels. Lymphatic spread

---

Table 24.5
FIGO Classification of cervical cancer

Stage I	Carcinoma confined to the cervix (extension to the corpus does not advance the stage):
	Stage IA: Divided into IA1, early stromal invasion only, and IA2, microinvasion – where the tumour extends less than 5 mm from the base of the epithelium with a horizontal spread of no more than 7 mm
	Stage IB Invasion of more than 5 mm depth or 7 mm area but is still confined to the cervix
Stage II	Carcinoma extends beyond the cervix but does not reach the pelvic side wall or lower third of the vagina:
	Stage IIA No obvious parametrial involvement, upper two-thirds of the vagina involved
	Stage IIB Obvious parametrial involvement but not reaching the pelvic side wall
Stage III	Carcinoma extends to the pelvic side wall or lower third of the vagina – includes all cases of hydronephrosis/non-functioning kidney unless this is known to be due to another cause:
	Stage IIIA Tumour extends to lower third of the vagina
	Stage IIIB Extension to pelvic side wall or hydronephrosis
Stage IV	Carcinoma extending beyond the true pelvis or involving the bladder or rectal mucosa:
	Stage IVA Involvement of bladder or rectum
	Stage IVB Spread to distant organs

occurs in approximately 0.5% of women with stage Ia1 disease rising to 5% for stage Ia2 and 40% of women with stage II disease. Preferential spread occurs to the external iliac, internal iliac and obturator nodes. Secondary spread may also occur to inguinal, sacral and aortic nodes. Blood-borne metastases occur in the lungs, liver, bone and bowel.

Clinical features

Stage Ia disease is asymptomatic at the time of presentation and is detected at the time of routine examination for cervical cytology. The common presenting symptoms from invasive carcinoma of the cervix include postcoital bleeding, foul-smelling discharge, which is thin and watery and sometimes blood-stained, and irregular vaginal bleeding when the tumour becomes necrotic. Lateral invasion into the parametrium may involve the ureters, leading eventually to ureteric obstruction and renal failure. Invasion of nerves and bone produces excruciating and persistent pain, and involvement of lymphatic channels may result in lymphatic occlusion with intractable oedema of the lower limbs.

The tumour may also spread anteriorly or posteriorly to involve the bladder or rectum respectively. Involvement of the bladder produces symptoms of frequency, dysuria and haematuria; if the bowel is involved, tenesmus, diarrhoea and rectal bleeding may occur. The neoplasm may initially grow within the endocervix, producing a cylindrical, barrel-shaped enlargement of the cervix with little external manifestation of the tumour.

The exophytic tumour grows over the vaginal portion of the cervix and appears as a cauliflower-like tumour (Fig. 24.14). The tumour eventually sloughs and replaces the normal cervical tissue and extends on to the vaginal walls.

Death occurs from uraemia following bilateral ureteric obstruction or from sepsis and haemorrhage with generalized cachexia and wasting.

Investigation

The diagnosis is established histologically by biopsy of the tumour, which should be greater than 5 mm in depth to distinguish between microinvasive and invasive disease. Careful evaluation and staging should be completed by vaginal and rectal examination and by cystoscopy, proctoscopy, intravenous urography, and lung and skeletal radiography (Table 24.5).

Treatment of invasive carcinoma

Treatment is by surgery or radiotherapy or a combination of both methods.

Local excision carried out by cone biopsy is an option for patients with stage IA lesions who wish to preserve fertility.

Extended hysterectomy or radiotherapy can be used to treat stage Ib–IIa. The cure rate is similar for both surgery and radiotherapy but the former is generally associated with less long-term morbidity from vaginal stenosis. Stage II–IV disease is usually treated with intracavity and external beam radiotherapy.

Surgery – radical hysterectomy and pelvic lymph node dissection

Radical hysterectomy (Wertheim's hysterectomy; Fig. 24.18) includes removal of the uterus, the upper third of the vagina, internal and external iliac and obturator lymph nodes. The ovaries may be conserved. This method of treatment is appropriate for patients with stage I disease. Complications include haemorrhage, infection, pelvic haematomas and damage to the ureters or bladder, which may result in fistula formation in 2–5% of cases. However, the incidence of vaginal stenosis is less than after radiotherapy, so coital function is better preserved, making it the treatment of choice in the younger woman.

Radiotherapy

This is to treat other stages of cervical cancer and those patients with bulky stage Ib disease or who are unfit for surgery. Survival stage for stage is similar to that for surgery. Adjuvant radiotherapy is also used for those patients who have been found to have lymph node involvement at the time of surgery.

Radiotherapy is administered by local insertion of a source of radium, caesium or cobalt-60 into the uterine cavity and the vaginal vault and external beam radiation to the pelvic side wall. Complications include the effects of excessive radiation on normal tissues, and may lead to radiation cystitis or proctitis, as well as fistula formation and vaginal stenosis.

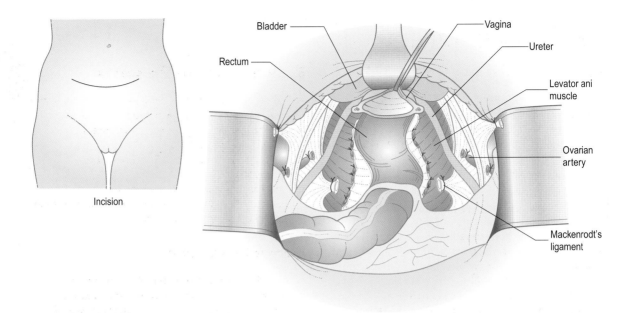

Incision

Bladder

Rectum

Vagina

Ureter

Levator ani muscle

Ovarian artery

Mackenrodt's ligament

Fig. 24.18 Wertheim's hysterectomy involves block dissection of the pelvic lymph nodes and excision of the uterus, tubes, ovaries and upper third of the vagina.

Prognosis

This depends mainly on the stage at diagnosis and lymph node status. The results for 5-year survival are:

- Stage I: 85%
- Stage II: 60%
- Stage III: 30%
- Stage IV: 10%.

The comparable survival figure for stage Ib using radical surgery is 90%.

A combination of limited radiation and subsequent radical surgery after 4–6 weeks has produced similar figures, with a 5-year survival in stage I disease of 77% and in stage IIa of 69%.

Recurrent cervical lesions occur in a third of cases and have a poor prognosis.

Where local recurrence involves the bladder or rectum but does not extend to other structures, curative excision may occasionally be achieved by radical excision or exenteration including total cystectomy and removal of the rectum.

VAGINAL AND CERVICAL CLEAR-CELL ADENOCARCINOMA

These tumours have been described in relation to diethylstilboestrol exposure and occur on both the vagina and the cervix. They are found in young girls born to women who received diethylstilboestrol during pregnancy. The tumours respond to radiation or radical surgery, and there is an overall 5-year survival rate of 70%. The tumour is commonly preceded by vaginal adenosis. The condition is rare in the UK.

ESSENTIAL INFORMATION

Benign vulval lesions

- Cause unknown/autoimmune
- Usually presents as pruritus
- Classified by appearance or histology
- Associated with malignant change in 5% cases
- Need to exclude malignancy, infection, diabetes and other systemic conditions

Malignant vulval lesions

- Commonest in sixth decade
- 2–3% of female cancers
- Majority are squamous (92%) or adenocarcinomas (5%)
- Present with pruritus, bleeding lesions
- Spreads by local invasion and via inguinal and femoral nodes
- Staged according to size, lymph node involvement and spread
- Good prognosis if confined to vulva at presentation

Vaginal tumours

- Benign tumours are commonly, embryological remnants, inclusion cysts or endometriotic
- Primary malignancy rare, squamous carcinomas arising in upper third
- Common site for spread from cervix and uterus
- Presents as pain, bleeding and fistula formation
- Spreads by local invasion and lymphatics
- Usually treated by radiotherapy
- Increased incidence in young women whose mothers were given diethylstilboestrol in pregnancy
- Premalignant changes associated with CIN

Benign lesions of the cervix

- Extension of the endocervical epithelium on to the ectocervix is a normal physiological variant
- Ectropion is cervical eversion revealing the endocervical mucosa
- Benign polyps commonly arise from the endocervix
- Fibroids may arise from the cervix
- Benign lesions may be asymptomatic or present as vaginal bleeding or discharge

Cervical screening

- 3-yearly intervals from 20 to 65 years of age
- Malignant change suggested by an increased nuclear–cytoplasmic ratio, mitotic figures and intense nuclear staining
- Dyskaryosis represents lesser degrees of abnormality
- Appearance of exfoliated cells varies with hormonal status and infection
- Abnormal cytology requires colposcopy

Cervical cancer

- More common in lower social class, smokers, early first intercourse and multiple partners
- Associated with herpes and human papilloma virus infection
- May be asymptomatic or present with vaginal bleeding, pain, and bowel or bladder symptoms
- Spreads by local invasion and iliac/obturator nodes
- Treatment is radical hysterectomy for early stage disease, radiotherapy otherwise
- 5-year survival varies from 10% to 90% depending on stage

25 Prolapse and disorders of the urinary tract

UTEROVAGINAL PROLAPSE

The position of the vagina and uterus depends on various fascial supports and ligaments derived from specific thickening of areas of the fascial support (Fig. 25.1).

The anterior vaginal wall is supported by the pubocervical fascia, which extends from the posterior surface of the pubic symphysis to the cervix and upper vagina. The posterior vaginal wall is supported by the fibrous tissue of the rectovaginal septum and the tonus of the pelvic floor and, in particular, the integrity of the levator ani.

The uterus is supported indirectly by the supports of the vaginal walls but directly by the cardinal or transverse cervical ligaments, which extend from the lateral pelvic wall to the upper part of the vagina and the lower part of the cervix. The uterosacral ligaments, which comprise the thickening of the pelvic floor fascia, extend from the sacrum to the lower parts of the cervix and the upper third of the vagina. The round and broad ligaments also provide weak support to the vagina and uterus. Indirect support of the vagina and uterus is provided by the integrity of the pelvic floor and the levator ani.

Definitions

Vaginal prolapse

Prolapse of the anterior vaginal wall may affect the urethra (*urethrocele*), and the bladder (*cystocele*; Fig. 25.2). On examination, the urethra and bladder can be seen to descend and bulge into the anterior vaginal wall and, in severe cases, will be visible at the introitus of the vagina. A *rectocele* is formed by a rectovaginal hernia, which can be seen as a visible bulge of the rectum through the posterior vaginal wall. It is often associated with deficiency and laxity of the pelvic floor.

An *enterocele* is formed by a prolapse of the recto-uterine pouch, i.e. the pouch of Douglas, through the upper part of the vaginal vault (Fig. 25.2) The condition may occur in isolation but usually occurs in association

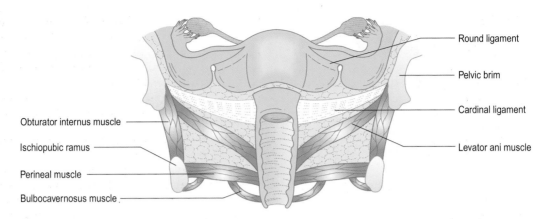

Fig. 25.1 Supports of the uterus, cervix and vagina.

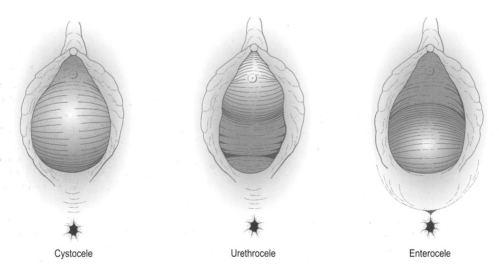

Cystocele Urethrocele Enterocele

Fig. 25.2 The clinical appearance of vaginal prolapse.

with uterine prolapse. An enterocele may also occur following hysterectomy when there is inadequate support of the vaginal vault.

Uterine prolapse

Descent of the uterus may occur in isolation from vaginal wall prolapse but more commonly occurs in conjunction with it. First-degree prolapse of the uterus often occurs in association with retroversion of the uterus and descent of the cervix within the vagina. If the cervix descends to the vaginal introitus, the prolapse is defined as second degree. The term procidentia is applied to where the cervix and the body of the uterus and the vagina walls protrude through the introitus. The word actually means 'prolapse' or 'falling' but is generally reserved for the description of total or third-degree prolapse (Fig. 25.3).

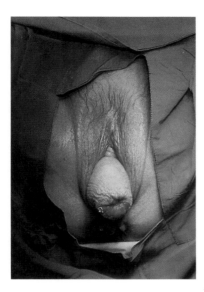

Fig. 25.3 Procidentia: a third-degree prolapse of the uterus and vaginal walls.

Symptoms and signs

 Mild degrees of prolapse are common in parous women and may be asymptomatic.

Symptoms generally depend on the severity and site of the prolapse.

There are some symptoms that are common to all forms of prolapse; these include:

- A sense of fullness in the vagina associated with dragging discomfort
- Visible protrusion of the cervix and vaginal walls
- Sacral backache.

Symptoms are often multiple and related to the nature of prolapse.

Urethrocele and cystocele

Specific symptoms relating to the urinary tract depend on the effect the prolapse has on the bladder neck. The loss of the posterior urethrovesical angle is often associated with stress incontinence, i.e. the involuntary loss of urine following raised intra-abdominal pressure. If the angle between the bladder and urethra becomes exaggerated, then there may be incomplete emptying of the bladder and this will be associated with double micturition, the desire to repeat micturition immediately after apparent completion of voiding, or recurrent urinary tract infection as a result of incomplete emptying of the bladder. The sensation of incomplete emptying or difficulty in initiating micturition can be relieved by replacing the cystocele digitally or by the use of a vaginal pessary or tampon.

The diagnosis is established by examination with a Sims' speculum so that the vaginal wall can be seen. When the patient is asked to strain, the bulge in the anterior vaginal wall can be seen and often appears at the introitus. It is important to culture a specimen of urine to exclude the presence of infection. The differential diagnosis is limited to cysts or tumours of the anterior vaginal wall, and diverticulum of the urethra or bladder.

Rectocele

The prolapse of the rectum through the posterior vaginal wall is commonly associated with a deficient pelvic floor, disruption of the perineal body and separation of the levator ani. It is predominantly a problem that results from overdistension of the introitus and pelvic floor during parturition.

The symptoms that relate in particular to rectocele are difficulties with evacuation of faeces and the awareness of a reducible mass bulging into the vagina and through the introitus.

Examination of the vulva usually shows a deficient perineum, a lax introitus, and the rectum bulging into the posterior vaginal wall.

Enterocele

Herniation of the pouch of Douglas usually occurs through the vaginal vault, either through the posterior fornix or through the vaginal vault if the uterus has been removed. It is often difficult to distinguish between a high rectocele and an enterocele as the symptoms of vaginal pressure are identical. Occasionally, but rarely, the enterocele occurs anterior to the vaginal vault and may mimic a cystocele.

A large enterocele may contain bowel and may be associated with incarceration and obstruction of the bowel.

Uterine prolapse

Descent of the uterus is initially associated with prolongation of the cervix and descent of the body of the uterus. The symptoms are those of pressure in the vagina and, ultimately, complete protrusion of the uterus through the introitus. At this stage, the prolapsed uterus may produce discomfort on sitting, and decubitus ulceration may result in haemorrhage (Fig. 25.4). Cervical prolongation often leads to confusion in staging the degree of prolapse as it may appear to be in a more advanced stage than it actually is.

Urinary tract infection may occur because of compression of the ureters and consequent hydronephrosis due to incomplete emptying of the bladder.

Pathogenesis of uterovaginal prolapse

Prolapse may be congenital or acquired:

- **Congenital:** Uterine prolapse in young or nulliparous women is due to weakness of the supports of the uterus and vaginal vault. There is a minimal degree of vaginal wall prolapse.
- **Acquired:** The commonest form of prolapse is acquired under the influence of multiple factors. This type of prolapse is both uterine and vaginal but

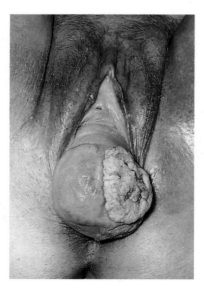

Fig. 25.4 Procidentia associated with dependent ulceration of the vaginal skin.

it must also be remembered that vaginal wall prolapse can also occur without any uterine descent. Predisposing factors include:

- *High parity:* Uterovaginal prolapse is a condition of parous women. The pelvic floor provides direct and indirect support for the vaginal walls and when this support is disrupted by laceration or overdistension it predisposes to vaginal wall prolapse.
- *Raised intra-abdominal pressure:* Tumours or ascites may result in raised intra-abdominal pressure, but a more common cause is a chronic cough.
- *Hormonal changes:* The symptoms of prolapse often worsen rapidly at the time of the menopause. Cessation of oestrogen production leads to thinning of the vaginal walls and the supports of the uterus. Although the prolapse is generally present before the menopause, it is at this time that the symptoms become noticeable and the degree of descent visibly worsens.

Management

The management of prolapse is medical or surgical.

Prevention

Good surgical technique in supporting the vaginal vault at the time of hysterectomy reduces the incidence of later vault prolapse. Avoiding a prolonged second stage of labour, encouraging pelvic floor exercises after delivery and the use of hormone replacement therapy after the menopause may all help to reduce the risk of prolapse in later life.

Medical treatment

Many women have minor degrees of uterovaginal prolapse, which are asymptomatic. If the recognition of the prolapse is a coincidental finding, the woman should be advised against any surgical treatment.

Minor degrees of prolapse are common after childbirth and should be treated by pelvic floor exercises or the use of a pessary. Operative intervention is contraindicated for at least 6 months after delivery, as the tissues remain vascular and may undergo further spontaneous improvement.

Symptoms associated with cystocele after the menopause are often improved by hormone replacement therapy.

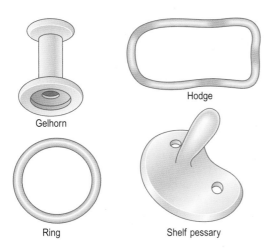

Gelhorn

Hodge

Ring

Shelf pessary

Fig. 25.5 Various types of vaginal pessary used in the conservative management of uterovaginal prolapse.

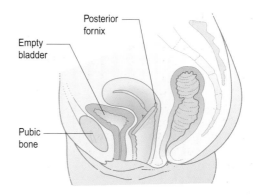

Fig. 25.6 Ring pessary in situ.

Where short-term support is required or the general health of the woman makes operative treatment dangerous, then both vaginal wall and uterine prolapse can be treated by using vaginal pessaries. It is, however, necessary to have some pelvic floor support if a pessary is to be retained.

The most widely used pessaries (Fig. 25.5) are.

- **Ring pessary:** This pessary consists of a malleable plastic ring, which may vary in diameter from 60 to 80 mm. The pessary is inserted in the posterior fornix and behind the pubic symphysis (Fig. 25.6). Distension of the vaginal walls tends to support the vaginal wall prolapse.
- **Hodge pessary:** This is a rigid, elongated, curved ovoid which is inserted in a similar way to the ring pessary and is principally useful in uterine retroversion.
- **Gelhorn pessary:** This pessary is shaped like a collar stud and is used in the treatment of severe degrees of prolapse.
- **Shelf pessary:** This is shaped like a coathook and is used mainly in the treatment of uterine or vaginal vault prolapse.

The main problem with long-term use of pessaries is ulceration of the vaginal vault. Pessaries should be replaced every 4–12 months and the vagina should be examined for any signs of ulceration.

Surgical treatment

Surgical treatment of a cystocele is by anterior colporrhaphy (Fig. 25.7). The operation consists of a surgical excision of the excess vaginal wall and buttressing of the pubocervical fascia. In the presence of stress incontinence due to loss of the posterior urethrovesical angle, this angle is reconstructed by placing buttressing sutures under the bladder neck. These are described as *Kelly's sutures*.

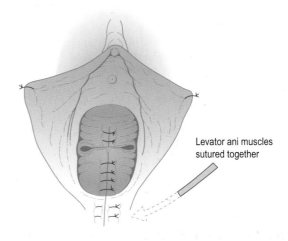

Levator ani muscles sutured together

Fig. 25.7 Anterior and posterior colporrhaphy.

Rectocele is repaired by posterior colpoperineorrhaphy with reconstruction of the pelvic floor, reapposition of the levator muscles and excision of the redundant vaginal skin.

Where there is an enterocele, the hernial sac is opened and transfixed at its neck, with excision of the redundant tissue.

The treatment of choice for uterine prolapse is vaginal hysterectomy with or without repair of the vaginal walls. If preservation of reproductive function is required, then the uterus can be conserved by simply excising the cervix and suturing the cardinal ligaments in front of the cervical stump. This procedure is known as a *Manchester* or *Fothergill repair*. The vaginal skin is then sutured into the cervical stump.

Vault prolapse occurring after hysterectomy can be treated by suspending the vaginal vault from the anterior longitudinal ligament of the sacrum using a synthetic mesh. This procedure is known as *sacrocolpopexy*.

Complications

The immediate complications of vaginal hysterectomy or repair include haemorrhage, haematoma formation, infection and urinary retention. The long-term complications are dyspareunia and vaginal stenosis. Inadequate supportive tissue may result in recurrence of the prolapse of the vaginal vault.

URINARY TRACT DISORDERS

Structure and physiology of the urinary tract

The urinary bladder is a hollow muscular organ with an outer adventitial layer, a smooth muscle layer known as the detrusor muscle and an inner layer of transitional epithelium.

The innervation of the bladder contains both sympathetic and parasympathetic components (Fig. 25.8). The sympathetic fibres arise from the lower two thoracic and upper two lumbar segments of the spinal cord, and the parasympathetic fibres from the second, third and fourth sacral segments. The urethra consists of a muscle coat lined by epithelium continuous with the bladder epithelium. The muscle coat consists of a mixture of smooth muscle with an outer sleeve of striated muscle. The bladder neck does not contain a smooth muscle sphincter. The majority of muscle fibres in the bladder

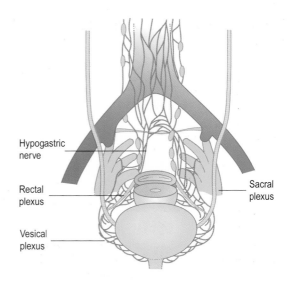

Hypogastric nerve

Rectal plexus

Vesical plexus

Sacral plexus

Fig. 25.8 Sympathetic and parasympathetic innervation of the bladder.

neck enter obliquely or longitudinally into the wall of the urethra.

During micturition, the pressure in the bladder rises to exceed the pressure within the urethral lumen and there is a fall in urethral resistance. The tonus of muscle fibres around the bladder neck is reduced by central inhibition of the motor neurones in the sacral plexus.

The ureter is 25 cm long. It runs along the transverse processes of the lumbar spine, anterior to the psoas muscle, is crossed by the ovarian vessels and enters the pelvis anterior to the bifurcation of the common iliacs. From there it runs anterior to the internal iliac vessels to the ischial spines where it turns medially to the cervix. It turns again anteriorly 1.5 cm lateral to the vaginal fornix, crossing below the uterine vessels to enter the posterior surface of the bladder.

The bladder fills at 1–6 ml/min. The intravesical pressure remains low because of compliance of the bladder wall as it stretches and reflex inhibition of the detrusor muscle. At the same time the internal urethral meatus is closed by tonic contraction of the rhabdosphincter and the tone of the urethral mucosa. During rises in intra-abdominal pressure such as coughing or sneezing, continence is maintained by transmission of the pressure rise to the proximal urethra (which lies normally within the intra-abdominal space) and an increase in the levator tone.

Common disorders of bladder function

The common symptoms of bladder dysfunction include:

- Urinary incontinence
- Frequency of micturition
- Dysuria
- Urinary retention.

Incontinence of urine

The involuntary loss of urine may be associated with bladder or urethral dysfunction or fistula formation. Types of incontinence are as follows.

- **True incontinence** is continuous loss of urine through the vagina; it is commonly associated with fistula formation but may occasionally be a manifestation of urinary retention with overflow.
- **Stress incontinence** – the involuntary loss of urine that occurs during a brief period of raised intra-abdominal pressure – is related to pelvic floor weakness and in 30% of cases to detrusor instability. Examination reveals the involuntary loss of urine during coughing, with descent of the anterior vaginal wall and reduction of the posterior urethrovesical angle. Digital elevation of the anterior vaginal wall leads to correction of the condition. Loss of support to the anterior vaginal wall is frequently associated with reduced pelvic floor support.
- **Urge incontinence** is the problem of sudden detrusor contraction, with uncontrolled loss of urine. The condition may be due to idiopathic detrusor instability or associated with urinary infection, obstructive uropathy, diabetes or neurological disease. It is particularly important to exclude urinary tract infection.
- **Mixed urge and stress incontinence:** A substantial number of women with urge incontinence also have true stress incontinence and, if the latter is corrected, the detrusor instability will disappear.

Urinary frequency

Urinary frequency is an insuppressible desire to void more than seven times a day or more than once a night. If affects 20% of women aged between 30 and 64 years, and can be caused by pregnancy, diabetes, pelvic masses, renal failure, diuretics, excess fluid intake or habit, although the most common cause is urinary tract infection.

However, enhanced bladder contractility may occur without the presence of infection. Reduced bladder capacity may also result in frequency of micturition.

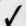 Patients may also develop frequency because of anxiety concerning involuntary loss of urine.

Dysuria

This symptom results from infection. Local urethral infection or trauma causes burning or scalding during micturition, but bladder infection is more likely to cause pain suprapubically after micturition has been completed. It is always advisable to perform a vaginal examination on any woman who complains of scalding on micturition because urethritis is associated with vaginitis and vaginal infection.

Urinary retention and outflow obstruction

Acute urinary retention is not in women the common problem that it is in the ageing male. It is, however, seen:

- After vaginal delivery and episiotomy
- Following operative delivery
- After vaginal repair procedures – particularly those operations that involve posterior colpoperineorrhaphy
- In the menopause – spontaneous obstructive uropathy is more likely to occur in menopausal women
- In pregnancy – a retroverted uterus may become impacted in the pelvis towards the end of the first trimester
- When inflammatory lesions of the vulva are present
- As a result of untreated over-distension of the bladder (such as following delivery), neuropathy or malignancy.

! Good bladder care is essential after delivery, especially those involving spinal or epidural anaesthesia. Neglected urinary retention in these circumstances can result in overdistension of the bladder, and the subsequent hypotonus of the bladder can lead to prolonged voiding difficulties.

Diagnosis

The diagnosis is initially indicated by the history. Continuous loss of urine indicates a fistula, but not all fistulas leak urine continuously. The fistulous communication usually occurs between the bladder and vagina, *vesicovaginal fistula*, and the ureter and vagina, *ureterovaginal fistula*. Fistula formation results from:

- Surgical trauma
- Obstetric trauma associated with obstructed labour
- Malignant disease
- Radiotherapy.

There are other types of fistula with communications between bowel and urinary tract and between bowel and vagina, but these are less common.

Rectovaginal fistulas have a similar pathogenesis, with the additional factor of perineal breakdown after a third-degree tear.

Urinary fistulas are localized by:

- Cystoscopy
- Intravenous urogram
- Instillation of methylene blue via a catheter into the bladder; the appearance of dye in the vagina indicates a vesicovaginal fistula.

The differential diagnosis between stress and urge incontinence is more difficult and is often unsatisfactory. Adequate preoperative assessment is important if the correct operation is to be employed or if surgery is to be avoided.

The cystometrogram

Pressure is measured intravesically and intrarectally, because intrarectal pressure represents intra-abdominal pressure and is subtracted from the intravesical pressure to give a measure of detrusor pressure. The volume of fluid in the bladder at which the first desire to void occurs is usually about 150 ml. A strong desire to void occurs at 400 ml in the normal bladder. High detrusor pressure at a lower volume reflects an abnormally sensitive bladder associated with chronic infection. There should be no detrusor contraction during filling, and any contraction that occurs under these circumstances indicates *detrusor instability*. An underactive detrusor shows no contraction on complete filling and indicates an abnormality of neurological control. The average bladder has a capacity of 250–550 ml, but capacity is a poor index of bladder function. Thus, cystometry is a useful method for assessing detrusor muscle function or detrusor instability, which may result in urge incontinence.

Pressure/flow studies (Fig. 25.9) enable a measurement to be made of the rate of flow in relation to intravesical pressure and hence indicate if there is any bladder neck obstruction. Normal flow may occur in the presence of a bladder neck obstruction if there is a powerful detrusor muscle.

Detrusor overactivity is indicated by high resting urethral pressure, good voluntary increase in urethral pressure, good ability to stop midstream, the presence of good detrusor muscle power, frequent strong bladder contractions and small volumes of urine on frequency/volume charts (Fig. 25.9b)

In the presence of urethral incompetence, there is low resting urethral pressure, no voluntary increase in urethral pressure, inability to stop midstream, decreased pressure transmission to the abdominal urethra and large volumes in the frequency/volume measurements. There is not always a clear-cut demarcation between the two conditions, as there may be a mixture of both stress and urge incontinence. Nevertheless, it is important to differentiate between the predominant influence of bladder neck weakness and stress incontinence, and detrusor instability and urge incontinence.

Management

Urinary tract fistula

In western European countries, most urinary tract fistulas result from surgical trauma. The commonest fistulas are vesicovaginal (Fig. 25.10a) or ureterovaginal and result from surgical trauma at the time of hysterectomy, or sometimes following caesarean section.

A vesicovaginal fistula will usually become apparent in the first postoperative week. If the fistula is small, closure may be achieved spontaneously.

The patient should be treated by catheterization and continuous drainage. If closure has not occurred after 2–3 months, the fistula is unlikely to close spontaneously and surgical closure is recommended. The timing of further surgery is still a subject of controversy. Until recently, a delay of 6 months was recommended but there is increasing evidence that good results can be obtained with early surgical intervention. However, the fistulous site should be free of infection.

Surgical closure may be achieved vaginally by meticulous separation of the edges of the fistula and closure

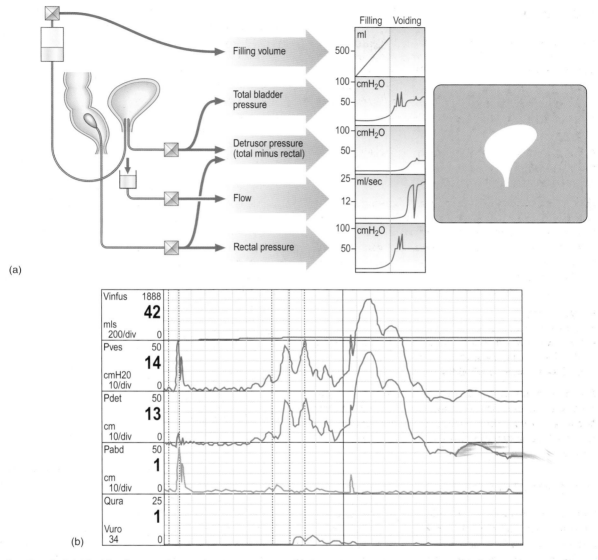

Fig. 25.9 (a) Bladder flow studies in the investigation of lower urinary tract symptoms. (b) Cystometrogram from a patient with idiopathic detrusor instability.

in layers of the bladder and vagina (Fig. 25.10b). Postoperative care includes continuous catheter drainage for 1 week and antibiotic cover. An abdominal approach to the fistula can also be used and has some advantages, allowing the interposition of omentum in cases where there is a large fistula.

Ureterovaginal fistulas are usually treated by reimplantation of the damaged ureter into the bladder.

Stress incontinence

> ! Surgical procedures for stress incontinence may worsen symptoms of detrusor instability.

Stress incontinence should be managed initially by pelvic floor physiotherapy. Surgical treatment is

(a)

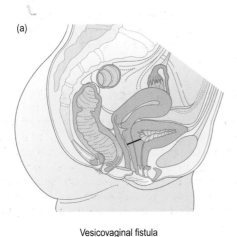

Vesicovaginal fistula

(b)

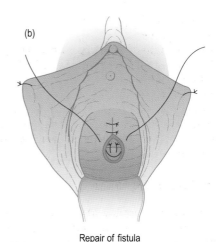

Repair of fistula

Fig. 25.10 True incontinence is associated with a fistulous opening between bladder and vagina – the vesicovaginal fistula (a); it can be closed by either the vaginal or the abdominal route (b).

indicated where there is a failure to respond to conservative management. In the presence of anterior vaginal wall prolapse, *anterior repair*, with the placement of buttressing sutures at the bladder neck, has the virtue of simplicity. It will certainly relieve the prolapse but the results are variable as far as the stress incontinence is concerned, with relief in about 40–50% of cases. It is of no value in the absence of evidence of prolapse.

Where there is minimal prolapse, the following procedures are used.

- **Marshall–Marchetti–Krantz procedure:** The bladder neck and trigone are elevated by suturing the paraurethral and paravesical tissues to the periosteum on the back of the pubic symphysis. This creates a valve-like effect at the bladder neck.
- **Burch colposuspension:** The bladder neck is elevated by suturing the upper lateral vaginal walls to the ilioinguinal ligaments (Fig. 25.11)
- **Laparoscopic colposuspension** involves bladder neck elevation by suturing the upper lateral vaginal walls to the iliopectineal ligaments under laparoscopic control.

All these procedures have a higher success rate in curing stress incontinence but have a significant surgical complication rate and often cause detrusor instability as well as other urinary symptoms due to incomplete bladder emptying.

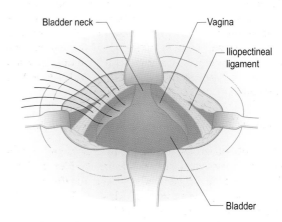

Fig. 25.11 Burch colposuspension.

- **Sling procedures:** Fascial strips from the anterior abdominal wall or inert synthetic materials attached to the anterior abdominal wall are placed in a sling under the bladder neck and cause urethral closure when the sling is stretched.
- **Stamey procedure.** A Mersilene strip is introduced per vaginam using a large specialized needle and is fixed to the anterior abdominal wall. The procedure has the advantage of simplicity, with the minimum

size of incision and rapid recovery with a short convalescence time.

- **Tension-free vaginal tape:** Bladder neck elevation can also be achieved by tension-free tape instead of a conventional Stamey suture. As this can be carried out under local anaesthetic the amount of bladder neck elevation can be adjusted until it is just sufficient to prevent leakage when the patient bears down. The long-term effectiveness of this treatment is not yet known.

The unstable bladder

The features of the unstable bladder are those of frequency of micturition and nocturia, urgency and urge incontinence. When confronted with this history, it is important to obtain some indication of the frequency as related to fluid intake and output. A chart should therefore be kept by the patient to clarify this aspect.

The assessment of predisposing factors includes urine culture, urinary flow rates and urodynamic studies.

Treatment will obviously be directed at the cause, so the presence of urinary tract infection necessitates the administration of the appropriate antibiotic therapy. Postmenopausal women with atrophic vaginal epithelium and symptoms of urgency and frequency often respond to replacement therapy with low-dose oestrogens.

Detrusor instability of unknown aetiology

If the problem arises at a cerebral level, then psychotherapeutic measures are indicated. Bladder drill involves a regime of gradually increasing the voiding interval on a recorded pattern. This is effective in the short term but the relapse rate is high.

The placebo response rate in detrusor instability is more than 40% and spontaneous remissions occur.

Drug treatment

The alternative approach is to use anticholinergic drugs that act at the level of the bladder wall. The most effective drugs are oxybutynin, propantheline and imipramine. The addition of tranquillizers and hypnotics may also help. Oxybutynin is prescribed in a dose of 5 mg three times daily and has a direct local anaesthetic effect on the bladder. As an anticholinergic drug, it also has side effects such as mouth dryness and blurring of vision.

Surgical treatments are not commonly used but include bladder over-distension, bladder transection and transvesical injection of 6% aqueous phenol into the trigone.

Bladder outlet obstruction

Primary bladder neck obstruction in the female probably results from the failure of the vesical neck to open during voiding, and can be treated either with alpha-adrenergic blocking agents or by urethral dilatation. Secondary outlet obstruction is usually associated with previous surgery for incontinence and may respond to urethral dilatation but the results are not particularly good.

The neuropathic bladder

Loss of bladder function may be associated with a variety of conditions that affect the central nervous system. These conditions may also be associated with alteration in bowel function, sexual dysfunction and loss of function of the lower limbs.

Presentation

The neuropathic bladder is a reflection of dyssynergy between the activity of the detrusor muscle and the bladder sphincter. This results in a variety of disorders ranging from the 'automatic bladder' through retention with overflow at high or low pressure to total stress incontinence. It may also be associated with renal failure.

Aetiology

The causation may be suprapontine, such as a cerebrovascular accident, Parkinson's disease or a cerebral tumour. Infrapontine causes include cord injuries or compression, multiple sclerosis and spina bifida. Peripheral autonomic neuropathies that affect bladder function may be idiopathic or diabetic and, occasionally, secondary to surgical injury.

Diagnosis

The diagnosis is established by a systematic search for the cause involving cystometry, urinary flow rate studies, neurological screening, brain scan, pyelography and renal isotope scans.

Management

The management clearly depends on establishing the cause, but symptomatically it also involves non-surgical management using absorptive pads and clean inter-mittent self-catheterization. Anticholinergic drugs also have a place for some patients. Surgical treatment includes the use of artificial sphincters and sacral nerve stimulators.

ESSENTIAL INFORMATION

Prolapse

- May involve anterior or posterior vaginal wall with varying degrees of uterine descent
- Predisposing factors include high parity, chronically raised intra-abdominal pressure and hormonal changes
- Symptoms depend on degree of prolapse and whether bowel or bladder neck involved
- May present as renal failure
- May undergo spontaneous improvement up to 6 months postpartum
- Treatment of choice is surgical repair ± hysterectomy
- No treatment required for asymptomatic minor degrees of prolapse

Stress incontinence

- Involuntary loss of urine causing social or hygienic problems and objectively demonstrable
- Commonly associated with prolapse of the bladder neck
- Associated with detrusor instability in up to 30% of cases
- Indicated by a low resting urethral pressure, decreased pressure transmission to abdominal urethra and inability to stop midstream during micturition

Detrusor instability

- Presents as frequency, urgency, nocturia and incontinence
- Usually idiopathic but needs to be distinguished from obstructive uropathy, diabetes, neurological disorders and infection
- May present as stress incontinence
- Associated with high resting urethral pressure and frequent strong bladder contractions at low volumes on cystometry
- Management includes bladder drill, anticholinergics and treatment of infection

Appendix: Medicolegal aspects of obstetrics and gynaecology

CONSENT

When a woman agrees to a surgical procedure, it is important that the implications of benefit and risk are explained to her before embarking on the procedure. Indeed, it is a fundamental law of medical and legal practice that a doctor must obtain consent from the patient for any particular medical or surgical treatment and that without appropriate consent a procedure may constitute an act of assault or trespass against the person.

Secondly, the patient must receive sufficient knowledge of any proposed treatment to make a valid choice about whether or not to consent. The consent form provides evidence that consent has been given for a particular procedure, but it only has meaning if it is evident that the patient did actually understand the nature and implications of the procedure.

In explaining the nature of a procedure to any woman, it is important to explain the purpose of the operation and the potential complications. Given that there may be a range of complications for any operation, the question arises as to how far it is necessary to go in explaining all the potential complications, given that this may induce disproportionate anxiety about a series of very remote risks.

In general terms, a risk in excess of a 1% chance should be explained to the patient, although this is a guideline rather than an absolute figure.

A common example that addresses the issues of informed consent is the information given to patients before sterilization about potential failure rates. During the 1980s a substantial number of legal actions were based on alleged failure to inform patients that there was a significant risk of failure and that pregnancy could follow any of the commonly used sterilization procedures. The patient bringing a claim would generally allege that no advice was given about the risk of failure and subsequent pregnancy and that, had such advice been given, either the woman would not have had the operation or she would have continued to use contraception after the sterilization procedure. It is now standard practice to advise all patients, both female and male that there is a risk of failure and to record a statement to the effect that such advice has been given.

The failure of a sterilization procedure in either sex may result from a method failure or recanalization. In the female, a clip may be applied to the wrong structure or may transect the tube during application. In this case, pregnancy usually occurs within 6 months of the procedure.

The second cause of failure is recanalization of the Fallopian tubes or, in men, the vas deferens. This may result in a pregnancy many years later and is an unavoidable risk of the procedure. Despite the signing of a consent form that records the risk of failure, errors of technique are generally indefensible.

> **!** A consent form does not protect either the patient or the surgeon if performance of the procedure is faulty.

It is important that consent is obtained by a member of staff who is medically qualified and who signs the consent form with the patient after explaining both the nature of the procedure and the potential complications.

> **!** Ideally, consent should be obtained by the surgeon who is performing the procedure. There are limitations as to what can be reasonably included in a consent form and it is common practice to include a general statement, either in the text of the consent form or in the patient's records, that the risks and the intended purpose of the procedure have been explained to the patient.

It is also important to ensure that the details concerning the patient's name and the description of the procedure to be performed are correct. For example, it is not sufficient to write 'sterilization' to describe the operation when the procedure may be tubal cautery, clip sterilization or tubal ligation. The actual procedure to be performed must be written on the consent form.

The consent from must always be available and must be checked in theatre before any operation is commenced.

LITIGATION IN OBSTETRICS AND GYNAECOLOGY

Litigation in obstetrics and gynaecology has had a profound effect on the provision of maternity services. In the UK, the problem has been masked to some extent by Crown indemnity. The government provides insurance cover for all doctors and midwives practising within the National Health Service. However, in countries such as the USA and Australia, closure of maternity units and the reduction of maternity services are common events. The costs of insurance either have to be passed on to the mothers or the services cannot survive. The reality of the situation is that, regardless of the issues of fault, unless damages are capped, maternity services are commercially uninsurable. Indeed, in many parts of the USA, obstetricians cannot actually purchase insurance cover as their specialty is considered to be too high-risk.

When a patient decides to make a claim against her doctor, she will approach her solicitor. If the solicitor considers there is justification, s/he will advance the action by issuing a summons, seek access to the relevant case note records and then lodge an application for a hearing. If the case is to proceed, in England and Wales it will be heard in the High Court by Masters of the Queen's Bench Division. Cases may also be heard in the County Court if the costs are below a certain figure. In the UK, cases are heard before a judge and not a jury. There tends to be a long time between the issuing of a summons and its hearing and between setting down a case for trial and the actual date of the trial.

Medical litigation is expensive and it is not therefore surprising that most plaintiffs in the UK are supported by Legal Aid. The statement of claim outlines the nature of the claim and it is up to the defendant to respond and either acknowledge or refute the allegations. The legally aided litigant has considerable advantages, as the Legal Aid fund meets all costs. There is no penalty for failure of a claim.

> **!** In an attempt to speed up the resolution of disputes in the UK, new regulations have been introduced through the Civil Procedures Rules and were implemented as guidance to expert witnesses as recently as April 2002.
> The rules specify that the primary responsibility of an expert is to the Court and that this